BST

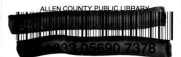

P9-EED-454

Injury & Trauma Sourcebook

Learning Disabilities Sourcebook, 2nd Edition

Leukemia Sourcebook

Liver Disorders Sourcebook

Lung Disorders Sourcebook

Medical Tests Sourcebook, 3rd Edition

Men's Health Concerns Sourcebook, 2nd
    Edition

Mental Health Disorders Sourcebook, 3rd
    Edition

Mental Retardation Sourcebook

Movement Disorders Sourcebook

Multiple Sclerosis Sourcebook

Muscular Dystrophy Sourcebook

Obesity Sourcebook

Osteoporosis Sourcebook

Pain Sourcebook, 3rd Edition

Pediatric Cancer Sourcebook

Physical & Mental Issues in Aging
    Sourcebook

Podiatry Sourcebook, 2nd Edition

Pregnancy & Birth Sourcebook, 2nd
    Edition

Prostate Cancer Sourcebook

Prostate & Urological Disorders Sourcebook

Reconstructive & Cosmetic Surgery
    Sourcebook

Rehabilitation Sourcebook

Respiratory Disorders Sourcebook, 2nd
    Edition

Sexually Transmitted Diseases Sourcebook,
    3rd Edition

Sleep Disorders Sourcebook, 2nd Edition

Smoking Concerns Sourcebook

Sports Injuries Sourcebook, 3rd Edition

Stress-Related Disorders Sourcebook, 2nd
    Edition

Stroke Sourcebook, 2nd Edition

Surgery Sourcebook, 2nd Edition

Thyroid Disorders Sourcebook

Transplantation Sourcebook

Traveler's Health Sourcebook

Urinary Tract & Kidney Diseases Sourcebook, 2nd Edition

Vegetarian Sourcebook

Women's Health Concerns Sourcebook, 2nd
    Edition

Workplace Health & Safety Sourcebook

Worldwide Health Sourcebook

Teen Health Series

Abuse and Violence Information for
    Teens

Alcohol Information for Teens

Allergy Information for Teens

Asthma Information for Teens

Body Information for Teens

Cancer Information for Teens

Complementary & Alternative
    Medicine Information for Teens

Diabetes Information for Teens

Diet Information for Teens, 2nd Edition

Drug Information for Teens, 2nd Edition

Eating Disorders Information for Teens

Fitness Information for Teens, 2nd
    Edition

Learning Disabilities Information for
    Teens

Mental Health Information for Teens,
    2nd Edition

Pregnancy Information for Teens

Sexual Health Information for Teens,
    2nd Edition

Skin Health Information for Teens

Sleep Information for Teens

Sports Injuries Information for Teens,
    2nd Edition

Stress Information for Teens

Suicide Information for Teens

Tobacco Information for Teens

Diabetes

SOURCEBOOK

Fourth Edition

Health Reference Series

Fourth Edition

Diabetes
SOURCEBOOK

Basic Consumer Health Information about Type 1 and Type 2 Diabetes Mellitus, Gestational Diabetes, Monogenic Forms of Diabetes, and Insulin Resistance, with Guidelines for Lifestyle Modifications and the Medical Management of Diabetes, Including Facts about Insulin, Insulin Delivery Devices, Oral Diabetes Medications, Self-Monitoring of Blood Glucose, Meal Planning, Physical Activity Recommendations, Foot Care, and Treatment Options for People with Kidney Failure

Along with a Section about Diabetes Complications and Co-Occurring Conditions, a Glossary of Related Terms, and Directories of Resources for Additional Help and Information

Edited by
Karen Bellenir

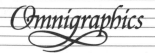

Omnigraphics

P.O. Box 31-1640, Detroit, MI 48231

Bibliographic Note

Because this page cannot legibly accommodate all the copyright notices, the Bibliographic Note portion of the Preface constitutes an extension of the copyright notice.

Edited by Karen Bellenir

Health Reference Series

Karen Bellenir, *Managing Editor*
David A. Cooke, M.D., *Medical Consultant*
Elizabeth Collins, *Research and Permissions Coordinator*
Cherry Stockdale, *Permissions Assistant*
EdIndex, Services for Publishers, *Indexers*

* * *

Omnigraphics, Inc.

Matthew P. Barbour, *Senior Vice President*
Kevin M. Hayes, *Operations Manager*

* * *

Peter E. Ruffner, *Publisher*

Copyright © 2008 Omnigraphics, Inc.

ISBN 978-0-7808-1005-1

Library of Congress Cataloging-in-Publication Data

Diabetes sourcebook : basic consumer health information about type 1 and type 2 diabetes mellitus, gestational diabetes, monogenic forms of diabetes, and insulin resistance, with guidelines for lifestyle modifications and the medical management of diabetes, including facts about insulin, insulin delivery devices, oral diabetes medications, self-monitoring of blood glucose, meal planning, physical activity recommendations, foot care, and treatment options for people with kidney failure; along with a section about diabetes complications and co-occurring conditions, a glossary of related terms, and directories of resources for additional help and information / edited by Karen Bellenir.-- 4th ed.
        p. cm. -- (Health reference series)
    Includes bibliographical references and index.
    Summary: "Provides updated basic consumer health information about treatment, management, and complications of Type 1 and Type 2 diabetes, including diet and exercise guidelines and coping strategies. Includes index, glossary of related terms, and other resources"--Provided by publisher.
    ISBN-13: 978-0-7808-1005-1 (hardcover : alk. paper) 1. Diabetes--Popular works. I. Bellenir, Karen.
    RC660.4.D56 2008
    616.4'62--dc22
                                                                    2008018819

This book is printed on acid-free paper meeting the ANSI Z39.48 Standard. The infinity symbol that appears above indicates that the paper in this book meets that standard.

Printed in the United States

Table of Contents

Visit www.healthreferencescries.com to view *A Contents Guide to the Health Reference Series*, a listing of more than 14,000 topics and the volumes in which they are covered.

Preface xi

Part I: About Diabetes

Chapter 1—What Is Diabetes? 3

Chapter 2—Diabetes Statistics 7

Section 2.1—One-Third of Adults with
Diabetes Still Don't Know
They Have It 8

Section 2.2—National Diabetes Statistics 11

Section 2.3—Groups Especially Affected by
Diabetes 15

Section 2.4—Diabetes Costs and Complications 18

Chapter 3—Type 1 Diabetes: What Is It? 23

Chapter 4—Insulin Resistance and Pre-Diabetes 29

Chapter 5—Type 2 Diabetes: The Most Common Form of
Diabetes 39

Chapter 6—Gestational Diabetes 47

Chapter 7—Monogenic Forms of Diabetes 55

Chapter 8—Steroid-Induced Diabetes 63

Chapter 9—Diabetes Insipidus 67

Part II: Lifestyle Issues and Diabetes Management

Chapter 10—Everyday Guidelines for Taking Care of Your Diabetes 75

Chapter 11—Dietary Guidelines for People with Diabetes 91

Chapter 12—Tips for Healthy Meal Planning 103

    Section 12.1—Recipe and Meal Planning Guide 104

    Section 12.2—How Does Fiber Affect Blood Glucose Levels? 108

    Section 12.3—Calorie Counting vs. Exchanges in Meal Planning ... 109

    Section 12.4—Carbohydrate Counting 111

    Section 12.5—Is the Glycemic Index a Helpful Tool? 118

    Section 12.6—Diabetes and Alcohol 119

    Section 12.7—Tips for Using Less Salt 122

    Section 12.8—Ordering Fast-Food Wisely 124

    Section 12.9—Buffet Table Tips for People with Diabetes 126

Chapter 13—Physical Activity Guidelines for People with Diabetes 127

Chapter 14—Take Care of Your Feet and Skin 135

Chapter 15—Take Care of Your Teeth and Gums 141

Chapter 16—Taking Care of Your Diabetes during Challenging Times 145

Chapter 17—Adjusting to Life with Diabetes 149

    Section 17.1—Feelings about Diabetes 150

    Section 17.2—Getting Your Diabetes Ready for Winter 152

    Section 17.3—Diabetes-Friendly Tips for Handling the Summer Heat ... 154

    Section 17.4—Driving when You Have Diabetes 156

    Section 17.5—Traveling with Diabetes 159

    Section 17.6—Diabetes and Work 162

    Section 17.7—Growing Older and Staying Healthy with Diabetes 165

Part III: Medical Interventions for Diabetes Management

Chapter 18—Managing Diabetes Is Your Responsibility 171

    Section 18.1—Keep Your Diabetes Under
           Control 172

    Section 18.2—Frequently Asked
           Questions about Diabetes
           Examinations and Tests 177

    Section 18.3—Diabetes Management
           Numbers At-a-Glance.............. 180

Chapter 19—Tests Used to Monitor Diabetes 183

    Section 19.1—Glucose Tolerance Testing 184

    Section 19.2—The ABCs of A1C Testing 191

    Section 19.3—Ketone Testing 194

    Section 19.4—Blood Urea Nitrogen (BUN) ... 196

    Section 19.5—Creatinine 199

    Section 19.6—Microalbumin and Micro-
           albumin/Creatinine Ratio 203

    Section 19.7—Glomerular Filtration Rate
           (GFR) 207

Chapter 20—Self-Monitoring of Blood Glucose 209

Chapter 21—Insulin 217

Chapter 22—Insulin Delivery Devices 225

    Section 22.1—Syringes, Pumps, Injectors,
           and More.................................. 226

    Section 22.2—Can I Reuse My Insulin
           Syringe? 250

    Section 22.3—Safe Needle Disposal 251

Chapter 23—Oral Medications for Type 2 Diabetes................. 255

    Section 23.1—Classes of Diabetes
           Medications 256

    Section 23.2—Metformin May Offer
           Important Advantages 262

    Section 23.3—Incretin-Based Therapy 264

    Section 23.4—Stronger Heart Warning on
           Some Diabetes Drugs 267

Chapter 24—Flu Shots and Other Vaccinations
          Recommended for People with Diabetes............. 269

Chapter 25—Complementary and Alternative Medical
        Therapies for Diabetes 273

**Part IV: Diabetes Complications and Co-Occurring
Conditions**

Chapter 26—Hypoglycemia 285

Chapter 27—Diabetes and Obesity 293

Chapter 28—Diabetes, Heart Disease, and Stroke 297

Chapter 29—Diabetic Vascular Disease 307

Chapter 30—Foot Ulcers 309

Chapter 31—Hypertension and Diabetes 315

Chapter 32—Diabetes and Kidney Disease 317

        Section 32.1—How Can Diabetes Damage
                the Kidneys? 318

        Section 32.2—Proteinuria 322

        Section 32.3—Amyloidosis 324

        Section 32.4—Nephrotic Syndrome 327

        Section 32.5—Glomerular Diseases 329

Chapter 33—Anemia and Diabetes 333

Chapter 34—Sexual and Urologic Problems of Diabetes 337

Chapter 35—Polycystic Ovary Syndrome 343

Chapter 36—Diabetic Neuropathies 347

Chapter 37—Gastroparesis 359

Chapter 38—Diabetic Retinopathy 365

Chapter 39—Diabetes and Bone-Related Concerns 375

Chapter 40—Diabetes and Depression 381

Part V: Diabetes and Kidney Failure

Chapter 41—Your Kidneys and How They Work 387

Chapter 42—Kidney Failure: Choosing a Treatment That's
        Right for You 399

Chapter 43—Understanding Hemodialysis 413

        Section 43.1—Hemodialysis for the
                Treatment of Kidney Failure 414

Section 43.2—Vascular Access for
                 Hemodialysis 418
Section 43.3—Hemodialysis Dose and
                 Adequacy 422
Section 43.4—Home Hemodialysis 426
Section 43.5—Eat Right to Feel Right on
                 Hemodialysis 429

Chapter 44—Understanding Peritoneal Dialysis 435
Section 44.1—Peritoneal Dialysis for the
                 Treatment of Kidney Failure ... 436
Section 44.2—Peritoneal Dialysis Dose
                 and Adequacy 444

Chapter 45—Skin and Hair Problems on Dialysis 447

Chapter 46—Kidney Transplantation 451

Chapter 47—Kidney and Pancreas Transplantation 457

Chapter 48—Pancreatic Islet Transplantation 461

Part VI: Diabetes-Related Research

Chapter 49—Diabetes Knowledge: Yesterday, Today, and
                 Tomorrow 469

Chapter 50—Diabetes Research: An Update 479

Chapter 51—Researching Diabetes Risk Factors 489
Section 51.1—Diabetes Risk Factors
                 Develop Earlier in Women 490
Section 51.2—Androgen Deprivation
                 Therapy May Increase Risk
                 of Diabetes 492
Section 51.3—Researchers Identify New
                 Genetic Risk Factors for
                 Type 2 Diabetes 494
Section 51.4—Long-Term Use of Selenium
                 Supplements and Risk for
                 Type 2 Diabetes 496
Section 51.5—Does Prenatal Exposure
                 to Viruses Place Children at
                 Risk for Diabetes? 498
Section 51.6—Does Hepatitis C Infection
                 Increase Risks for Diabetes? 501

Section 51.7—Greater Diabetes Risk in
Patients Taking High Blood
Pressure Medications 504

Chapter 52—Stress and Diabetes: A Review of the Links 505

Chapter 53—Diabetes Prevention Program 525

Part VII: Additional Help and Information

Chapter 54—Diabetes Dictionary 533

Chapter 55—Cookbooks for People with Diabetes or
Kidney Failure 555

Chapter 56—Directory of Diabetes Organizations 559

Chapter 57—Diabetes Research and Training Centers'
Prevention and Control Divisions 565

Chapter 58—Getting High Quality Medical Care in a
Changing Healthcare Landscape 577

Chapter 59—Financial Help for Diabetes Care or Kidney
Failure 587

Index 601

Preface

About This Book

According to the Centers for Disease Control and Prevention (CDC), the number of people in the United States with diagnosed diabetes has more than doubled in the last 15 years, but many cases—an estimated one in three—remain undiagnosed. Recent statistics suggest that a total of nearly 21 million Americans have diabetes, and another 54 million U.S. adults have prediabetes, placing them at high risk for developing the disorder. Diabetes is one of the leading causes of death and disability in the United States, and its long-term complications can affect almost every part of the body. Although there is no known cure, proper management, including lifestyle changes, early detection, and education about diabetes self-management, can help prevent the onset of diabetes among adults at high risk and reduce the burden of diabetes complications.

Diabetes Sourcebook, Fourth Edition contains updated information for people seeking to understand the risk factors, complications, and management of type 1 diabetes, type 2 diabetes, gestational diabetes, and monogenic forms of diabetes—those that result from mutations in a single gene. It offers information about lifestyle modifications related to delaying the onset of diabetes and managing its course after it has been diagnosed. It discusses medical interventions, including the use of insulin and oral diabetes medications, self-monitoring of blood glucose, and complementary and alternative therapies. Diabetes complications, including eye disease, gum disease, nerve damage, and kidney problems, are also addressed. The book concludes with a glossary of related terms and directories of information for people with diabetes or kidney failure.

How to Use This Book

This book is divided into parts and chapters. Parts focus on broad areas of interest. Chapters are devoted to single topics within a part.

Part I: About Diabetes describes the three major forms of diabetes—type 1 diabetes (formerly known as juvenile diabetes), type 2 diabetes (formerly known as adult-onset diabetes), and gestational diabetes—as well as other lesser-known varieties. It also offers statistical data about the prevalence of diabetes and its complications.

Part II: Lifestyle Issues and Diabetes Management discusses everyday tactics that can be used to maintain wellness and avoid or slow the progression of diabetes-related complications. Strategies include following a meal plan, being physically active, caring for the feet, skin, teeth, and gums, and dealing with challenges related to lifestyle adjustments.

Part III: Medical Interventions for Diabetes Management provides facts about tests and procedures used in the diagnosis and control of diabetes, including glucose tolerance testing, tests of kidney functioning, and self-monitoring of blood glucose. It also describes the use of insulin, insulin delivery devices, and oral diabetes medications. The part concludes with information about complementary and alternative therapies sometimes used by people with diabetes.

Part IV: Diabetes Complications and Co-Occurring Conditions describes some of the most common medical concerns among people with diabetes, including hypoglycemia, obesity, heart and vascular disease, foot ulcers, and hypertension. It also describes the diabetic processes that can lead to kidney disease, sexual and urologic problems, nerve problems, vision loss, and other impairments.

Part V: Diabetes and Kidney Failure explains hemodialysis, peritoneal dialysis, kidney transplantation, and other procedures that may be considered if the kidneys stop working. It discusses the advantages, disadvantages, and complications of the various options, and it provides facts about medical circumstances and lifestyle preferences that may influence treatment decisions.

Part VI: Diabetes-Related Research describes current research initiatives regarding the diagnosis, treatment, and prevention of diabetes and its complications.

Part VII: Additional Help and Information includes supplementary resources for people with diabetes. It offers a glossary, a list of cookbooks, directories of organizations and research centers, and suggestions for those who need help navigating the healthcare system or finding financial assistance.

Bibliographic Note

This volume contains documents and excerpts from publications issued by the following U.S. government agencies: Agency for Healthcare Research and Quality; Centers for Disease Control and Prevention (CDC); Equal Employment Opportunity Commission; National Center for Chronic Disease Prevention and Health Promotion; National Center for Complementary and Alternative Medicine; National Diabetes Education Program; National Diabetes Information Clearinghouse; National Digestive Diseases Information Clearinghouse; National Eye Institute; National Heart, Lung, and Blood Institute; National Highway Traffic Safety Administration; National Institute of Child Health and Human Development; National Institute of Diabetes and Digestive and Kidney Diseases; National Institutes of Health (NIH); National Institute of Arthritis and Musculoskeletal and Skin Diseases; National Kidney and Urologic Diseases Information Clearinghouse; National Kidney Disease Education Program; NIH Clinical Center; Office of Minority Health; U.S. Department of Health and Human Services; U.S. Department of Veterans' Affairs; U.S. Environmental Protection Agency; and the U.S. Food and Drug Administration.

In addition, this volume contains copyrighted documents from the following organizations: American Association for Clinical Chemistry; American Association of Kidney Patients; American College of Physicians; American Diabetes Association; American Podiatric Medical Association; CancerConsultants; Cleveland Clinic Foundation; Hepatitis C Support Project; Hormone Foundation; International Diabetes Federation; International Pemphigus and Pemphigoid Foundation; Joslin Diabetes Center; Life Options Rehabilitation Program; LifeMed Media, Inc.; Michigan Diabetes Research and Training Center; National Anemia Action Council; Nemours Foundation; and the University at Buffalo (State University of New York).

Full citation information is provided on the first page of each chapter or section. Every effort has been made to secure all necessary rights to reprint the copyrighted material. If any omissions have been made, please contact Omnigraphics to make corrections for future editions.

Acknowledgements

In addition to the organizations who have contributed to this *Sourcebook*, special thanks go to editorial assistants Nicole Salerno and Elizabeth Bellenir, research and permissions coordinator Liz Collins, and permissions assistant Cherry Stockdale.

About the Health Reference Series

The *Health Reference Series* is designed to provide basic medical information for patients, families, caregivers, and the general public. Each volume takes a particular topic and provides comprehensive coverage. This is especially important for people who may be dealing with a newly diagnosed disease or a chronic disorder in themselves or in a family member. People looking for preventive guidance, information about disease warning signs, medical statistics, and risk factors for health problems will also find answers to their questions in the *Health Reference Series*. The *Series*, however, is not intended to serve as a tool for diagnosing illness, in prescribing treatments, or as a substitute for the physician/patient relationship. All people concerned about medical symptoms or the possibility of disease are encouraged to seek professional care from an appropriate health care provider.

A Note about Spelling and Style

Health Reference Series editors use *Stedman's Medical Dictionary* as an authority for questions related to the spelling of medical terms and the *Chicago Manual of Style* for questions related to grammatical structures, punctuation, and other editorial concerns. Consistent adherence is not always possible, however, because the individual volumes within the *Series* include many documents from a wide variety of different producers and copyright holders, and the editor's primary goal is to present material from each source as accurately as is possible following the terms specified by each document's producer. This sometimes means that information in different chapters or sections may follow other guidelines and alternate spelling authorities.

For example, occasionally a copyright holder may require that epony-
mous terms be shown in possessive forms (Crohn's disease *vs.* Crohn
disease) or that British spelling norms be retained (leukaemia *vs.* leukemia).

Locating Information within the Health Reference Series

The *Health Reference Series* contains a wealth of information about
a wide variety of medical topics. Ensuring easy access to all the fact
sheets, research reports, in-depth discussions, and other material con-
tained within the individual books of the *Series* remains one of our
highest priorities. As the *Series* continues to grow in size and scope,
however, locating the precise information needed by a reader may
become more challenging.

A *Contents Guide to the Health Reference Series* was developed to
direct readers to the specific volumes that address their concerns. It
presents an extensive list of diseases, treatments, and other topics of
general interest compiled from the Tables of Contents and major index headings. To access *A Contents Guide to the Health Reference Series*, visit www.healthreferenceseries.com.

Medical Consultant

Medical consultation services are provided to the *Health Reference
Series* editors by David A. Cooke, M.D. Dr. Cooke is a graduate of
Brandeis University, and he received his M.D. degree from the University of Michigan. He completed residency training at the University of Wisconsin Hospital and Clinics. He is board-certified in Internal
Medicine. Dr. Cooke currently works as part of the University of Michigan Health System and practices in Ann Arbor, MI. In his free time,
he enjoys writing, science fiction, and spending time with his family.

Our Advisory Board

We would like to thank the following board members for providing guidance to the development of this *Series*:

- Dr. Lynda Baker,
  Associate Professor of Library and Information Science,
  Wayne State University, Detroit, MI

- Nancy Bulgarelli,
  William Beaumont Hospital Library, Royal Oak, MI

- Karen Imarisio,
  Bloomfield Township Public Library, Bloomfield Township, MI

- Karen Morgan,
  Mardigian Library, University of Michigan-Dearborn,
  Dearborn, MI

- Rosemary Orlando,
  St. Clair Shores Public Library, St. Clair Shores, MI

Health Reference Series *Update Policy*

The inaugural book in the *Health Reference Series* was the first edition of *Cancer Sourcebook* published in 1989. Since then, the *Series* has been enthusiastically received by librarians and in the medical community. In order to maintain the standard of providing high-quality health information for the layperson the editorial staff at Omnigraphics felt it was necessary to implement a policy of updating volumes when warranted.

Medical researchers have been making tremendous strides, and it is the purpose of the *Health Reference Series* to stay current with the most recent advances. Each decision to update a volume is made on an individual basis. Some of the considerations include how much new information is available and the feedback we receive from people who use the books. If there is a topic you would like to see added to the update list, or an area of medical concern you feel has not been adequately addressed, please write to:

Editor
Health Reference Series
Omnigraphics, Inc.
P.O. Box 31-1640
Detroit, MI 48231-1640
E-mail: editorial@omnigraphics.com

Part One

About Diabetes

Chapter 1

What Is Diabetes?

Diabetes means your blood glucose (often called blood sugar) is too high. Your blood always has some glucose in it because your body needs glucose for energy to keep you going. But too much glucose in the blood isn't good for your health.

How do you get high blood glucose?

Glucose comes from the food you eat and is also made in your liver and muscles. Your blood carries the glucose to all the cells in your body. Insulin is a chemical (a hormone) made by the pancreas. The pancreas releases insulin into the blood. Insulin helps the glucose from food get into your cells. If your body doesn't make enough insulin, or if the insulin doesn't work the way it should, glucose can't get into your cells. It stays in your blood instead. Your blood glucose level then gets too high, causing pre-diabetes or diabetes.

What is pre-diabetes?

Pre-diabetes is a condition in which blood glucose levels are higher than normal but not high enough for a diagnosis of diabetes. People with pre-diabetes are at increased risk for developing type 2 diabetes and for heart disease and stroke. The good news is, if you have

From "Your Guide to Diabetes: Type 1 and Type 2," National Diabetes Information Clearinghouse, National Institute of Diabetes and Digestive and Kidney Diseases, NIH Pub. 07-4016, October 2006.

pre-diabetes, you can reduce your risk of getting diabetes. With modest weight loss and moderate physical activity, you can delay or prevent type 2 diabetes and even return to normal glucose levels.

What are the signs of diabetes?

The following are signs diabetes:

- being very thirsty
- urinating often
- feeling very hungry or tired
- losing weight without trying
- having sores that heal slowly
- having dry, itchy skin
- losing the feeling in your feet or having tingling in your feet
- having blurry eyesight

You may have had one or more of these signs before you found out you had diabetes. Or you may have had no signs at all. A blood test to check your glucose levels will show if you have pre-diabetes or diabetes.

What kind of diabetes do you have?

People can get diabetes at any age. There are three main kinds. Type 1 diabetes, formerly called juvenile diabetes or insulin-dependent diabetes, is usually first diagnosed in children, teenagers, or young adults. With this form of diabetes, the beta cells of the pancreas no longer make insulin because the body's immune system has attacked and destroyed them. Treatment for type 1 diabetes includes taking insulin, making wise food choices, being physically active, taking aspirin daily (for some), and controlling blood pressure and cholesterol.

Type 2 diabetes, formerly called adult-onset diabetes or noninsulin-dependent diabetes, is the most common form of diabetes. People can develop type 2 diabetes at any age—even during childhood. This form of diabetes usually begins with insulin resistance, a condition in which fat, muscle, and liver cells do not use insulin properly. At first, the pancreas keeps up with the added demand by producing more insulin. In time, however, it loses the ability to secrete enough insulin in response to meals. Being overweight and inactive increases the chances of developing type 2 diabetes. Treatment includes using diabetes medicines,

4

making wise food choices, being physically active, taking aspirin daily, and controlling blood pressure and cholesterol.

Some women develop gestational diabetes during the late stages of pregnancy. Although this form of diabetes usually goes away after the baby is born, a woman who has had it is more likely to develop type 2 diabetes later in life. Gestational diabetes is caused by the hormones of pregnancy or a shortage of insulin.

Why do you need to take care of your diabetes?

After many years, diabetes can lead to serious problems with your eyes, kidneys, nerves, and gums and teeth. But the most serious problem caused by diabetes is heart disease. When you have diabetes, you are more than twice as likely as people without diabetes to have heart disease or a stroke.

If you have diabetes, your risk of a heart attack is the same as someone who has already had a heart attack. Both women and men with diabetes are at risk. You may not even have the typical signs of a heart attack.

You can reduce your risk of developing heart disease by controlling your blood pressure and blood fat levels. If you smoke, talk with your doctor about quitting. Remember that every step toward your goals helps!

The best way to take care of your health is to work with your health care team to keep your blood glucose, blood pressure, and cholesterol in your target range.

What's a desirable blood glucose level?

Everyone's blood has some glucose in it. In people who don't have diabetes, the normal range is about 70 to 120. Blood glucose goes up after eating but 1 or 2 hours later returns to the normal range.

Ask your health care team when you should check your blood glucose with a meter. Talk about whether the typical blood glucose targets are best for you. Then make your own targets.

Table 1.1. Blood Glucose Targets for Most People with Diabetes

When	Target Levels
Before meals	90 to 130
1 to 2 hours after the start of a meal	Less than 180

5

It may be hard to reach your target range all of the time. But the closer you get to your goal, the more you will reduce your risk of diabetes-related problems and the better you will feel. Every step helps.

Chapter 2

Diabetes Statistics

Chapter Contents

Section 2.1—One-Third of Adults with Diabetes Still
  Don't Know They Have It 8
Section 2.2—National Diabetes Statistics 11
Section 2.3—Groups Especially Affected by Diabetes 15
Section 2.4—Diabetes Costs and Complications 18

Section 2.1

One-Third of Adults with Diabetes Still Don't Know They Have It

Excerpted from, "One-Third of Adults with Diabetes Still Don't Know They Have It," Office of Minority Health, U.S. Department of Health and Human Services, May 26, 2006.

The prevalence of diagnosed diabetes in U.S. adults age 20 and older has risen from about 5.1 percent to 6.5 percent, according to researchers at the National Institutes of Health (NIH) and the Centers for Disease Control and Prevention (CDC), who analyzed national survey data from two periods—1988 to 1994 and 1999 to 2002. However, the percentage of adults with undiagnosed diabetes did not change significantly over the years studied. About 2.8 percent of U.S. adults—one-third of those with diabetes—still don't know they have it.

The study, published in the June 2006 issue of *Diabetes Care*, notes that type 2 diabetes accounts for up to 95 percent of all diabetes cases and virtually all undiagnosed diabetes cases. Diabetes is a group of diseases marked by high levels of blood glucose resulting from defects in insulin production, insulin action, or both. It is the most common cause of blindness, kidney failure, and amputations in adults and a major cause of heart disease and stroke.

Over the years studied, about 26 percent of adults age 20 and older continued to have impaired fasting glucose (IFG), a form of pre-diabetes. IFG, in which blood glucose measured after an overnight fast is high but not yet diagnostic of diabetes, increases the risk of heart disease as well as the risk of developing type 2 diabetes.

The researchers also found the following:

- Nearly 22 percent of people age 65 and older had diabetes.

- About 13 percent of non-Hispanic blacks age 20 and older had diabetes. Diabetes was twice as common in non-Hispanic blacks compared to non-Hispanic whites.

8

- About 13 percent of non-Hispanic blacks age 20 and older had diabetes. Diabetes was twice as common in non-Hispanic blacks compared to non-Hispanic whites.

- About 8 percent of Mexican Americans age 20 and older had diabetes.

Because the average age of Mexican Americans is younger than for other groups, the age-and sex-adjusted prevalence of diabetes in Mexican Americans is twice that of non-Hispanic whites and about equal to that of non-Hispanic blacks.

- IFG and undiagnosed diabetes were about 70 percent more common in men than in women, especially in non-Hispanic white men.

- Nearly 40 percent of people age 65 and older had IFG, which becomes more common with age.

In the study, the researchers compared two slices of data, one from 1988 to 1994 and the other from 1999 to 2002. The data were derived from a national sample of U.S. adults age 20 years and older who took part in the National Health and Nutrition Examination Survey (NHANES) conducted by the CDC's National Center for Health Statistics. Survey participants were interviewed in their homes and received a physical exam with a blood test, which included a glucose reading taken after an overnight fast. The NHANES is unique because it includes a blood test that detects undiagnosed diabetes and IFG.

"This study updates and generally corroborates earlier analyses that were based on two years of NHANES data," said lead author Cathcrine Cowie, Ph.D., of the National Institute of Diabetes and Digestive and Kidney Diseases (NIDDK). "We're seeing a rising prevalence of diagnosed diabetes that is not substantially offset by a drop in the rate of undiagnosed—about one-third of adults with diabetes still don't know they have it. Another 26 percent of adults have a form of pre-diabetes."

Pre-diabetes, which usually causes no symptoms, is serious because many people with the condition develop type 2 diabetes in the next 10 years. Also, pre-diabetes substantially raises the risk of a heart attack or stroke even if type 2 diabetes does not develop.

People with pre-diabetes may have IFG or impaired glucose tolerance (IGT) or both.

- In IFG, blood glucose is high (100 to 125 milligrams per deciliter or mg/dL) after an overnight fast but not high enough to be diagnostic of diabetes.

- In IGT, blood glucose is high (140 to 199 mg/dL) two hours after drinking a sugary drink in an oral glucose tolerance test but not high enough to be diagnostic of diabetes.

In the current study, researchers did not assess the prevalence of IGT because an oral glucose tolerance test was not a part of the survey.

People with pre-diabetes can often prevent or delay diabetes if they lose a modest amount of weight by cutting calories in their diet and increasing physical activity (for example, walking 30 minutes a day five days a week). A major study of people with IGT has shown that lifestyle changes leading to a 5 to 7 percent weight loss lowered diabetes onset by 58 percent.

If you are over age 45, you should consult your health care provider about testing for pre-diabetes or diabetes. If you are younger than 45, overweight, and have another risk factor, you should ask about testing.

Section 2.2

National Diabetes Statistics

Excerpted from "National Diabetes Statistics," National Diabetes
Information Clearinghouse, National Institute of Diabetes and Digestive and Kidney Diseases, NIH Pub. No. 06-3892, November 2005.

Total Prevalence of Diabetes in the United States, All Ages, 2005

- **Total:** 20.8 million people—7 percent of the population—have diabetes.

- **Diagnosed:** 14.6 million people

- **Undiagnosed:** 6.2 million people

Prevalence of Diagnosed Diabetes in People Aged 20 Years or Younger, United States, 2005

- About 176,500 people aged 20 years or younger have diabetes. This group represents 0.22 percent of all people in this age group.

- About one in every 400 to 600 children and adolescents has type 1 diabetes.

- Although type 2 diabetes can occur among youth, the nationally representative data that would be needed to monitor diabetes trends in youth by type are not available. Clinically based reports and regional studies suggest that type 2 diabetes, although still rare, is being diagnosed more frequently in children and adolescents, particularly in American Indians, African Americans, and Hispanic/Latino Americans.

Note: The CDC's National Health Interview Survey (NHIS) is the only source of national data on diabetes in children and adolescents. Because diabetes is relatively rare in this age group and the NHIS sample size is small, prevalence estimates for diabetes in youth vary considerably from year to year. To reduce this variability, prevalence estimates in this report are based on five years of NHIS data instead of three, resulting in a lower estimate of diabetes in youth than the estimate for 2003. CDC and the National Institutes of Health are funding a five-year study, SEARCH for Diabetes in Youth, which is examining the incidence and prevalence of diabetes in youth in six geographical regions of the United States. When completed, the SEARCH study will provide more reliable estimates of diabetes in youth.

Total Prevalence of Diabetes among People Aged 20 Years or Older, United States, 2005

- **Age 20 years or older:** 20.6 million; 9.6 percent of all people in this age group have diabetes.

- **Age 60 years or older:** 10.3 million; 20.9 percent of all people in this age group have diabetes.

- **Men:** 10.9 million; 10.5 percent of all men aged 20 years or older have diabetes.

- **Women:** 9.7 million; 8.8 percent of all women aged 20 years or older have diabetes.

Total Prevalence of Diabetes by Race/Ethnicity among People Aged 20 Years or Older, United States, 2005

- **Non-Hispanic whites:** 13.1 million; 8.7 percent of all non-Hispanic whites aged 20 years or older have diabetes.

- **Non-Hispanic blacks:** 3.2 million; 13.3 percent of all non-Hispanic blacks aged 20 years or older have diabetes. After adjusting for population age differences, non-Hispanic blacks are 1.8 times as likely to have diabetes as non-Hispanic whites of similar age.

- **Hispanic/Latino Americans:** After adjusting for population age differences, Mexican Americans, the largest Hispanic/Latino subgroup, are 1.7 times as likely to have diabetes as non-Hispanic whites. If the prevalence of diabetes among Mexican Americans was applied to the total Hispanic/Latino population, about 2.5 million (9.5 percent) Hispanic/Latino Americans aged 20 years or older would have diabetes. Sufficient data are not available to derive estimates of the total prevalence of diabetes (both diagnosed and undiagnosed diabetes) for other Hispanic/Latino groups.

However, residents of Puerto Rico are 1.8 times as likely to have diagnosed diabetes as non-Hispanic whites in the United Sates.

- **American Indians and Alaska Natives who receive care from the Indian Health Service (IHS):** 99,500; 12.8 percent of American Indians and Alaska Natives aged 20 years or older who received care from the Indian Health Service (IHS) in 2003 had diagnosed diabetes. Applying the rate of undiagnosed diabetes in the total U.S. population to the American Indians and Alaska Natives who receive care from IHS gives an estimate of 118,000 (15.1 percent) American Indians and Alaska Natives aged 20 years or older with diabetes (both diagnosed and undiagnosed diabetes). After adjusting for population age differences, the total prevalence of diabetes in this group is lowest among Alaska Natives (8.1 percent) and highest among American Indians in the southern United States (26.7 percent) and in southern Arizona (27.6 percent). Taking into account population age differences, American Indians and Alaska Natives are 2.2 times as likely to have diabetes as non-Hispanic whites.

- **Asian Americans and Native Hawaiian or other Pacific Islanders:** The total prevalence of diabetes (both diagnosed and undiagnosed diabetes) is not available for Asian Americans or Pacific Islanders. In Hawaii, however, Asians, Native Hawaiians, and other Pacific Islanders aged 20 years or older are more than two times as likely to have diagnosed diabetes as whites after adjusting for population age differences. Similarly in California, Asians were 1.5 times as likely to have diagnosed diabetes as non-Hispanic whites. Other groups within these populations also have increased risk for diabetes.

Incidence of Diabetes, United States, 2005

- 1.5 million new cases of diabetes were diagnosed in people aged 20 years or older in 2005.

Deaths among People with Diabetes, United States, 2002

- Diabetes was the sixth leading cause of death listed on U.S. death certificates in 2002. This ranking is based on the 73,249 death certificates in which diabetes was listed as the underlying cause of death. According to death certificate reports, diabetes contributed to a total of 224,092 deaths.

- Diabetes is likely to be underreported as a cause of death. Studies have found that only about 35 to 40 percent of decedents with diabetes have diabetes listed anywhere on the death certificate and only about 10 to 15 percent had it listed as the underlying cause of death.

- Overall, the risk for death among people with diabetes is about twice that of people without diabetes of similar age.

Pre-Diabetes: Impaired Glucose Tolerance and Impaired Fasting Glucose

- In a cross-section sample of U.S. adults aged 40 to 74 years (tested from 1988 to 1994), 33.8 percent had IFG, 15.4 percent had IGT, and 40.1 percent had pre-diabetes (IGT or IFG or both). Applying these percentages to the entire U.S. population in 2000, an estimated 35 million adults aged 40 to 74 years had IFG, 16 million had IGT, and 41 million had pre-diabetes (there is overlap between the IFG and IGT groups).

- More recent estimates from 1999–2002 indicate that, among U.S. adults age 20 years and older, 26 percent had IFG, which was similar to the prevalence in 1988–1994 (25 percent). Applying this percentage to the entire U.S. population, 54 million American adults had IFG in 2002. Because IGT was not measured in 1999–2002, these data suggest that at least 54 million American adults had pre-diabetes in 2002.

- Progression to diabetes among those with pre-diabetes is not inevitable. Studies have shown that people with pre-diabetes who lose weight and increase their physical activity can prevent or delay diabetes and even return their blood glucose levels to normal.

Treating Diabetes

- To survive, people with type 1 diabetes must have insulin delivered by injections or a pump.

- Many people with type 2 diabetes can control their blood glucose by following a healthy meal plan and exercise program, losing excess weight, and taking oral medication.

- Many people with diabetes also need to take medications to control their cholesterol and blood pressure.

- Diabetes self-management education is an integral component of medical care.

- Among adults with diagnosed diabetes, 16 percent take insulin only, 12 percent take both insulin and oral medication, 57 percent take oral medication only, and 15 percent do not take either insulin or oral medications.

Section 2.3

Groups Especially Affected by Diabetes

Excerpted from "Frequently Asked Questions: Groups Especially Affected by Diabetes," National Center for Chronic Disease Prevention and Health Promotion, Centers for Disease Control and Prevention, June 2007.

How are women especially affected by diabetes?

Of the 20.8 million people with diabetes in the United States, 9.7 million are women. The risk of heart disease, the most common complication of diabetes, is more serious among women than men. Among people with diabetes who have had a heart attack, women have lower survival rates and a poorer quality of life than men. Women with diabetes have a shorter life expectancy than women without diabetes, and women are at greater risk of blindness from diabetes than men. Death rates for women aged 25–44 years with diabetes are more than three times the rate for women without diabetes.

Women with diabetes must also plan childbearing carefully. It is especially important to keep blood glucose levels as near to normal as possible before and during pregnancy, to protect both mother and baby. Pregnancy itself may affect insulin levels, as well as diabetes-related eye and kidney problems.

What is gestational diabetes?

Gestational diabetes is a type of diabetes, or high blood sugar, that only pregnant women get. If a woman gets high blood sugar when she's pregnant, but she never had high blood sugar before, she has gestational diabetes.

Managing gestational diabetes is very important in order to protect the baby. Babies born to mothers with uncontrolled gestational diabetes can be overly large at birth, making delivery more dangerous. These babies can also have breathing problems. Moreover, children exposed to diabetes in the womb are more likely to become obese during childhood and adolescence, and develop type 2 diabetes later in life.

Usually, gestational diabetes goes away after the baby is born. However, women who have had gestational diabetes are at higher risk for developing type 2 diabetes later in life, so healthy eating, physical activity, and weight maintenance are important steps to prevention.

What racial and ethnic groups are especially affected by diabetes?

African Americans, Hispanic/Latino Americans, American Indians, Asian Americans, and Pacific Islander Americans are at particularly high risk for type 2 diabetes. In addition, gestational diabetes occurs more frequently in African Americans, Hispanic/Latino Americans, and American Indians than in other groups.

Why do some racial and ethnic groups have higher rates of diabetes?

Diabetes can indeed "run in families," meaning that heredity often makes someone more likely to develop diabetes. Researchers believe that certain genes affecting immune response can play a role in the development of type 1 diabetes, while genes affecting insulin function can contribute to the development of type 2 diabetes. While African Americans, Hispanic/Latino Americans, American Indians, Asian Americans, and Pacific Islander Americans have a slightly lower rate of type 1 diabetes, they are at a higher risk for type 2 diabetes than the rest of the population.

Many researchers think that some African Americans, Hispanic/Latino Americans, American Indians, Asian Americans, and Pacific Islander Americans inherited a "thrifty gene" which helped their ancestors store food energy better during times when food was plentiful, to survive during times when food was scarce. Now that "feast or famine" situations rarely occur for most people in the United States, the gene which was once helpful may now put these groups at a higher risk for type 2 diabetes.

In addition, poverty, lack of access to health care, cultural attitudes, and behaviors are barriers to preventive and diabetes management care for some minority Americans.

How are children especially affected by diabetes?

Type 1 diabetes, which used to be called juvenile diabetes, is usually first diagnosed in children, teens, or young adults. In type 1 diabetes, the body's immune system attacks and destroys beta cells in the pancreas, so that they no longer make insulin. People with type 1 diabetes must take insulin every day. Approximately one of every 400 to 500 children and adolescents has type 1 diabetes.

Type 2 diabetes, a disease usually diagnosed in adults aged 40 years or older, is now becoming more common among children and adolescents, particularly in American Indians, African Americans, and Hispanic/Latinos.

Among youth, obesity, physical inactivity, and prenatal exposure to diabetes in the mother have become widespread, and may contribute to the increased development of type 2 diabetes during childhood and adolescence.

How are older adults especially affected by diabetes?

As we age, our risk for developing diabetes increases. Approximately half of all diabetes cases occur in people aged 60 years or older. Approximately 20.9% (10.3 million) of people in the United States aged 60 years or older have diabetes. Diabetes often leads to chronic conditions that eventually result in death, such as heart disease and kidney disease. Thus, diabetes is often responsible for, but not listed as, the cause of many deaths.

How are some veterans affected by diabetes?

Vietnam veterans exposed to the herbicide Agent Orange may be at increased risk for developing type 2 diabetes. In the year 2000, the Veterans Administration announced that it would recognize diabetes as a Vietnam service-related disease.

Section 2.4

Diabetes Costs and Complications

Excerpted from "National Diabetes Statistics," National Diabetes
Information Clearinghouse, National Institute of Diabetes and Digestive and Kidney Diseases, NIH Pub. No. 06-3892, November 2005.

Cost of Diabetes in the United States, 2002

- Total (direct and indirect): $132 billion

- Direct medical costs: $92 billion

- Indirect costs: $40 billion (disability, work loss, premature mor-
tality)

These data are based on a study conducted by the Lewin Group, Inc.,
for the American Diabetes Association and are 2002 estimates of both
the direct costs (cost of medical care and services) and indirect costs
(costs of short-term and permanent disability and of premature death)
attributable to diabetes. This study uses a specific cost-of-disease meth-
odology to estimate the health care costs that are due to diabetes.

Complications of Diabetes in the United States

Heart Disease and Stroke

- Heart disease and stroke account for about 65 percent of deaths
in people with diabetes.

- Adults with diabetes have heart disease death rates about two
to four times higher than adults without diabetes.

- The risk for stroke is two to four times higher among people
with diabetes.

High Blood Pressure

- About 73 percent of adults with diabetes have blood pressure
greater than or equal to 130/80 mm Hg or use prescription medications for hypertension.

Blindness

- Diabetes is the leading cause of new cases of blindness among adults aged 20 to 74 years.

- Diabetic retinopathy causes 12,000 to 24,000 new cases of blindness each year.

Kidney Disease

- Diabetes is the leading cause of kidney failure, accounting for 44 percent of new cases in 2002.

- In 2002 in the United States and Puerto Rico, 44,400 people with diabetes began treatment for end-stage kidney disease.

- In 2002 in the United States and Puerto Rico, 153,730 people with end-stage kidney disease due to diabetes were living on chronic dialysis or with a kidney transplant.

Nervous System Disease

- About 60 to 70 percent of people with diabetes have mild to severe forms of nervous system damage. The results of such damage include impaired sensation or pain in the feet or hands, slowed digestion of food in the stomach, carpal tunnel syndrome, and other nerve problems.

- Almost 30 percent of people with diabetes aged 40 years or older have impaired sensation in the feet (that is, at least one area that lacks feeling).

- Severe forms of diabetic nerve disease are a major contributing cause of lower-extremity amputations.

Amputations

- More than 60 percent of nontraumatic lower-limb amputations occur among people with diabetes.

- In 2002, about 82,000 nontraumatic lower-limb amputations were performed in people with diabetes.

Dental Disease

- Periodontal (gum) disease is more common in people with diabetes. Among young adults, those with diabetes have about twice the risk of those without diabetes.

- Almost one-third of people with diabetes have severe periodontal diseases with loss of attachment of the gums to the teeth measuring 5 millimeters or more.

Complications of Pregnancy

- Poorly controlled diabetes before conception and during the first trimester of pregnancy can cause major birth defects in 5 to 10 percent of pregnancies and spontaneous abortions in 15 to 20 percent of pregnancies.

- Poorly controlled diabetes during the second and third trimesters of pregnancy can result in excessively large babies, posing a risk to both mother and child.

Other Complications

- Uncontrolled diabetes often leads to biochemical imbalances that can cause acute life-threatening events, such as diabetic ketoacidosis and hyperosmolar (nonketotic) coma.

- People with diabetes are more susceptible to many other illnesses and, once they acquire these illnesses, often have worse prognoses. For example, they are more likely to die with pneumonia or influenza than people who do not have diabetes.

Prevention of Diabetes Complications

Diabetes can affect many parts of the body and can lead to serious complications such as blindness, kidney damage, and lower-limb amputations. Working together, people with diabetes and their health care providers can reduce the occurrence of these and other diabetes complications by controlling the levels of blood glucose, blood pressure, and blood lipids and by receiving other preventive care practices in a timely manner.

- **Glucose control:** Studies in the United States and abroad have found that improved glycemic control benefits people with either type 1 or type 2 diabetes. In general, every percentage point drop in A1C blood test results (for example, from 8 to 7 percent) reduces the risk of microvascular complications (eye, kidney, and nerve disease) is reduced by 40 percent.

- **Blood pressure control:** Blood pressure control reduces the risk of cardiovascular disease (heart disease or stroke) among persons with diabetes by 33 to 50 percent, and the risk of micro-vascular complications (eye, kidney, and nerve disease) by about 33 percent. In general, for every 10 mm Hg reduction in systolic blood pressure, the risk for any complication related to diabetes is reduced by 12 percent.

- **Control of blood lipids:** Improved control of cholesterol or blood lipids (for example, HDL, LDL, and triglycerides) can reduce cardiovascular complications by 20 to 50 percent.

Preventive Care Practices for Eyes, Kidneys, and Feet

- Detecting and treating diabetic eye disease with laser therapy can reduce the development of severe vision loss by an estimated 50 to 60 percent.

- Comprehensive foot care programs can reduce amputation rates by 45 to 85 percent.

- Detecting and treating early diabetic kidney disease by lowering blood pressure can reduce the decline in kidney function by 30 to 70 percent. Treatment with ACE inhibitors and angiotensin receptor blockers (ARBs) are more effective in reducing the decline in kidney function than other blood pressure-lowering drugs.

Chapter 3

Type 1 Diabetes: What Is It?

If you have a child who has been diagnosed with diabetes, you're not alone. Every year in the United States, 13,000 children are diagnosed with type 1 diabetes, and more than 1 million American kids and adults deal with the disease every day.

Diabetes is a chronic condition that needs close attention, but with some practical knowledge, you can become your child's most important ally in learning to live with the disease.

What Is Diabetes?

Diabetes is a disease that affects how the body uses glucose, the main type of sugar in the blood. Glucose comes from the foods we eat and is the major source of energy needed to fuel the body's functions.

After you eat a meal, your body breaks down the foods you eat into glucose and other nutrients, which are then absorbed into the bloodstream from the gastrointestinal tract. The glucose level in the blood rises after a meal and triggers the pancreas to make the hormone insulin and release it into the bloodstream. But in people with diabetes, the body either can't make or can't respond to insulin properly.

Insulin works like a key that opens the doors to cells and allows the glucose in. Without insulin, glucose can't get into the cells (the doors

"Type 1 Diabetes: What Is It?" March 2005, reprinted with permission from www.kidshealth.org. Copyright © 2005 The Nemours Foundation. This information was provided by KidsHealth, one of the largest resources online for medically reviewed health information written for parents, kids, and teens. For more articles like this one, visit www.KidsHealth.org, or www.TeensHealth.org.

are "locked" and there is no key) and so it stays in the bloodstream. As a result, the level of sugar in the blood remains higher than normal. High blood sugar levels are a problem because they can cause a number of health problems.

What Is Type 1 Diabetes?

There are two major types of diabetes: type 1 and type 2. Both type 1 and type 2 diabetes cause blood sugar levels to become higher than normal. However, they cause it in different ways.

Type 1 diabetes (formerly called insulin-dependent diabetes or juvenile diabetes) results when the pancreas loses its ability to make the hormone insulin. In type 1 diabetes, the person's own immune system attacks and destroys the cells in the pancreas that produce insulin. Once those cells are destroyed, they won't ever make insulin again.

Although no one knows for certain why this happens, scientists think it has something to do with genes. But just getting the genes for diabetes isn't usually enough. A person probably would then have to be exposed to something else—like a virus—to get type 1 diabetes.

Type 1 diabetes can't be prevented, and there is no practical way to predict who will get it. There is nothing that either a parent or the child did to cause the disease. Once a person has type 1 diabetes, it does not go away and requires lifelong treatment. Children and teens with type 1 diabetes depend on daily insulin injections or an insulin pump to control their blood glucose levels.

Type 2 diabetes (formerly called non-insulin-dependent diabetes or adult-onset diabetes) is different from type 1 diabetes. Type 2 diabetes results from the body's inability to respond to insulin normally. Unlike people with type 1 diabetes, most people with type 2 diabetes can still produce insulin, but not enough to meet their body's needs.

Signs and Symptoms of Type 1 Diabetes

A person can have diabetes without knowing it because the symptoms aren't always obvious and they can take a long time to develop. Type 1 diabetes may come on gradually or suddenly.

Parents of a child with typical symptoms of type 1 diabetes may notice that their child:

- urinates frequently. The kidneys respond to high levels of glucose in the bloodstream by flushing out the extra glucose in urine. A child with diabetes needs to urinate more frequently and in larger volumes.

- is abnormally thirsty. Because the child is losing so much fluid from peeing so much, he or she becomes very thirsty to help avoid becoming dehydrated. A child who has developed diabetes drinks a lot in an attempt to keep the level of body water normal.

- loses weight (or fails to gain weight as he or she grows) in spite of a good appetite. Kids and teens who develop type 1 diabetes may have an increased appetite, but often lose weight. This is because the body breaks down muscle and stored fat in an attempt to provide fuel to the hungry cells.

- often feels tired because the body can't use glucose for energy properly.

But in some cases, other symptoms may be the signal that something is wrong. Sometimes the first sign of diabetes is bedwetting in a child who has been dry at night. The possibility of diabetes should also be suspected if a vaginal yeast infection (also called a *Candida* infection) occurs in a girl who hasn't started puberty yet.

If these early symptoms of diabetes aren't recognized and treatment isn't started, chemicals called ketones can build up in the child's blood and cause stomach pain, nausea, vomiting, fruity-smelling breath, breathing problems, and even loss of consciousness. Sometimes these symptoms are mistaken for the flu or appendicitis. Doctors call this serious condition diabetic ketoacidosis, or DKA.

In addition to short-term problems like those listed above, diabetes can also cause long-term complications in some people, including heart disease, stroke, vision impairment, and kidney damage. Diabetes can also cause other problems throughout the body in the blood vessels, nerves, and gums. These problems don't usually show up in kids or teens with type 1 diabetes who have had the disease for only a few years. However, these health problems can occur in adulthood in some people with diabetes, particularly if they haven't managed or controlled their diabetes properly.

There's good news, though—proper treatment can stop or control these diabetes symptoms and reduce the risk of long-term problems. Doctors can say for sure if a person has diabetes by testing urine and blood samples for glucose. If you think your child has symptoms of diabetes, talk to your child's doctor. If the diagnosis of diabetes is suspected or confirmed, the doctor may refer your child to a pediatric endocrinologist, a doctor who specializes in the diagnosis and treatment of children with diseases of the endocrine system, such as diabetes and growth disorders.

Living with Type 1 Diabetes

Children and teens with diabetes need to monitor and control their glucose levels. They need to:

- check blood sugar levels a few times a day by testing a small blood sample;

- give themselves insulin injections, have an adult give them injections, or use an insulin pump;

- eat a balanced, healthy diet and pay special attention to the amounts of sugars and starches in the food they eat and the timing of their meals;

- get regular exercise to help control blood sugar levels and help avoid some of the long-term health problems that diabetes can cause, like heart disease;

- work closely with their doctor and diabetes health care team to help achieve the best possible control of their diabetes and be monitored for signs of diabetes complications and other health problems that occur more frequently in children with type 1 diabetes.

Living with diabetes is a challenge, no matter what a child's age, but young children and teens often have special issues to deal with. Young children may not understand why the blood samples and insulin injections are necessary. They may be scared, angry, and uncooperative.

Teens may feel different from their peers and may want to live a more spontaneous lifestyle than their diabetes allows. Even when they faithfully follow their treatment schedule, teens with diabetes may feel frustrated when the natural adolescent body changes during puberty may make their diabetes somewhat harder to control.

Having a child with diabetes may seem overwhelming at times, but you're not alone. Your child's diabetes care team is not only a great resource for dealing with blood sugar control and medical issues, but also for supporting and helping you and your child cope and live with diabetes.

What's New in the Treatment of Type 1 Diabetes?

Doctors and researchers are developing new equipment and treatments to help children cope with the special problems of growing up with diabetes.

Some kids and teens are already using new devices that make blood glucose testing and insulin injections easier, less painful, and more effective. One of these devices is the insulin pump, a mechanical device which can be used to deliver insulin more like the pancreas does. There's also been progress toward the development of a wearable or implantable "artificial pancreas." This device consists of an insulin pump linked to a device that measures the person's blood glucose level continuously.

Doctors and scientists are also investigating a potential cure for diabetes. This involves transplanting insulin-producing cells into the body of a person with diabetes. Researchers are also testing ways to stop diabetes before it starts. For example, scientists are studying whether diabetes can be prevented in those who may have inherited an increased risk for the disease.

Until scientists have perfected ways to better treat and possibly even prevent or cure diabetes, parents can help their children lead happier, healthier lives by giving constant encouragement, arming themselves with diabetes information, and making sure their children eat properly, exercise, and stay on top of blood sugar control every day. Doing so will enable kids to do all the things that other children do while helping them grow up to be healthy, well-adjusted, productive adults.

Chapter 4

Insulin Resistance and Pre-Diabetes

Insulin resistance is a silent condition that increases the chances of developing diabetes and heart disease. Learning about insulin resistance is the first step you can take toward making lifestyle changes that will help you prevent diabetes and other health problems.

What does insulin do?

After you eat, the food is broken down into glucose, the simple sugar that is the main source of energy for the body's cells. But your cells cannot use glucose without insulin, a hormone produced by the pancreas. Insulin helps the cells take in glucose and convert it to energy. When the pancreas does not make enough insulin or the body is unable to use the insulin that is present, the cells cannot use glucose. Excess glucose builds up in the bloodstream, setting the stage for diabetes.

Being obese or overweight affects the way insulin works in your body. Extra fat tissue can make your body resistant to the action of insulin, but exercise helps insulin work well.

How are insulin resistance, pre-diabetes, and type 2 diabetes linked?

If you have insulin resistance, your muscle, fat, and liver cells do not use insulin properly. The pancreas tries to keep up with the demand

"Insulin Resistance and Pre-Diabetes," National Diabetes Information Clearinghouse, National Institute of Diabetes and Digestive and Kidney Diseases, NIH Pub. 06-4893, August 2006.

for insulin by producing more. Eventually, the pancreas cannot keep up with the body's need for insulin, and excess glucose builds up in the bloodstream. Many people with insulin resistance have high levels of blood glucose and high levels of insulin circulating in their blood at the same time.

People with blood glucose levels that are higher than normal but not yet in the diabetic range have "pre-diabetes." Doctors sometimes call this condition impaired fasting glucose (IFG) or impaired glucose tolerance (IGT), depending on the test used to diagnose it. Pre-diabetes is becoming more common in the United States, according to new estimates provided by the U.S. Department of Health and Human Services. About 40 percent of U.S. adults ages 40 to 74—or 41 million people—had pre-diabetes in 2000. New data suggest that at least 54 million U.S. adults had pre-diabetes in 2002.

If you have pre-diabetes, you have a higher risk of developing type 2 diabetes, formerly called adult-onset diabetes or noninsulin-dependent diabetes. Studies have shown that most people with pre-diabetes go on to develop type 2 diabetes within 10 years, unless they lose 5 to 7 percent of their body weight—which is about 10 to 15 pounds for someone who weighs 200 pounds—by making modest changes in their diet and level of physical activity. People with pre-diabetes also have a higher risk of heart disease.

Type 2 diabetes is sometimes defined as the form of diabetes that develops when the body does not respond properly to insulin, as opposed to type 1 diabetes, in which the pancreas makes no insulin at all. At first, the pancreas keeps up with the added demand by producing more insulin. In time, however, it loses the ability to secrete enough insulin in response to meals.

Insulin resistance can also occur in people who have type 1 diabetes, especially if they are overweight.

What causes insulin resistance?

Because insulin resistance tends to run in families, we know that genes are partly responsible. Excess weight also contributes to insulin resistance because too much fat interferes with muscles' ability to use insulin. Lack of exercise further reduces muscles' ability to use insulin.

Many people with insulin resistance and high blood glucose have excess weight around the waist, high LDL (bad) blood cholesterol levels, low HDL (good) cholesterol levels, high levels of triglycerides (another fat in the blood), and high blood pressure, all conditions that also put the heart at risk. This combination of problems is referred to as the metabolic syndrome, or the insulin resistance syndrome (formerly called Syndrome X).

Metabolic Syndrome

Metabolic syndrome is defined by the National Cholesterol Education Program as the presence of any three of the following conditions:

- excess weight around the waist (waist measurement of more than 40 inches for men and more than 35 inches for women)
- high levels of triglycerides (150 mg/dL or higher)
- low levels of HDL, or "good," cholesterol (below 40 mg/dL for men and below 50 mg/dL for women
- high blood pressure (130/85 mm Hg or higher)
- high fasting blood glucose levels (110 mg/dL or higher)

What are the symptoms of insulin resistance and pre-diabetes?

Insulin resistance and pre-diabetes usually have no symptoms. You may have one or both conditions for several years without noticing anything. If you have a severe form of insulin resistance, you may get dark patches of skin, usually on the back of your neck. Sometimes people get a dark ring around their neck. Other possible sites for these dark patches include elbows, knees, knuckles, and armpits. This condition is called acanthosis nigricans.

If you have a mild or moderate form of insulin resistance, blood tests may show normal or high blood glucose and high levels of insulin at the same time.

Do you have insulin resistance or pre-diabetes?

Anyone 45 years or older should consider getting tested for diabetes. If you are overweight and aged 45 or older, it is strongly recommended that you get tested. You should consider getting tested if you are younger than 45, overweight, and have one or more of the following risk factors:

- family history of diabetes
- low HDL cholesterol and high triglycerides

- high blood pressure

- history of gestational diabetes (diabetes during pregnancy) or gave birth to a baby weighing more than 9 pounds

- minority group background (African American, American Indian, Hispanic American/Latino, or Asian American/Pacific Islander)

Diabetes and pre-diabetes can be detected with one of the following tests:

A fasting glucose test measures your blood glucose after you have gone overnight without eating. This test is most reliable when done in the morning. Fasting glucose levels of 100 to 125 mg/dL are above normal but not high enough to be called diabetes. This condition is called pre-diabetes or impaired fasting glucose, and it suggests that you have probably had insulin resistance for some time. IFG is considered a pre-diabetic state, meaning that you are more likely to develop diabetes but do not have it yet.

A glucose tolerance test measures your blood glucose after an overnight fast and two hours after you drink a sweet liquid provided by the doctor or laboratory. If your blood glucose falls between 140 and 199 mg/dL two hours after drinking the liquid, your glucose tolerance is above normal but not high enough for diabetes. This condition, also a form of pre-diabetes, is called impaired glucose tolerance and, like IFG, it points toward a history of insulin resistance and a risk for developing diabetes.

These tests give only indirect evidence of insulin resistance. The test that most accurately measures insulin resistance is too complicated and expensive to use as a screening tool in most doctors' offices. The test, called the euglycemic clamp, is a research tool that helps scientists learn more about sugar metabolism problems. Insulin resistance can also be assessed with measurement of fasting insulin. If conventional tests show that you have IFG or IGT, your doctor may suggest changes in diet and exercise to reduce your risk of developing diabetes.

If your blood glucose is higher than normal but lower than the diabetes range, have your blood glucose checked in one to two years.

Lab Tests and What They Show

- *Blood glucose:* High blood glucose may be a sign that your body does not have enough insulin or does not use it well. However, a fasting measurement or oral glucose tolerance test gives more precise information.

- *Insulin:* An insulin measurement helps determine whether a high blood glucose reading is the result of insufficient insulin or poor use of insulin.

- *Fasting glucose:* Your blood glucose level should be lower after several hours without eating. After an overnight fast, the normal level is below 100 mg/dL. If it is in the 100 to 125 mg/dL range, you have impaired fasting glucose or pre-diabetes. A result of 126 or higher, if confirmed on a repeat test, indicates diabetes.

- *Glucose tolerance:* Your blood glucose level will be higher after drinking a sugar solution, but it should still be below 140 mg/dL two hours after the drink. If it is higher than normal (in the 140 to 199 mg/dL range) two hours after drinking the solution, you have IGT or pre-diabetes, which is another strong indication that your body has trouble using glucose. A level of 200 or higher, if confirmed, means diabetes is already present.

Can you reverse insulin resistance?

Yes. Physical activity and weight loss make the body respond better to insulin. By losing weight and being more physically active, you may avoid developing type 2 diabetes. In fact, a major study has verified the benefits of healthy lifestyle changes and weight loss. In 2001, the National Institutes of Health completed the Diabetes Prevention Program (DPP), a clinical trial designed to find the most effective ways of preventing type 2 diabetes in overweight people with pre-diabetes. The researchers found that lifestyle changes reduced the risk of diabetes by 58 percent. Also, many people with pre-diabetes returned to normal blood glucose levels.

The main goal in treating insulin resistance and pre-diabetes is to help your body relearn to use insulin normally. You can do several things to help reach this goal.

Be Active and Eat Well

Physical activity helps your muscle cells use blood glucose because they need it for energy. Exercise makes those cells more sensitive to insulin.

The DPP confirmed that people who follow a low-fat, low-calorie diet and who increase activities such as walking briskly or riding a

33

bike for 30 minutes, five times a week, have a far smaller risk of developing diabetes than people who do not exercise regularly. The DPP also reinforced the importance of a low-calorie, low-fat diet. Following a low-calorie, low-fat diet can provide two benefits. If you are overweight, one benefit is that limiting your calorie and fat intake can help you lose weight. DPP participants who lost weight were far less likely to develop diabetes than others in the study who remained at an unhealthy weight. Increasing your activity and following a low-calorie, low-fat diet can also improve your blood pressure and cholesterol levels and has many other health benefits.

Scientists have established some numbers to help people set goals that will reduce their risk of developing glucose metabolism problems.

- *Weight:* Body mass index (BMI) is a measure used to evaluate body weight relative to height. You can use the BMI Table (Table 4.1) to find out whether you are underweight, normal weight, overweight, or obese.

  - Find your height in the left-hand column.

  - Move across in the same row to the number closest to your weight.

  - The number at the top of that column is your BMI. Check the word above your BMI to see whether you are normal weight, overweight, or obese. If you are overweight or obese, talk with your doctor about ways to lose weight to reduce your risk of diabetes.

- *Blood pressure:* Blood pressure is expressed as two numbers that represent pressure in your blood vessels when your heart is beating (systolic pressure) and when it is resting (diastolic pressure). The numbers are usually written with a slash—for example, 140/90, which is expressed as "140 over 90." For the general population, blood pressure below 130/85 is considered normal, although people whose blood pressure is slightly elevated and who have no additional risk factors for heart disease may be advised to make lifestyle changes—that is, diet and exercise—rather than take blood pressure medicines. People who have diabetes, however, should take whatever steps necessary, including lifestyle changes and medicine, to reach a blood pressure goal of below 130/80.

- *Cholesterol:* Your cholesterol is usually reported with three values: low density lipoprotein (LDL) cholesterol, high density lipoprotein (HDL) cholesterol, and total cholesterol. LDL cholesterol

Table 4.1. Body Mass Index

Height (inches)	Normal						Overweight					Obese										Extreme Obesity														
BMI	19	20	21	22	23	24	25	26	27	28	29	30	31	32	33	34	35	36	37	38	39	40	41	42	43	44	45	46	47	48	49	50	51	52	53	54
												Body Weight (pounds)																								
58	91	96	100	105	110	115	119	124	129	134	138	143	148	153	158	162	167	172	177	181	186	191	196	201	205	210	215	220	224	229	234	239	244	248	253	258
59	94	99	104	109	114	119	124	128	133	138	143	148	153	158	163	168	173	178	183	188	193	198	203	208	212	217	222	227	232	237	242	247	252	257	262	267
60	97	102	107	112	118	123	128	133	138	143	148	153	158	163	168	174	179	184	189	194	199	204	209	215	220	225	230	235	240	245	250	255	261	266	271	276
61	100	106	111	116	122	127	132	137	143	148	153	158	164	169	174	180	185	190	195	201	206	211	217	222	227	232	238	243	248	254	259	264	269	275	280	285
62	104	109	115	120	126	131	136	142	147	153	158	164	169	175	180	186	191	196	202	207	213	218	224	229	235	240	246	251	256	262	267	273	278	284	289	295
63	107	113	118	124	130	135	141	146	152	158	163	169	175	180	186	191	197	203	208	214	220	225	231	237	242	248	254	259	265	270	278	282	287	293	299	304
64	110	116	122	128	134	140	145	151	157	163	169	174	180	186	192	197	204	209	215	221	227	232	238	244	250	256	262	267	273	279	285	291	296	302	308	314
65	114	120	126	132	138	144	150	156	162	168	174	180	186	192	198	204	210	216	222	228	234	240	246	252	258	264	270	276	282	288	294	300	306	312	318	324
66	118	124	130	136	142	148	155	161	167	173	179	186	192	198	204	210	216	223	229	235	241	247	253	260	266	272	278	284	291	297	303	309	315	322	328	334
67	121	127	134	140	146	153	159	166	172	178	185	191	198	204	211	217	223	230	236	242	249	255	261	268	274	280	287	293	299	306	312	319	325	331	338	344
68	125	131	138	144	151	158	164	171	177	184	190	197	203	210	216	223	230	236	243	249	256	262	269	276	282	289	295	302	308	315	322	328	335	341	348	354
69	128	135	142	149	155	162	169	176	182	189	196	203	209	216	223	230	236	243	250	257	263	270	277	284	291	297	304	311	318	324	331	338	345	351	358	365
70	132	139	146	153	160	167	174	181	188	195	202	209	216	222	229	236	243	250	257	264	271	278	285	292	299	306	313	320	327	334	341	348	355	362	369	376
71	136	143	150	157	165	172	179	186	193	200	208	215	222	229	236	243	250	257	265	272	279	286	293	301	308	315	322	329	338	343	351	358	365	372	379	386
72	140	147	154	162	169	177	184	191	199	206	213	221	228	235	242	250	258	265	272	279	287	294	302	309	316	324	331	338	346	353	361	368	375	383	390	397
73	144	151	159	166	174	182	189	197	204	212	219	227	235	242	250	257	265	272	280	288	295	302	310	318	325	333	340	348	355	363	371	378	386	393	401	408
74	148	155	163	171	179	186	194	202	210	218	225	233	241	249	256	264	272	280	287	295	303	311	319	326	334	342	350	358	365	373	381	389	396	404	412	420
75	152	160	168	176	184	192	200	208	216	224	232	240	248	256	264	272	279	287	295	303	311	319	327	335	343	351	359	367	375	383	391	399	407	415	423	431
76	156	164	172	180	189	197	205	213	221	230	238	246	254	263	271	279	287	295	304	312	320	328	336	344	353	361	369	377	385	394	402	410	418	426	435	443

Source: Adapted from *Clinical Guidelines on the Identification, Evaluation, and Treatment of Overweight and Obesity in Adults: The Evidence Report.*

is sometimes called "bad" cholesterol, while HDL cholesterol is called "good" cholesterol. To lower your risk of cardiovascular problems if you have diabetes, you should try to keep your LDL cholesterol below 100 and your total cholesterol below 200.

If you have metabolic syndrome, your doctor may recommend weight loss with diet and exercise, as well as medication to lower your cholesterol and blood pressure levels.

Stop Smoking

In addition to increasing your risk of cancer and cardiovascular disease, smoking contributes to insulin resistance. Quitting smoking is not easy, but it could be the single smartest thing you can do to improve your health. You will reduce your risk for respiratory problems, lung cancer, and diabetes.

Can medicines help?

Two classes of drugs can improve response to insulin and are used by prescription for type 2 diabetes—biguanides and thiazolidinediones. Other medicines used for diabetes act by other mechanisms. Alpha-glucosidase inhibitors restrict or delay the absorption of carbohydrates after eating, resulting in a slower rise of blood glucose levels. Sulfonylureas and meglitinides increase insulin production.

The DPP showed that the diabetes drug metformin, a biguanide, reduced the risk of diabetes in those with pre-diabetes but was much less successful than losing weight and increasing activity. In another study, treatment with troglitazone, a thiazolidinedione later withdrawn from the market following reports of liver toxicity, delayed or prevented type 2 diabetes in Hispanic women with a history of gestational diabetes. Acarbose, an alpha-glucosidase inhibitor, has been effective in delaying development of type 2 diabetes. Additional studies using other diabetes medicines and some types of blood pressure medicines to prevent diabetes are under way. No drug has been approved by the Food and Drug Administration (FDA) specifically for insulin resistance or pre-diabetes.

What research is being done?

Researchers sponsored by the National Institute of Diabetes and Digestive and Kidney Diseases conducted the DPP to find the most effective ways to prevent or delay the onset of type 2 diabetes. Volunteers were recruited from groups known to be at particularly high risk for IGT and type 2 diabetes. The study was designed to compare the effectiveness of lifestyle changes (weight loss through exercise and diet) with drug therapy (metformin). A control group received a placebo and information on diet and exercise. Participants assigned to the intensive lifestyle intervention reduced their risk of getting type 2 diabetes by 58 percent over three years. Participants treated with metformin reduced their risk by 31 percent. Metformin is not currently approved for use in preventing diabetes, but the FDA may determine whether to make diabetes prevention an added indication for this drug. In any event, the DPP demonstrates that a healthy diet and exercise are the most effective treatment for insulin resistance and the pre-diabetic states of IFG and IGT.

Chapter 5

Type 2 Diabetes: The Most Common Form of Diabetes

What is type 2 diabetes?

Diabetes is a disease in which blood glucose levels are above normal. People with diabetes have problems converting food to energy. After a meal, food is broken down into a sugar called glucose, which is carried by the blood to cells throughout the body. Cells use the hormone insulin, made in the pancreas, to help them process blood glucose into energy.

People develop type 2 diabetes because the cells in the muscles, liver, and fat do not use insulin properly. Eventually, the pancreas cannot make enough insulin for the body's needs. As a result, the amount of glucose in the blood increases while the cells are starved of energy. Over the years, high blood glucose damages nerves and blood vessels, leading to complications such as heart disease, stroke, blindness, kidney disease, nerve problems, gum infections, and amputation.

Can type 2 diabetes be prevented?

Research has demonstrated that people at risk for type 2 diabetes can prevent or delay developing type 2 diabetes by losing a little weight. The results of the Diabetes Prevention Program (DPP) showed that moderate diet changes and physical activity can delay and prevent type

From "Am I at Risk for Type 2 Diabetes," National Diabetes Information Clearinghouse, National Institute of Diabetes and Digestive and Kidney Diseases, NIH Pub. 07-4805, December 2006.

2 diabetes. Participants in this federally funded study of 3,234 people at high risk for diabetes experienced a 5- to 7-percent weight loss. For example, a 5- to 7-percent weight loss for a 200-pound person would be 10 to 14 pounds.

Study participants were overweight and had higher than normal levels of blood glucose, a condition called pre-diabetes, also called impaired glucose tolerance. Both pre-diabetes and obesity are strong risk factors for type 2 diabetes. Because of the high risk for diabetes among some minority groups, about half of the DPP participants were African American, American Indian, Asian American, Pacific Islander, or Hispanic/Latino.

DPP participants also included others at high risk for developing type 2 diabetes, such as women with a history of gestational diabetes and individuals aged 60 and older.

The DPP tested two approaches to preventing diabetes: lifestyle change—a program of healthy eating and exercise—and the diabetes drug metformin. People in the lifestyle change group exercised about 30 minutes a day 5 days a week, usually by walking, and lowered their intake of fat and calories. Those who took the diabetes drug metformin received information on exercise and diet. A third group only received information on exercise and diet.

The results showed that people in the lifestyle change group reduced their risk of getting type 2 diabetes by 58 percent. In the first year of the study, people lost an average of 15 pounds. Lifestyle change was even more effective in those aged 60 and older. They reduced their risk by 71 percent. People receiving metformin reduced their risk by 31 percent.

What are the signs and symptoms of type 2 diabetes?

More than 6 million people in the United States have type 2 diabetes and do not know it. Many have no signs or symptoms. Symptoms can also be so mild that you might not even notice them. Some people have symptoms but do not suspect diabetes.

Symptoms include the following:

- increased thirst
- increased hunger
- fatigue
- increased urination, especially at night
- weight loss

- blurred vision
- sores that do not heal

Many people do not find out they have the disease until they have diabetes complications, such as blurry vision or heart trouble. If you find out early that you have diabetes, then you can get treatment to prevent damage to the body.

Should I be tested for diabetes?

Anyone 45 years old or older should consider getting tested for diabetes. If you are 45 or older and overweight—see the BMI chart on page 35—getting tested is strongly recommended. If you are younger than 45, overweight, and have one or more of the risk factors, you should consider getting tested. Ask your doctor for a fasting blood glucose test or an oral glucose tolerance test. Your doctor will tell you if you have normal blood glucose, pre-diabetes, or diabetes.

What does having pre-diabetes mean?

Pre-diabetes means your blood glucose is higher than normal but lower than the diabetes range. It also means you are at risk for getting type 2 diabetes and heart disease. However, you can reduce the risk of getting diabetes and even return to normal blood glucose levels with modest weight loss and moderate physical activity. If you are told you have pre-diabetes, have your blood glucose checked again in one to two years.

Besides being older and overweight, what other factors increase my risk for type 2 diabetes?

To find out your risk for type 2 diabetes, consider each item and if it applies to you.

- I have a parent, brother, or sister with diabetes.
- My family background is Alaska Native, American Indian, African American, Hispanic/Latino, Asian American, or Pacific Islander.
- I have had gestational diabetes, or I gave birth to at least one baby weighing more than 9 pounds.
- My blood pressure is 140/90 mm Hg or higher, or I have been told that I have high blood pressure.

41

- My cholesterol levels are not normal. My HDL cholesterol—"good" cholesterol—is below 35 mg/dL, or my triglyceride level is above 250 mg/dL.

- I am fairly inactive. I exercise fewer than three times a week.

- I have polycystic ovary syndrome, also called PCOS—women only.

- On previous testing, I had impaired glucose tolerance (IGT) or impaired fasting glucose (IFG).

- I have other clinical conditions associated with insulin resistance, such as acanthosis nigricans.

- I have a history of cardiovascular disease.

The more items that apply to you, the higher your risk.

How can I reduce my risk?

You can do a lot to lower your chances of getting diabetes. Exercising regularly, reducing fat and calorie intake, and losing a little weight can help you reduce your risk of developing type 2 diabetes. Lowering blood pressure and cholesterol levels also helps you stay healthy.

If you are overweight:

- Reach and maintain a reasonable body weight;
- Make wise food choices most of the time;
- Be physically active every day.

If you are fairly inactive:

- Be physically active every day.

If your blood pressure is too high:

- Reach and maintain a reasonable body weight;
- Make wise food choices most of the time;
- Reduce your intake of sodium and alcohol;
- Be physically active every day;
- Talk with your doctor about whether you need medicine to control your blood pressure.

If your cholesterol or triglyceride levels are too high

- Make wise food choices most of the time;
- Be physically active every day;
- Talk with your doctor about whether you need medicine to control your cholesterol levels.

How can I make changes to lower my risk?

Making big changes in your life is hard, especially if you are faced with more than one change. You can make it easier by taking these steps:

- Make a plan to change behavior.
- Decide exactly what you will do and when you will do it.
- Plan what you need to get ready.
- Think about what might prevent you from reaching your goals.
- Find family and friends who will support and encourage you.
- Decide how you will reward yourself when you do what you have planned.
- Your doctor, a dietitian, or a counselor can help you make a plan. Consider making changes to lower your risk of diabetes.

Reach and Maintain a Reasonable Body Weight

Your weight affects your health in many ways. Being overweight can keep your body from making and using insulin properly. Excess body weight can also cause high blood pressure.

Body mass index (BMI) is a measure of body weight relative to height. You can use BMI to see whether you are underweight, normal weight, overweight, or obese. Use a Body Mass Index Table to find your BMI. (A copy of the BMI Table is available in Chapter 4, Figure 4.1 on page 35.)

If you are overweight or obese, choose sensible ways to get in shape.

- Avoid crash diets. Instead, eat less of the foods you usually have. Limit the amount of fat you eat.

- Increase your physical activity. Aim for at least 30 minutes of exercise most days of the week.

- Set a reasonable weight-loss goal, such as losing one pound a week. Aim for a long-term goal of losing five to seven percent of your total body weight.

Make Wise Food Choices Most of the Time

What you eat has a big impact on your health. By making wise food choices, you can help control your body weight, blood pressure, and cholesterol.

- Take a look at the serving sizes of the foods you eat. Reduce serving sizes of main courses such as meat, desserts, and foods high in fat. Increase the amount of fruits and vegetables.

- Limit your fat intake to about 25 percent of your total calories. For example, if your food choices add up to about 2,000 calories a day, try to eat no more than 56 grams of fat. Your doctor or a dietitian can help you figure out how much fat to have. You can also check food labels for fat content.

- Limit your sodium intake to less than 2,300 mg—about one teaspoon of salt—each day.

- Talk with your doctor about whether you may drink alcoholic beverages. If you choose to drink alcoholic beverages, limit your intake to one drink—for women—or two drinks—for men—per day.

- You may also wish to reduce the number of calories you have each day. People in the DPP lifestyle change group lowered their daily calorie total by an average of about 450 calories. Your doctor or dietitian can help you with a meal plan that emphasizes weight loss.

- Keep a food and exercise log. Write down what you eat, how much you exercise—anything that helps keep you on track.

- When you meet your goal, reward yourself with a nonfood item or activity, like watching a movie.

Be Physically Active Every Day

Regular exercise tackles several risk factors at once. It helps you lose weight, keeps your cholesterol and blood pressure under control, and helps your body use insulin. People in the DPP who were physically active for 30 minutes a day, five days a week, reduced their risk of type 2 diabetes. Many chose brisk walking for exercise.

If you are not very active, you should start slowly. Talk with your doctor first about what kinds of exercise would be safe for you. Make a plan to increase your activity level toward the goal of being active at least 30 minutes a day most days of the week.

Choose activities you enjoy. Some ways to work extra activity into your daily routine include the following:

- Take the stairs rather than an elevator or escalator.
- Park at the far end of the parking lot and walk.
- Get off the bus a few stops early and walk the rest of the way.
- Walk or bicycle whenever you can.

Take Your Prescribed Medications

Some people need medication to help control their blood pressure or cholesterol levels. If you do, take your medicines as directed. Ask your doctor about medicines to prevent type 2 diabetes.

What research is being done?

We now know that many people can prevent type 2 diabetes through weight loss, regular exercise, and lowering their intake of fat and calories. Researchers are intensively studying the genetic and environmental factors that underlie the susceptibility to obesity, pre-diabetes, and diabetes. As they learn more about the molecular events that lead to diabetes, they will develop ways to prevent and cure the different stages of this disease. People with diabetes and those at risk for it now have easier access to clinical trials that test promising new approaches to treatment and prevention. For information about current studies, see http://clinicaltrials.gov.

Chapter 6

Gestational Diabetes

What is gestational diabetes?

Gestational diabetes is diabetes that is found for the first time when a woman is pregnant. Out of every 100 pregnant women in the United States, three to eight get gestational diabetes. Diabetes means that your blood glucose (also called blood sugar) is too high. Your body uses glucose for energy. But too much glucose in your blood can be harmful. When you are pregnant, too much glucose is not good for your baby.

This chapter is for women with gestational diabetes. If you have type 1 or type 2 diabetes and are considering pregnancy, call the National Diabetes Information Clearinghouse at 800-860-8747 for more information and consult your health care team before you get pregnant.

What causes gestational diabetes?

Changing hormones and weight gain are part of a healthy pregnancy. But both changes make it hard for your body to keep up with its need for a hormone called insulin. When that happens, your body doesn't get the energy it needs from the food you eat.

From "What I Need to Know about Gestational Diabetes," National Diabetes Information Clearinghouse, National Institute of Diabetes and Digestive and Kidney Diseases, NIH Pub. No. 06-5129, April 2006.

What is my risk of gestational diabetes?

To learn your risk for gestational diabetes, consider each item that applies to you. Talk with your doctor about your risk at your first prenatal visit.

- I have a parent, brother, or sister with diabetes.
- I am African American, American Indian, Asian American, Hispanic/Latino, or Pacific Islander.
- I am 25 years old or older.
- I am overweight.
- I have had gestational diabetes before, or I have given birth to at least one baby weighing more than 9 pounds.
- I have been told that I have "pre-diabetes," a condition in which blood glucose levels are higher than normal, but not yet high enough for a diagnosis of diabetes. Other names for it are "impaired glucose tolerance" and "impaired fasting glucose."

If any of these apply to you, ask your health care team about testing for gestational diabetes.

- You are at high risk if you are very overweight, have had gestational diabetes before, have a strong family history of diabetes, or have glucose in your urine.
- You are at average risk if you one or more of the risk factors apply to you.
- You are at low risk if none of the risk factors apply to you.

When will I be checked for gestational diabetes?

Your doctor will decide when you need to be checked for diabetes depending on your risk factors.

- If you are at high risk, your blood glucose level may be checked at your first prenatal visit. If your test results are normal, you will be checked again sometime between weeks 24 and 28 of your pregnancy.
- If you have an average risk for gestational diabetes, you will be tested sometime between weeks 24 and 28 of pregnancy.

- If you are at low risk, your doctor may decide that you do not need to be checked.

How is gestational diabetes diagnosed?

Your health care team will check your blood glucose level. Depending on your risk and your test results, you may have one or more of the following tests.

Fasting blood glucose or random blood glucose test: Your doctor may check your blood glucose level using a test called a fasting blood glucose test. Before this test, your doctor will ask you to fast, which means having nothing to eat or drink except water for at least eight hours. Or your doctor may check your blood glucose at any time during the day. This is called a random blood glucose test.

These tests can find gestational diabetes in some women, but other tests are needed to be sure diabetes is not missed.

Screening glucose challenge test: For this test, you will drink a sugary beverage and have your blood glucose level checked an hour later. This test can be done at any time of the day. If the results are above normal, you may need further tests.

Oral glucose tolerance test: If you have this test, your health care provider will give you special instructions to follow. For at least three days before the test, you should eat normally. Then you will fast for at least eight hours before the test.

The health care team will check your blood glucose level before the test. Then you will drink a sugary beverage. The staff will check your blood glucose levels one hour, two hours, and three hours later. If your

Table 6.1. Above-Normal Results for the Oral Glucose Tolerance Test*

Fasting	95 or higher
At 1 hour	180 or higher
At 2 hours	155 or higher
At 3 hours	140 or higher

Note: Some labs use other numbers for this test.

*These numbers are for a test using a drink with 100 grams of glucose.

levels are above normal at least twice during the test, you have gestational diabetes.

How will gestational diabetes affect my baby?

Untreated or uncontrolled gestational diabetes can mean problems for your baby, such as the following:

- being born very large and with extra fat; this can make delivery difficult and more dangerous for your baby
- low blood glucose right after birth
- breathing problems

If you have gestational diabetes, your health care team may recommend some extra tests to check on your baby, such as the following:

- an ultrasound exam, to see how your baby is growing
- "kick counts" to check your baby's activity (the time between the baby's movements) or special "stress" tests

Working closely with your health care team will help you give birth to a healthy baby. Both you and your baby are at increased risk for type 2 diabetes for the rest of your lives.

How will gestational diabetes affect me?

Often, women with gestational diabetes have no symptoms. However, gestational diabetes may have the following impacts:

- increase your risk of high blood pressure during pregnancy
- increase your risk of a large baby and the need for cesarean section at delivery

The good news is your gestational diabetes will probably go away after your baby is born. However, you will be more likely to get type 2 diabetes later in your life. You may also get gestational diabetes again if you get pregnant again.

Some women wonder whether breastfeeding is OK after they have had gestational diabetes. Breastfeeding is recommended for most babies, including those whose mothers had gestational diabetes.

Gestational diabetes is serious, even if you have no symptoms. Taking care of yourself helps keep your baby healthy.

How is gestational diabetes treated?

Treating gestational diabetes means taking steps to keep your blood glucose levels in a target range. You will learn how to control your blood glucose using these tools:

- a meal plan
- physical activity
- insulin (if needed)

Meal plan: You will talk with a dietitian or a diabetes educator who will design a meal plan to help you choose foods that are healthy for you and your baby. Using a meal plan will help keep your blood glucose in your target range. The plan will provide guidelines on which foods to eat, how much to eat, and when to eat. Choices, amounts, and timing are all important in keeping your blood glucose levels in your target range.

You may be advised to do the following:

- limit sweets
- eat three small meals and one to three snacks every day
- be careful about when and how much carbohydrate-rich food you eat; your meal plan will tell you when to eat carbohydrates and how much to eat at each meal and snack
- include fiber in your meals in the form of fruits, vegetables, and whole-grain crackers, cereals, and bread

Physical activity: Physical activity, such as walking and swimming, can help you reach your blood glucose targets. Talk with your health care team about the type of activity that is best for you. If you are already active, tell your health care team what you do.

Physical activity can help you reach your blood glucose targets.

Insulin: Some women with gestational diabetes need insulin, in addition to a meal plan and physical activity, to reach their blood glucose targets. If necessary, your health care team will show you how to give yourself insulin. Insulin is not harmful for your baby. It cannot move from your bloodstream to the baby's.

51

How will I know whether my blood glucose levels are on target?

Your health care team may ask you to use a small device called a blood glucose meter to check your levels on your own. You will learn the following:

- how to use the meter
- how to prick your finger to obtain a drop of blood
- what your target range is
- when to check your blood glucose

You may be asked to check your blood glucose at these times:

- when you wake up
- just before meals
- one or two hours after breakfast
- one or two hours after lunch
- one or two hours after dinner

The following chart shows blood glucose targets for most women with gestational diabetes. Talk with your health care team about whether these targets are right for you.

Table 6.2. Blood Glucose Targets for Most Women with Gestational Diabetes

On awakening	not above 95
One hour after a meal	not above 140
Two hours after a meal	not above 120

Each time you check your blood glucose, write down the results in a record book. Take the book with you when you visit your health care team. If your results are often out of range, your health care team will suggest ways you can reach your targets.

Will I need to do other tests on my own?

Your health care team may teach you how to test for ketones in your morning urine or in your blood. High levels of ketones are a sign that your body is using your body fat for energy instead of the food you eat. Using fat for energy is not recommended during pregnancy. Ketones may be harmful for your baby.

If your ketone levels are high, your health care providers may suggest that you change the type or amount of food you eat. Or you may need to change your meal times or snack times.

After I have my baby, how can I find out whether my diabetes is gone?

You will probably have a blood glucose test 6 to 12 weeks after your baby is born to see whether you still have diabetes. For most women, gestational diabetes goes away after pregnancy. You are, however, at risk of having gestational diabetes during future pregnancies or getting type 2 diabetes later.

How can I prevent or delay getting type 2 diabetes later in life?

You can do a lot to prevent or delay type 2 diabetes.

- Reach and maintain a reasonable weight. Even if you stay above your ideal weight, losing five to seven percent of your body weight is enough to make a big difference. For example, if you weigh 200 pounds, losing 10 to 14 pounds can greatly reduce your chance of getting diabetes.

- Be physically active for 30 minutes most days. Walk, swim, exercise, or go dancing.

- Follow a healthy eating plan. Eat more grains, fruits, and vegetables. Cut down on fat and calories. A dietitian can help you design a meal plan.

Remind your health care team to check your blood glucose levels regularly. Women who have had gestational diabetes should continue to be tested for diabetes or pre-diabetes every one to two years. Diagnosing diabetes or pre-diabetes early can help prevent complications such as heart disease later.

Your child's risk for type 2 diabetes may be lower if you breastfeed your baby and if your child maintains a healthy weight.

Chapter 7

Monogenic Forms of Diabetes

The most common forms of diabetes, type 1 and type 2, are polygenic, meaning the risk of developing these forms of diabetes is related to multiple genes. Environmental factors, such as obesity in the case of type 2 diabetes, also play a part in the development of polygenic forms of diabetes. Polygenic forms of diabetes often run in families. Doctors diagnose polygenic forms of diabetes by testing blood glucose in individuals with risk factors or symptoms of diabetes.

Genes provide the instructions for making proteins within the cell. If a gene has a mutation, the protein may not function properly. Genetic mutations that cause diabetes affect proteins that play a role in the ability of the body to produce insulin or in the ability of insulin to lower blood glucose. People have two copies of most genes; one gene is inherited from each parent.

Some rare forms of diabetes result from mutations in a single gene and are called monogenic. Monogenic forms of diabetes account for about one to five percent of all cases of diabetes in young people. In most cases of monogenic diabetes, the gene mutation is inherited; in the remaining cases the gene mutation develops spontaneously. Most mutations in monogenic diabetes reduce the body's ability to produce insulin, a protein produced in the pancreas that helps the body use glucose for energy. Neonatal diabetes mellitus (NDM) and maturity-onset diabetes of the young (MODY) are the two main forms of monogenic diabetes.

From "Monogenic Forms of Diabetes: Neonatal Diabetes Mellitus and Maturity-Onset Diabetes of the Young," National Institute of Diabetes and Digestive and Kidney Diseases, NIH Pub. No. 07-6141, March 2007.

MODY is much more common than NDM. NDM first occurs in newborns and young infants; MODY usually first occurs in children or adolescents but may be mild and not detected until adulthood.

Genetic testing can diagnose most forms of monogenic diabetes. If genetic testing is not performed, people with monogenic diabetes may appear to have one of the polygenic forms of diabetes. When hyperglycemia is first detected in adulthood, type 2 is often diagnosed instead of monogenic diabetes. Some monogenic forms of diabetes can be treated with oral diabetes medications while other forms require insulin injections. A correct diagnosis that allows the proper treatment to be selected should lead to better glucose control and improved health in the long term. Testing of other family members may also be indicated to determine whether they are at risk for diabetes.

What is neonatal diabetes mellitus (NDM)?

NDM is a monogenic form of diabetes that occurs in the first six months of life. It is a rare condition occurring in only one in 100,000 to 500,000 live births. Infants with NDM do not produce enough insulin, leading to an increase in blood glucose. NDM can be mistaken for the much more common type 1 diabetes, but type 1 diabetes usually occurs later than the first six months of life. In about half of those with NDM, the condition is lifelong and is called permanent neonatal diabetes mellitus (PNDM). In the rest of those with NDM, the condition is transient and disappears during infancy but can reappear later in life; this type of NDM is called transient neonatal diabetes mellitus (TNDM). Specific genes that can cause NDM have been identified.

Symptoms of NDM include thirst, frequent urination, and dehydration. NDM can be diagnosed by finding elevated levels of glucose in blood or urine. In severe cases, the deficiency of insulin may cause the body to produce an excess of acid, resulting in a potentially life-threatening condition called ketoacidosis. Most fetuses with NDM do not grow well in the womb and newborns are much smaller than those of the same gestational age, a condition called intrauterine growth restriction. After birth, some infants fail to gain weight and grow as rapidly as other infants of the same age and sex. Appropriate therapy improves and may normalize growth and development.

What is maturity-onset diabetes of the young (MODY)?

MODY is a monogenic form of diabetes that usually first occurs during adolescence or early adulthood. However, MODY sometimes remains undiagnosed until later in life. A number of different gene mutations have been shown to cause MODY, all of which limit the ability of the pancreas to produce insulin. This process leads to the high blood glucose levels characteristic of diabetes and, in time, may damage body tissues, particularly the eyes, kidneys, nerves, and blood vessels. MODY accounts for about one to five percent of all cases of diabetes in the United States. Family members of people with MODY are at greatly increased risk for the condition.

People with MODY may have only mild or no symptoms of diabetes and their hyperglycemia may only be discovered during routine blood tests. MODY may be confused with type 1 or type 2 diabetes. People with MODY are generally not overweight and do not have other risk factors for type 2 diabetes, such as high blood pressure or abnormal blood fat levels. While both type 2 diabetes and MODY can run in families, people with MODY typically have a family history of diabetes in multiple successive generations, meaning that MODY is present in a grandparent, a parent, and a child. Unlike people with

Table 7.1. Monogenic Forms of Diabetes

Type	How Common	Gene Involved*
Neonatal diabetes mellitus (NDM)	rare; occurs in about one of every 100,000 to 500,000 live births	
Permanent neonatal diabetes mellitus (PNDM)	50% of all cases of NDM	KCNJ11; ABCC8; GCK; IPF1 (also known as PDX1); PTF1A; FOXP3 (IPEX syndrome); EIF2AK3 (Wolcott-Rallison syndrome)
Transient neonatal diabetes mellitus (TNDM)	50% of all cases of NDM	ZAC/HYMAI; ABCC8; KCNJ11; HNF1 β (beta), also known as HNF1B
Maturity-onset diabetes of the young	1 to 5% of all cases of diabetes in the United States	HNF4A; GCK; TCF1; IPF1, (also known as PDX1); TCF2; NeuroD1 (or BETA2)

*Gene involved: The name of the gene with the mutation. Each of the genes listed has been identified as a cause of diabetes.

type 1 diabetes who always require insulin, people with MODY can often be treated with oral diabetes medications. Treatment varies depending on the genetic mutation that has caused the MODY.

What do I need to know about genetic testing and counseling?

Testing for monogenic diabetes involves providing a blood sample from which DNA is isolated. The DNA is analyzed for changes in the genes that cause monogenic diabetes. Abnormal results can determine the gene responsible for diabetes in a particular individual or show whether someone is likely to develop a monogenic form of diabetes in the future. Genetic testing can also be helpful in selecting the most appropriate treatment for individuals with monogenic diabetes. Prenatal testing can diagnose these conditions in unborn children.

Most forms of monogenic diabetes are caused by dominant mutations, meaning that the condition can be passed on to children when

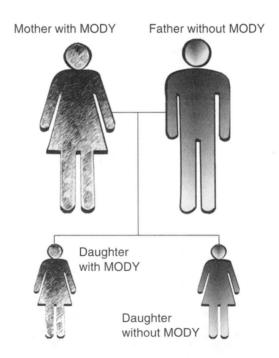

Figure 7.1. *Each child of a parent with MODY has a 50 percent chance of inheriting the disease.*

only one parent is affected. In contrast, if the mutation is a recessive mutation, a disease gene must be inherited from both parents for diabetes to occur. For recessive forms of monogenic diabetes, testing can indicate whether parents or siblings without disease are carriers for recessive genetic conditions that could be inherited by their children.

If you suspect that you or a member of your family may have a monogenic form of diabetes, you should seek help from health care professionals—physicians and genetic counselors—who have specialized knowledge and experience in this area. They can determine whether genetic testing is appropriate, select the genetic tests that should be performed, and provide information about the basic principles of genetics, genetic testing options, and confidentiality issues. They also can review the test results with the patient or parent after testing, make recommendations about how to proceed, and discuss testing options for other family members.

Hope through Research

Researchers are studying the genetic causes of and metabolic processes related to diabetes. Discoveries about monogenic forms of diabetes may contribute to the search for the causes of and treatments for type 1 and type 2 diabetes. For information about clinical trials related to diabetes and genetics, see www.clinicaltrials.gov.

Points to Remember

- Mutations in single genes can cause rare forms of diabetes.
- Genetic testing can identify many forms of monogenic diabetes.
- A physician evaluates whether genetic testing is appropriate.
- A correct diagnosis aided by genetic testing can lead to optimal treatment.
- Recent research results show that people with certain forms of monogenic diabetes can be treated with oral diabetes medications instead of insulin injections.

For More Information

National Human Genome Research Institute
Genetic and Rare Diseases Information Center
P.O. Box 8126
Gaithersburg, MD 20898-8126

Phone: 888-205-2311
Fax: 240-632-9164
Website: www.genome.gov/health
E-mail: gardinfo@nih.gov

Online Sources

The GeneTests website (www.genetests.org) provides information about medical genetics, an international directory of genetic testing laboratories, and an international directory of genetics clinics providing genetic evaluation and genetic counseling.

The Genetics Home Reference website (www.ghr.nlm.nih.gov) provides consumer-friendly information about genetic conditions. A service of the National Library of Medicine (NLM), NIH.

The Online Mendelian Inheritance in Man database (www.ncbi.nlm .nih.gov/entrez/query.fcgi?db=OMIM) is a catalog of human genes and genetic disorders with references and related links. A service of the National Center for Biotechnology Information, NLM, NIH.

Entrez Gene (www.ncbi.nlm.nih.gov/entrez/query.fcgi?db=gene) is a searchable database of genes with extensive information and related links. A service of the National Center for Biotechnology Information, NLM, NIH.

The Diabetes Research department and the Centre for Molecular Genetics at the Peninsula Medical School and Royal Devon and Exeter Hospital, Exeter, United Kingdom (www.diabetesgenes.org) provides information for patients and health care professionals about genetic forms of diabetes.

The International Society for Pediatric and Adolescent Diabetes (www.ispad.org) is an international society for health care professionals and others interested in childhood diabetes. They publish consensus guidelines; see the list of selected references.

Selected References

Babenko AP, Polak M, Cavé H, Busiah K, Czernichow P, Scharfmann R, Bryan J, Aguilar-Bryan L, Vaxillaire M, Froguel P. Activating mutations in the ABCC8 gene in neonatal diabetes mellitus. New *England Journal of Medicine*. 2006;355(5):456–466.

Colombo C, Delvecchio M, Zecchino C, Falenza MF, Cavallo L, Barbetti F. Transient neonatal diabetes mellitus is associated with a recurrent (R201H) KCNJ11 (Kir6.2) mutation. *Diabetologia*. 2005;48:2439–2441.

Craig ME, Hattersley A, Donaghue K. International Society for Pediatric and Adolescent Diabetes (ISPAD) Clinical Practice Consensus Guidelines 2006–2007. Definition, epidemiology and classification. *Pediatric Diabetes*. 2006;7:343–351.

Fajans SS, Bell GI, Polonsky KS. Molecular mechanisms and clinical pathophysiology of maturity-onset diabetes of the young. *New England Journal of Medicine*. 2001;345(13):971–980.

Gloyn AL, Pearson ER, Antcliff JF, Proks P, Bruining GJ, Slingerland AS, Howard N, Srinivasan S, Silva JM, Molnes J, Edghill EL, Frayling TM, Temple IK, Mackay D, Shield JP, Sumnik Z, van Rhijn A, Wales JK, Clark P, Gorman S, Aisenberg J, Ellard S, Njølstad PR, Ashcroft FM, Hattersley AT. Activating mutations in the gene encoding the ATP-sensitive potassium-channel subunit Kir6.2 and permanent neonatal diabetes. *New England Journal of Medicine*. 2004;350(18):1838–1849.

Hattersley A, Bruining J, Shield J, Njølstad P, Donaghue K. International Society for Pediatric and Adolescent Diabetes (ISPAD) Clinical Practice Consensus Guidelines 2006–2007. The diagnosis and management of monogenic diabetes in children. *Pediatric Diabetes*. 2006;7:352–360.

Hattersley AT. Beyond the beta cell in diabetes. *Nature Genetics*. 2006;38(1):12–13.

Hattersley AT, Ashcroft FM. Activating mutations in Kir6.2 and neonatal diabetes: new clinical syndromes, new scientific insights, and new therapy. *Diabetes*. 2005;54:2503–2513.

Hattersley AT, Pearson, ER. Minireview: pharmacogenetics and beyond: the interaction of therapeutic response, beta-cell physiology, and genetics in diabetes. *Endocrinology*. 2006;147:2657–2663.

National Center for Biotechnology Information, National Library of Medicine, National Institutes of Health, National Institute of Diabetes and Digestive and Kidney Diseases. The genetic landscape of diabetes.

Available at: www.ncbi.nlm.nih.gov/books/bv.fcgi?call=bv.View..Show TOC&rid=diabetes.TOC&depth=2. Posted 2004. Accessed January 2, 2007.

Pearson ER, Flechtner I, Njølstad PR, Malecki MT, Flanagan SE, Larkin B, Ashcroft FM, Klimes I, Codner E, Iotova V, Slingerland AS, Shield J, Robert JJ, Holst JJ, Clark PM, Ellard S, Søvik O, Polak M, Hattersley AT for the Neonatal Diabetes International Collaborative Group. Switching from insulin to oral sulfonylureas in patients with diabetes due to Kir6.2 mutations. *New England Journal of Medicine.* 2006;355(5):467–477.

Ræder H, Johansson S, Holm PI, Haldorsen IS, Mas E, Sbarra V, Nermoen I, Eide SA, Grevle L, Bjorkhaug L, Sagen JV, Aksnes L, Søvik O, Lombardo D, Molven A, Njølstad PR. Mutations in the CEL VNTR cause a syndrome of diabetes and pancreatic exocrine dysfunction. *Nature Genetics.* 2006;38(1):54–62.

Sperling MA. ATP-sensitive potassium channels—neonatal diabetes mellitus and beyond. *New England Journal of Medicine.* 2006;355(5): 507–510.

Sperling MA. Neonatal diabetes mellitus: from understudy to center stage. *Current Opinion in Pediatrics.* 2005;17:512–518.

Vaxillaire M, Froguel P. Genetic basis of maturity-onset diabetes of the young. *Endocrinology and Metabolism Clinics of North America.* 2006;35:371–384.

Chapter 8

Steroid-Induced Diabetes

Steroids are commonly used in medicine, and their effects on blood sugar are often seriously underestimated. To give the bottom line first, steroids seriously increase the blood sugar level of people who have diabetes, and they cause or uncover diabetes in many people who don't yet have it.

While there are several kinds of steroids, such as the ones used in muscle building ("anabolic or androgenic steroids"), in this discussion we are talking about the group called corticosteroids or glucocorticoids, exemplified by the medications hydrocortisone, prednisone, or dexamethasone.

For people who don't think every day about steroids, blood sugar, insulin, diabetes, or steroids, a few basic comments may help:

Corticosteroids are essential hormones, made in the adrenal glands, and part of the "fight or flight" response that also includes adrenalin. Like many hormones, they must be present in the right amount: lack of corticosteroids (Addison disease) and excessive corticosteroids (Cushing disease) are each fatal if left untreated.

Corticosteroids are also used quite often medically, not only as a replacement drug in the setting of Addison disease but to take advantage of their strong effect in suppressing inflammation and suppressing various immune problems. So they are taken to treat many illnesses, from poison ivy to severe asthma to pemphigus. Doctors always want to use them in the lowest dose possible and for the shortest time possible, because the corticosteroids have significant side effects, collectively known as "Cushing syndrome."

One strong effect of corticosteroids is that they counteract insulin. So let's talk about insulin, since it, too, may be beyond your everyday experience: Insulin is another hormone we all have, unless we have type 1 diabetes. Made in the pancreas, insulin helps the body burn sugar for energy. Without enough insulin, the sugar accumulates in the blood, the blood sugar goes too high, and that is called diabetes.

So when corticosteroids counteract the effect of insulin, this means that whatever amount of insulin your pancreas makes normally, when you take steroids, it has to make a lot more to hold the blood sugar normal.[1] If your pancreas is strong and able, it rises to the occasion and makes more insulin when your doctor prescribes steroids. Your blood sugar stays normal. But if your pancreas is not so strong (call it "insulin challenged"), it can't put out enough insulin to overcome the resistance caused by the steroids, not enough to do the job of keeping blood sugar normal. That's when the blood sugar goes up, and you have steroid-induced diabetes. [2]

If you have ever had a cardiac stress test, you know that they look at your cardiogram when you are at rest and it may be fine. But then they want to know whether it stays normal when your heart is stressed by heavy exercise. In the same way, your pancreas may be fine normally, but not up to the stress of steroid treatment. Other such "stress tests" of the pancreas include pregnancy and, the most common, obesity. In each of these situations, the person may have diabetes caused by the stress (diabetes during pregnancy), that is removed by getting out from that stress (diabetes being cured by delivery of the baby).

Steroid-induced diabetes, then, is a sign that your pancreas is not entirely normal, that it may be fine when not challenged by steroids, but is limited when you do have to take the steroids. Steroids are a "stress test" for the pancreas.

The symptoms of steroid-induced diabetes are the same as when diabetes is caused by any other problem: thirst, frequent urination, and unintentional weight loss. Or, the doctor may pick it up by doing a blood glucose test (over 125 mg/dl when you have fasted over eight hours being diabetic.)

Also, the management of steroid-induced diabetes may be similar to the management of other causes of diabetes: a more healthy diet, pills, or even insulin. But the good news is that when the dose of steroids is reduced or they are stopped altogether, the diabetes may well go away. Having had diabetes once during steroid treatment, though, your pancreas has declared itself borderline.[3] You are at much higher risk of getting it again later, especially if you start steroids again.

Notes from Omnigraphics' Medical Advisor

1. Some individuals have significant resistance to insulin, even without taking steroids. Risk factors for this include obesity, inactivity, and family history of diabetes. If you have insulin resistance to begin with, adding steroids will make this far worse.

2. When insulin resistance is present, the pancreas will try to step up insulin production to overcome it. People with insulin resistance often produce higher than normal insulin levels, and are therefore able to maintain normal blood sugars. However, if you now add in steroids, you increase the insulin resistance even farther, and the pancreas may not be able to keep up any more. Blood sugars rise, and this leads to steroid-induced diabetes.

3. Having diabetes during steroid treatment shows that your body has abnormal glucose metabolism and that your risk of getting diabetes again is much higher.

Chapter 9

Diabetes Insipidus

What is diabetes insipidus?

Diabetes insipidus is a rare disorder of water metabolism. This means that the balance between how much water or fluid you drink is not balanced with the fluid you urinate. Diabetes insipidus is caused by a lack of, or nonresponse to, the antidiuretic hormone vasopressin. This hormone controls water balance by concentrating urine. Patients with diabetes insipidus urinate too much, so they need to drink a lot to replace the fluid they lose.

Vasopressin is made by the cells of the hypothalamus (located in the brain) and is stored and secreted by another part of the brain called the posterior pituitary gland. The antidiuretic hormone is then released into the bloodstream where it causes tubules within the kidney to reabsorb water. Water that cannot be reabsorbed is passed out of the body in the form of urine. Decreased secretion of vasopressin causes less water to be reabsorbed and more urine to be formed. When vasopressin is present at normal levels, more water is reabsorbed and less urine is formed.

You should not confuse diabetes insipidus with the metabolic disease, diabetes mellitus. Diabetes mellitus is a different disease caused by a lack of, or an impaired response to, the hormone insulin. This hormone is made by the pancreas and helps in carbohydrate metabolism.

Without insulin, a person cannot make use of the carbohydrates he or she takes in, such as sugar. The hormone insulin affects sugar

"Diabetes Insipidus," NIH Clinical Center, National Institutes of Health, 2006.

so that it can enter the body's cells and be used for energy. When insulin is insufficient or not present, an abnormally high amount of sugar will be in the blood and urine.

There are two types of diabetes insipidus. While the symptoms of these two disorders are similar, the causes are different. The next sections describe central diabetes insipidus and nephrogenic diabetes insipidus.

Central Diabetes Insipidus

If you have been diagnosed with central diabetes insipidus, there are some things you should know about how the disorder is caused and what you and your doctor can do about it.

What causes it?

In central diabetes insipidus, the antidiuretic hormone vasopressin is either missing or present at a low level. This low level or lack of vasopressin is due to a malfunction in the part of your brain, the posterior pituitary gland, which releases the hormone into your bloodstream. Injury to the head, tumors, neurosurgical operations, infections, or bleeding can affect your brain's ability to release the right amount of vasopressin.

What are the symptoms?

- Excessive urination (polyuria)
- Excessive thirst (polydipsia)

Patients with central diabetes insipidus are often extremely tired because they cannot get enough sleep uninterrupted by the need to urinate. Their urine is very clear and odorless. These symptoms can appear at any time. Because they lose so much water from urination, they also feel very thirsty. If this disorder is untreated, they could become seriously dehydrated, and their bodies will not have enough water to function properly.

Nephrogenic Diabetes Insipidus

Nephrogenic diabetes insipidus is much less common than central diabetes insipidus. If you have been diagnosed with nephrogenic diabetes insipidus, your doctor or nurse will discuss the disorder and its treatment with you.

What cauoco it?

Nephrogenic diabetes insipidus may be caused by kidney diseases that make the kidneys unable to respond to vasopressin. While there is enough vasopressin in the body (unlike in central diabetes insipidus), the kidneys cannot respond to the hormone's signal to reabsorb water. The disease may be acquired or inherited by male children.

What are the symptoms?

The symptoms of nephrogenic diabetes insipidus are similar to central diabetes insipidus; that is, excessive urination (polyuria) followed by excessive thirst (polydipsia).

How is it treated?

The first step in treating thio diooaoo io oorroot diagnosis. In addition to the medications available, balancing your water or fluid intake with your urine output is also part of treatment. If this disorder is untreated, you could become seriously dehydrated, and your body will not have enough water to function.

Questions and Answers about Diabetes Insipidus

What tests can find out if I have central diabetes insipidus or nephrogenic diabetes insipidus?

The two most common tests used to diagnose diabetes insipidus are the following:

- Water deprivation test/vasopressin test
- Hypertonic saline infusion test

Other tests which may be used are the urine specific gravity test and the serum or urine osmolality test. These tests measure the concentration of solid particles in your urine. Patients with diabetes insipidus have urine with fewer solids than that of people without the disease.

With the water deprivation test, you will be asked not to drink any fluids. Your doctor will tell you how long you must abstain from drinking. Then, laboratory tests will be done to show any change in the amount and concentration of particles in your urine.

The vasopressin test is done if the water deprivation test does not result in sufficiently concentrated urine. Vasopressin is given by the doctor or nurse by injection to test your body's reaction to the hormone.

During the hypertonic saline infusion test, you will receive a mixture of salt and water by intravenous infusion. Your doctor or nurse will then draw blood from you which will be tested for osmolality and vasopressin content.

The serum or urine osmolality test is done to find out the concentration of particles in your blood or urine.

The urine specific gravity test is also a way to find out the concentration of solid particles in urine. Patients with diabetes insipidus have fewer particles in urine, so their specific gravity measurements will be below normal.

What is the therapy for central diabetes insipidus?

If you are treated for central diabetes insipidus, you will sniff a drug called DDAVP (desmopressin), a derivative of vasopressin. You will be shown the right way to use this drug by your physician, nurse, or pharmacist.

What is the therapy for nephrogenic diabetes insipidus?

If you have nephrogenic diabetes insipidus, water pills (thiazide diuretics) may be prescribed by your doctor. You may be confused as to why you need to take diuretics for this disorder. Thiazide diuretics have been shown to stimulate the production of a hormone that helps your body retain salt. This added amount of salt keeps you from losing too much water.

What should I do while I am being treated for diabetes insipidus?

It is very important that you balance your water intake with your urinary output. However, it is also very important that you do not drink too much water. If you drink too much water, this could cause very serious side effects. This is the reason why it is so important for you and your physician to discuss a specific plan to meet your individual needs.

Call your doctor or nurse when you notice that you cannot balance your urinary output with your water intake. A sign of this imbalance is that you will urinate a large amount of clear, odorless fluid. After urination, you will be very thirsty and feel the need to drink a large amount of water.

Call your doctor or nurse if you have side effects from the medications that were ordered for you. Your physician, nurse, or pharmacist will discuss with you how the drugs work, how and when to take them, and their side effects. You may also want to refer to any written information they give you.

And of course, always feel free to ask your doctor or nurse any questions you have about your diagnosis and treatment.

Comparison of Diabetes Insipidus and Diabetes Mellitus

How common is the disease?

- **Central diabetes insipidus:** Uncommon
- **Nephrogenic diabetes insipidus:** Uncommon
- **Diabetes mellitus:** Common

What causes the disease?

- **Central diabetes insipidus:** The mechanism for secreting vasopressin malfunctions.

- **Nephrogenic diabetes insipidus:** The kidneys are unable to respond to the diuretic hormone vasopressin. It is acquired or may be inherited by male children.

- **Diabetes mellitus:** Enough of the hormone insulin is not secreted, or the body's cells do not respond to it. Heredity, obesity, pregnancy, and drugs can also lead to diabetes mellitus.

What do these hormones do and why they important?

- **Central diabetes insipidus:** Vasopressin is a hormone that controls water metabolism. It is made in the hypothalamus (a part of the brain) and is stored and secreted by the posterior pituitary gland (also in the brain).

- **Nephrogenic diabetes insipidus:** Vasopressin causes tubules within the kidney to reabsorb water. Water that is not absorbed is released as urine.

- **Diabetes mellitus:** Insulin is made in the pancreas, where it controls carbohydrate metabolism. It controls sugar (glucose) levels in the body.

What are the signs and symptoms of the disease?

- **Central diabetes insipidus:** Sudden or gradual urination of large amounts of clear, colorless fluid, followed by excessive thirst (polydipsia). Dehydration can occur if fluid balance is not maintained.

- **Nephrogenic diabetes insipidus:** Same as central diabetes insipidus: polyuria followed by polydipsia.

- **Diabetes mellitus:** Excessive urination (polyuria), excessive thirst (polydipsia), and excessive appetite (polyphagia). May be sudden or gradual with no symptoms. Tiredness, weight gain or loss, skin infections that do not heal.

What diagnostic tests detect the disease?

- **Central diabetes insipidus:** Water deprivation test/vasopressin test or hypertonic saline infusion test

- **Nephrogenic diabetes insipidus:** Water deprivation test/vasopressin test or hypertonic saline infusion test

- **Diabetes mellitus:** Fasting blood sugar, 2-hour post-prandial test, blood sugar test, glucose tolerance test, hemoglobin A1C blood test

What treatments combat the disease?

- **Central diabetes insipidus:** Balance fluid intake and urine output or replace antidiuretic hormone, vasopressin; find, if possible, underlying cause of disease

- **Nephrogenic diabetes insipidus:** Balance urine output with fluid intake or diuretics

- **Diabetes mellitus:** Correct sugar/insulin intake, prevent progression of disease, diet, or oral or injectable medication

Part Two

Lifestyle Issues and Diabetes Management

Chapter 10

Everyday Guidelines for Taking Care of Your Diabetes

Taking Care of Your Diabetes Every Day

Do four things every day to lower high blood glucose:

- Follow your meal plan.
- Be physically active.
- Take your diabetes medicine.
- Check your blood glucose.

Experts say most people with diabetes should try to keep their blood glucose level as close as possible to the level of someone who doesn't have diabetes. The closer to normal your blood glucose is, the lower your chances are of developing serious health problems. Check with your doctor about the right range for you.

Your health care team will help you learn how to reach your target blood glucose range. Your main health care providers are your doctor, nurse, diabetes educator, and dietitian.

A diabetes educator is a health care worker who teaches people how to manage their diabetes. Your educator may be a nurse, a dietitian, or other kind of health care worker.

From "Your Guide to Diabetes: Type 1 and Type 2," National Diabetes Information Clearinghouse, National Institute of Diabetes and Digestive and Kidney Diseases, NIH Pub. 07-4016, October 2006.

A dietitian is someone who's specially trained to help people plan their meals.

The next sections of this chapter will tell you more about the four main ways you take care of your diabetes: Follow Your Meal Plan, Be Physically Active, Take Your Diabetes Medicine, and Check Your Blood Glucose.

Follow Your Meal Plan

People with diabetes should have their own meal plan. Ask your doctor to give you the name of a dietitian who can work with you to develop a meal plan. Your dietitian can help you plan meals that include foods that you and your family like to eat and that are good for you too. Ask your dietitian to include foods that are heart-healthy to reduce your risk of heart disease.

Your diabetes meal plan will include breads, cereals, rice, and grains; fruits and vegetables; meat and meat substitutes; dairy products; and fats. People with diabetes don't need to eat special foods. The foods on your meal plan are good for everyone in your family. Making wise food choices will help you with the following goals:

- reach and stay at a weight that's good for your body
- keep your blood glucose, blood pressure, and cholesterol under control
- prevent heart and blood vessel disease

Action Steps

If You Use Insulin

- Follow your meal plan.
- Don't skip meals, especially if you've already taken your insulin, because your blood glucose may go too low.

If You Don't Use Insulin

- Follow your meal plan.
- Don't skip meals, especially if you take diabetes medicine, because your blood glucose may go too low. It may be better to eat several small meals during the day instead of one or two big meals.

Be Physically Active

Physical activity is good for your diabetes. Walking, swimming, dancing, riding a bicycle, playing baseball, and bowling are all good ways to be active. You can even get exercise when you clean house or work in your garden. Physical activity is especially good for people with diabetes because it helps with the following:

- helps keep weight down
- helps insulin work better to lower blood glucose
- is good for your heart and lungs
- gives you more energy

Before you begin exercising, talk with your doctor. Your doctor may check your heart and your feet to be sure you have no special problems. If you have high blood pressure or eye problems, some exercises like weightlifting may not be safe. Your health care team can help you find safe exercises.

Try to be active almost every day for a total of about 30 minutes. If you haven't been very active lately, begin slowly. Start with 5 to 10 minutes, and then add more time. Or exercise for 10 minutes, three times a day.

If your blood glucose is less than 100 to 120, have a snack before you exercise.

When you exercise, carry glucose tablets or a carbohydrate snack with you in case you get hypoglycemia. Wear or carry an identification tag or card saying that you have diabetes.

Action Steps

If You Use Insulin

- See your doctor before starting a physical activity program.

- Check your blood glucose before, during, and after exercising. Don't exercise when your blood glucose is over 240 or if you have ketones in your urine.

- Don't exercise right before you go to sleep because it could cause hypoglycemia during the night.

If You Don't Use Insulin

- See your doctor before starting a physical activity program.

77

Take Your Diabetes Medicine Every Day

Three kinds of diabetes medicine can help you reach your blood glucose targets: pills, insulin, and other injectable medicines.

If You Take Diabetes Pills

If your body makes insulin, but the insulin doesn't lower your blood glucose, you may need diabetes pills. Some pills are taken once a day, and others are taken more often. Ask your health care team when you should take your pills.

Be sure to tell your doctor if your pills make you feel sick or if you have any other problems. Remember, diabetes pills don't lower blood glucose by themselves. You'll still want to follow a meal plan and be active to help lower your blood glucose.

Sometimes, people who take diabetes pills may need insulin for a while. If you get sick or have surgery, the diabetes pills may no longer work to lower your blood glucose.

You may be able to stop taking diabetes pills if you lose weight. (Always check with your doctor before you stop taking your diabetes pills.) Losing 10 or 15 pounds can sometimes help you reach your target blood glucose level.

If You Use Insulin

You need insulin if your body has stopped making insulin or if it doesn't make enough. Everyone with type 1 diabetes needs insulin, and many people with type 2 diabetes do too. Some women with gestational diabetes also need to take insulin.

There are five ways to take insulin:

- Taking shots, also called injections. You'll use a needle attached to a syringe—a hollow tube with a plunger—that you fill with a dose of insulin. Some people use an insulin pen, a pen-like device with a needle and a cartridge of insulin.

- Using an insulin pump. A pump is a small device, worn on a belt or in a pocket, that holds insulin. The pump connects to a small plastic tube and a very small needle. The needle is inserted under the skin and stays in for several days.

- Using an insulin jet injector. This device sends a fine spray of insulin through the skin with high-pressure air instead of a needle.

- Using an insulin infuser. A small tube is inserted just beneath the skin and remains in place for several days. Insulin is injected into the end of the tube instead of through the skin.

- Using inhaled insulin. You'll use a special device to breathe in powdered insulin through the mouth.

If You Use Other Injectable Medicines

Some people with diabetes use other injectable medicines to reach their blood glucose targets. These medicines are not substitutes for insulin.

If You Don't Use Pills, Insulin, or Other Injectable Medicines

Many people with type 2 diabetes don't need diabetes medicines. They can take care of their diabetes by using a meal plan and exercising regularly.

Check Your Blood Glucose as Recommended

You'll want to know how well you're taking care of your diabetes. The best way to find out is to check your blood to see how much glucose is in it. If your blood has too much or too little glucose, you may need a change in your meal plan, exercise plan, or medicine.

Ask your doctor how often you should check your blood glucose. Some people check their blood glucose once a day. Others do it three or four times a day. You may check before and after eating, before bed, and sometimes in the middle of the night.

Your doctor or diabetes educator will show you how to check your blood using a blood glucose meter. Your health insurance or Medicare may pay for the supplies and equipment you need.

Take Other Tests for Your Diabetes

Urine tests: You may need to check your urine if you're sick or if your blood glucose is over 240. A urine test will tell you if you have ketones in your urine. Your body makes ketones when there isn't enough insulin in your blood. Ketones can make you very sick. Call your doctor right away if you find moderate or large amounts of ketones, along with high blood glucose levels, when you do a urine test. You may have a serious condition called ketoacidosis. If it isn't treated, it can cause death. Signs of ketoacidosis are vomiting, weakness, fast breathing, and a sweet smell on the breath. Ketoacidosis is more likely to develop in people with type 1 diabetes.

You can buy strips for testing ketones at a drug store. Your doctor or diabetes educator will show you how to use them.

The A1C test: Another test for blood glucose, the A1C, also called the hemoglobin A1C test, shows what your overall blood glucose was for the past 3 months. It shows how much glucose is sticking to your red blood cells. The doctor does this test to see what your blood glucose is most of the time. Have this test done at least twice a year.

Ask your doctor what your A1C test showed. A result of under 7 usually means that your diabetes treatment is working well and your blood glucose is under control. If your A1C is 8 or above, your blood glucose may be too high. You'll then have a greater risk of having diabetes problems, like kidney damage. You may need a change in your meal plan, physical activity plan, or diabetes medicine.

Talk with your doctor about what your target should be. Even if your A1C is higher than your target, remember that every step toward your goal helps reduce your risk of diabetes problems.

Keep Daily Records

Make copies of the Daily Diabetes Record Page (see Figure 10.1). Then write down the results of your blood glucose checks every day. You may also want to write down what you ate, how you felt, and whether you exercised.

By keeping daily records of your blood glucose checks, you can tell how well you're taking care of your diabetes. Show your blood glucose records to your health care team. They can use your records to see whether you need changes in your diabetes medicines or your meal plan. If you don't know what your results mean, ask your health care team.

Write things down every day in your record book:

- results of your blood glucose checks
- your diabetes medicines: times and amounts taken
- if your blood glucose was very low
- if you ate more or less food than you usually do
- if you were sick
- if you found ketones in your urine
- what kind of physical activity you did and for how long

80

Figure 10.1. Daily Diabetes Record Page. (Note: A person who doesn't use diabetes medicines will leave the medicine columns blank.)

Day	Other blood glucose	Breakfast blood glucose	Medicine	Lunch blood glucose	Medicine	Dinner blood glucose	Medicine	Bedtime blood glucose	Medicine	Notes: Special events, sick days, physical activity)
Mon										
Tue										
Wed										
Thur										
Fri										
Sat										
Sun										

Action Steps

If You Use Insulin

- Keep a daily record of your blood glucose numbers, the times of the day you took your insulin, the amount and type of insulin you took, and whether you had ketones in your urine.

If You Don't Use Insulin

- Keep a daily record of your blood glucose numbers, the times of the day you took your diabetes medicines, and your physical activity.

When Your Blood Glucose Is Too High or Too Low

Sometimes, no matter how hard you try to keep your blood glucose in your target range, it's too high or too low. Blood glucose that's too high or too low can make you very sick. Here's how to handle these emergencies.

What You Need to Know about Hyperglycemia

If your blood glucose stays over 180, it may be too high. High blood glucose means you don't have enough insulin in your body. High blood glucose, or "hyperglycemia," can happen if you miss taking your diabetes medicine, eat too much, or don't get enough exercise. Sometimes, the medicines you take for other problems cause high blood glucose. Be sure to tell your doctor about other medicines you take.

Having an infection, being sick, or under stress can also make your blood glucose too high. That's why it's very important to check your blood glucose and keep taking your diabetes medicines when you're sick.

If you're very thirsty and tired, have blurry vision, and have to go to the bathroom often, your blood glucose may be too high. Very high blood glucose may also make you feel sick to your stomach.

If your blood glucose is high much of the time, or if you have symptoms of high blood glucose, call your doctor. You may need a change in your diabetes medicines, or a change in your meal plan.

What You Need to Know about Hypoglycemia

Hypoglycemia happens if your blood glucose drops too low. It can come on fast. It's caused by taking too much diabetes medicine, missing a meal, delaying a meal, exercising more than usual, or drinking alcoholic beverages. Sometimes, medicines you take for other health problems can cause blood glucose to drop.

Hypoglycemia can make you feel weak, confused, irritable, hungry, or tired. You may sweat a lot or get a headache. You may feel shaky. If your blood glucose drops lower, you could pass out or have a seizure.

If you have any of these symptoms, check your blood glucose. If the level is 70 or below, have one of the following right away:

- 3 or 4 glucose tablets
- 1 serving of glucose gel (equal to 15 grams of carbohydrate)
- ½ cup (4 ounces) of any fruit juice
- 1 cup (8 ounces) of milk
- ½ cup (4 ounces) of a regular (not diet) soft drink
- 5 or 6 pieces of hard candy
- 1 tablespoon of sugar or honey

After 15 minutes, check your blood glucose again to make sure your level is 70 or above. Repeat these steps as needed. Once your blood glucose is stable, if it will be at least an hour before your next meal, have a snack.

If you take diabetes medicines that can cause hypoglycemia, always carry food for emergencies. It's a good idea also to wear a medical identification bracelet or necklace.

If you take insulin, keep a glucagon kit at home and at a few other places where you go often. Glucagon is given as an injection with a syringe and quickly raises blood glucose. Show your family, friends, and co-workers how to give you a glucagon injection if you pass out because of hypoglycemia.

You can prevent hypoglycemia by eating regular meals, taking your diabetes medicine, and checking your blood glucose often. Checking will tell you whether your glucose level is going down. You can then take steps, like drinking fruit juice, to raise your blood glucose.

Action Steps

If You Use Insulin

- Tell your doctor if you have hypoglycemia often, especially at the same time of the day or night several times in a row.

- Tell your doctor if you've passed out from hypoglycemia.

- Ask your doctor about glucagon. Glucagon is a medicine that raises blood glucose. If you pass out from hypoglycemia, someone should call 911 and give you a glucagon shot.

If You Don't Take Insulin

- Tell your doctor if you have hypoglycemia often, especially at the same time of the day or night several times in a row.

- Be sure to tell your doctor about other medicines you are taking.

- Some diabetes pills can cause hypoglycemia. Ask your doctor whether your pills can cause hypoglycemia.

Why Taking Care of Your Diabetes Is Important

Taking care of your diabetes every day will help keep your blood glucose in your target range and help prevent other health problems that diabetes can cause over the years. This part of the chapter describes those problems. We tell you about them not to scare you, but to help you understand what you can do to keep them from happening.

Diabetes and Your Heart and Blood Vessels

The biggest problem for people with diabetes is heart and blood vessel disease. Heart and blood vessel disease can lead to heart attacks and strokes. It also causes poor blood flow (circulation) in the legs and feet.

To check for heart and blood vessel disease, your health care team will do some tests. At least once a year, have a blood test to see how much cholesterol is in your blood. Your health care provider should take your blood pressure at every visit. Your provider may also check the circulation in your legs, feet, and neck.

The best way to prevent heart and blood vessel disease is to take good care of yourself and your diabetes.

- Eat foods that are low in fat and salt.

- Keep your blood glucose on track. Know your A1C. The target for most people is under 7.

- If you smoke, quit.

- Be physically active.

- Lose weight if you need to.

- Ask your health care team whether you should take an aspirin every day.

- Keep your blood pressure on track. The target for most people is under 130/80. If needed, take medicine to control your blood pressure.

- Keep your cholesterol level on track. The target for LDL cholesterol for most people is under 100. If needed, take medicine to control your blood fat levels.

Blood Pressure Levels

Blood pressure levels tell how hard your blood is pushing against the walls of your blood vessels. Your pressure is given as two numbers: The first is the pressure as your heart beats and the second is the pressure as your heart relaxes. If your blood pressure is higher than your target, talk with your health care team about changing your meal plan, exercising, or taking medicine.

What Are Desirable Blood Fat Levels?

Cholesterol, a fat found in the body, appears in different forms. If your LDL cholesterol ("bad" cholesterol) is 100 or above, you are at increased risk of heart disease and may need treatment. A high level of total cholesterol also means a greater risk of heart disease. But HDL cholesterol ("good" cholesterol) protects you from heart disease, so the higher it is, the better. It's best to keep triglyceride (another type of fat) levels under 150. All of these target numbers are important for preventing heart disease.

Diabetes and Your Eyes

Have your eyes checked once a year. You could have eye problems that you haven't noticed yet. It is important to catch eye problems early when they can be treated. Treating eye problems early can help prevent blindness.

High blood glucose can make the blood vessels in the eyes bleed. This bleeding can lead to blindness. You can help prevent eye damage by keeping your blood glucose as close to normal as possible. If your eyes are already damaged, an eye doctor may be able to save your sight with laser treatments or surgery.

The best way to prevent eye disease is to have a yearly eye exam. In this exam, the eye doctor puts drops in your eyes to dilate your pupils. When the pupils are dilated, or big, the doctor can see into the back of the eye. This is called a dilated eye exam and it doesn't hurt. If you've never had this kind of eye exam before, you should have one now, even if you haven't had any trouble with your eyes. Be sure to tell your eye doctor that you have diabetes.

Here are some tips for taking care of your eyes:

- For adults and adolescents (10 years old and older) with type 1 diabetes: Have your eyes examined within three to five years of being diagnosed with diabetes. Then have an exam every year.

- For people with type 2 diabetes: Have an eye exam every year.

- For women planning to have a baby: Have an eye exam before becoming pregnant.

- If you smoke, quit.

- Keep your blood glucose and blood pressure as close to normal as possible.

Tell your eye doctor right away if you have any problems like blurry vision or seeing dark spots, flashing lights, or rings around lights.

Diabetes and Your Kidneys

Your kidneys help clean waste products from your blood. They also work to keep the right balance of salt and fluid in your body.

Too much glucose in your blood is very hard on your kidneys. After a number of years, high blood glucose can cause the kidneys to stop working. This condition is called kidney failure. If your kidneys stop working, you'll need dialysis (using a machine or special fluids to clean your blood) or a kidney transplant.

Make sure you have the following tests at least once a year to make sure your kidneys are working well:

- a urine test for protein, called the microalbumin test

- a blood test for creatinine

Some types of blood pressure medicines can help prevent kidney damage. Ask your doctor whether these medicines could help you. You can also help prevent kidney problems by doing the following:

- Take your medicine if you have high blood pressure.

- Ask your doctor or your dietitian whether you should eat less protein (meat, poultry, cheese, milk, fish, and eggs).

- See your doctor right away if you get a bladder or kidney infection. Signs of bladder or kidney infections are cloudy or bloody urine, pain or burning when you urinate, and having to urinate often or in a hurry. Back pain, chills, and fever are also signs of kidney infection.

- Keep your blood glucose and blood pressure as close to normal as possible.

- If you smoke, quit.

Diabetes and Your Nerves

Over time, high blood glucose can harm the nerves in your body. Nerve damage can cause you to lose the feeling in your feet or to have painful, burning feet. It can also cause pain in your legs, arms, or hands or cause problems with eating, going to the bathroom, or having sex.

Nerve damage can happen slowly. You may not even realize you have nerve problems. Your doctor should check your nerves at least once a year. Part of this exam should include tests to check your sense of feeling and the pulses in your feet.

Tell the doctor about any problems with your feet, legs, hands, or arms. Also, tell the doctor if you have trouble digesting food, going to the bathroom, or having sex, or if you feel dizzy sometimes.

Nerve damage to the feet can lead to amputations. You may not feel pain from injuries or sore spots on your feet. If you have poor circulation because of blood vessel problems in your legs, the sores on your feet can't heal and might become infected. If the infection isn't treated, it could lead to amputation.

Ask your doctor whether you already have nerve damage in your feet. If you do, it is especially important to take good care of your feet. To help prevent complications from nerve damage, check your feet every day.

Here are some ways to take care of your nerves:

- Keep your blood glucose and blood pressure as close to normal as possible.

- Limit the amount of alcohol you drink.

- Check your feet every day.
- If you smoke, quit.

Foot Care Tips

You can do a lot to prevent problems with your feet. Keeping your blood glucose in your target range and taking care of your feet can help protect them.

- Check your bare feet every day. Look for cuts, sores, bumps, or red spots. Use a mirror or ask a family member for help if you have trouble seeing the bottoms of your feet.

- Wash your feet in warm—not hot—water every day, but don't soak them. Use mild soap. Dry your feet with a soft towel, and dry carefully between your toes.

- After washing your feet, cover them with lotion before putting your shoes and socks on. Don't put lotion or cream between your toes.

- File your toenails straight across with an emery board. Don't leave sharp edges that could cut the next toe.

- Don't try to cut calluses or corns off with a razor blade or knife, and don't use wart removers on your feet. If you have warts or painful corns or calluses, see a podiatrist, a doctor who treats foot problems.

- Wear thick, soft socks. Don't wear mended stockings or stockings with holes or seams that might rub against your feet.

- Check your shoes before you put them on to be sure they have no sharp edges or objects in them.

- Wear shoes that fit well and let your toes move. Break new shoes in slowly. Don't wear flip-flops, shoes with pointed toes, or plastic shoes. Never go barefoot.

- Wear socks if your feet get cold at night. Don't use heating pads or hot water bottles on your feet.

- Have your doctor check your feet at every visit. Take your shoes and socks off when you go into the examining room. This will remind the doctor to check your feet.

- See a podiatrist for help if you can't take care of your feet yourself.

Diabetes and Your Gums and Teeth

Diabetes can lead to infections in your gums and the bones that hold your teeth in place. Like all infections, gum infections can cause blood glucose to rise. Without treatment, teeth may become loose and fall out.

Help prevent damage to your gums and teeth by doing the following:

- See your dentist twice a year. Tell your dentist that you have diabetes.

- Brush and floss your teeth at least twice a day.

- If you smoke, quit.

- Keep your blood glucose as close to normal as possible.

Keeping your blood glucose in your target range, brushing and flossing your teeth every day, and having regular dental checkups are the best ways to prevent gum and teeth problems when you have diabetes.

Chapter 11

Dietary Guidelines for People with Diabetes

Eating and Diabetes

You can take good care of yourself and your diabetes by learning what to eat, how much to eat, and when to eat. Making wise food choices can help you feel good every day, lose weight if you need to, and lower your risk for heart disease, stroke, and other problems caused by diabetes.

Healthful eating, along with physical activity and, if needed, diabetes medicines, helps keep your blood glucose in your target range. The diabetes target range is the level suggested by diabetes experts for good health. You can help prevent health problems by keeping your blood glucose levels on target.

Blood Glucose Levels

What should my blood glucose levels be?

The following are target blood glucose levels for people with diabetes:

- before meals: 90 to 130

- one to two hours after the start of a meal: less than 180

From "What I Need to Know about Eating and Diabetes," National Diabetes Information Clearinghouse, National Institute of Diabetes and Digestive and Kidney Diseases, NIH Pub. No. 06-5043, May 2006.

Ask your doctor how often you should check your blood glucose on your own. Also ask your doctor for an A1C test at least twice a year. Your A1C number gives your average blood glucose for the past three months. The results from your blood glucose checks and your A1C test will tell you whether your diabetes care plan is working.

How can I keep my blood glucose levels on target?

You can keep your blood glucose levels on target by making wise food choices, being physically active, and taking medicines if needed.

For people taking certain diabetes medicines, following a schedule for meals, snacks, and physical activity is best. However, some diabetes medicines allow for more flexibility. You'll work with your health care team to create a diabetes plan that's best for you.

Your Diabetes Medicines

What you eat and when you eat affects how your diabetes medicines work. Talk with your doctor or diabetes teacher about when to take your diabetes medicines. Fill in the names of your diabetes medicines, when to take them, and how much to take. Draw hands on the clocks to show when to take your medicines.

Your Physical Activity Plan

What you eat and when also depend on how much you exercise. Physical activity is an important part of staying healthy and controlling your blood glucose. Keep these points in mind:

- Talk with your doctor about what types of exercise are safe for you.

- Make sure your shoes fit well and your socks stay clean and dry. Check your feet for redness or sores after exercising. Call your doctor if you have sores that do not heal.

- Warm up and stretch for five to ten minutes before you exercise. Then "cool down" for several minutes after you exercise. For example, walk slowly at first, stretch, and then walk faster. Finish up by walking slowly again.

- Check your blood glucose before you exercise. Do not exercise if your fasting blood glucose level is above 250 and you have ketones in your urine. If your blood glucose is below 100, eat a small snack.

- Know the signs of low blood glucose, also called hypoglycemia

- Always carry food or glucose tablets to treat low blood glucose.

- Always wear your medical identification or other ID.

- Find an exercise buddy. Many people find they are more likely to do something active if a friend joins them.

Low Blood Glucose (Hypoglycemia)

Low blood glucose can make you feel shaky, weak, confused, irritable, hungry, or tired. You may sweat a lot or get a headache. If you have these symptoms, check your blood glucose. If it is 70 or lower, have one of the following right away:

- three or four glucose tablets
- one serving of glucose gel (check the label—you'll want the amount equal to 15 grams of carbohydrate)
- ½ cup (4 ounces) of any fruit juice
- ½ cup of a regular (not diet) soft drink
- 1 cup (8 ounces) of milk
- five or six pieces of hard candy
- 1 tablespoon of sugar or honey

After 15 minutes, check your blood glucose again. If it's still too low, have another serving. Repeat until your blood glucose level is 70 or higher. If it will be an hour or more before your next meal, have a snack.

The Food Pyramid

The food pyramid can help you make wise food choices. It divides foods into groups, based on what they contain. Eat more from the groups at the bottom of the pyramid and less from the groups at the top. Foods from the starches, fruits, vegetables, and milk groups are highest in carbohydrate. They affect your blood glucose levels the most.

How much should I eat each day?

Have about 1,200 to 1,600 calories a day if you are a small woman who exercises, small or medium-sized woman who wants to lose weight, or medium-sized woman who does not exercise much. Choose this many servings from these food groups to have 1,200 to 1,600 calories a day:

93

- six starches
- two milks
- three vegetables
- four to six ounces meat and meat substitutes
- two fruits
- up to three fats

Talk with your diabetes teacher about how to make a meal plan that fits the way you usually eat, your daily routine, and your diabetes medicines. Then make your own plan.

Have about 1,600 to 2,000 calories a day if you are a large woman who wants to lose weight, small man at a healthy weight, medium-sized man who does not exercise much, or medium-sized or large man who wants to lose weight. Choose this many servings from these food groups to have 1,600 to 2,000 calories a day:

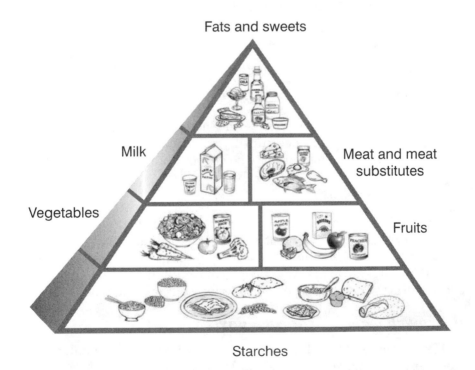

Figure 11.1. *The Food Pyramid. Eat more from the groups at the bottom of the pyramid and less from the groups at the top.*

- eight starches
- two milks
- four vegetables
- four to six ounces meat and meat substitutes
- three fruits
- up to four fats

Talk with your diabetes teacher about how to make a meal plan that fits the way you usually eat, your daily routine, and your diabetes medicines. Then make your own plan.

Have about 2,000 to 2,400 calories a day if you are a medium-sized or large man who exercises a lot or has a physically active job, large man at a healthy weight, or medium-sized or large woman who exercises a lot or has a physically active job.

Choose this many servings from these food groups to have 2,000 to 2,400 calories a day:

- ten starches
- two milks
- four vegetables
- five to seven ounces meat and meat substitutes
- four fruits
- up to five fats

Talk with your diabetes teacher about how to make a meal plan that fits the way you usually eat, your daily routine, and your diabetes medicines. Then make your own plan.

Starches

Starches are bread, grains, cereal, pasta, and starchy vegetables like corn and potatoes. They provide carbohydrate, vitamins, minerals, and fiber. Whole grain starches are healthier because they have more vitamins, minerals, and fiber.

Eat some starches at each meal. Eating starches is healthy for everyone, including people with diabetes. Examples of starches are bread, pasta, corn, pretzels, potatoes, rice, crackers, cereal, tortillas, beans, yams, and lentils.

Examples of one serving of a starch include one slice of bread, one small potato, one-half cup cooked cereal, three-quarters cup of dry cereal flakes, or one 6-inch tortilla. One small potato plus a small ear of corn is an example of two servings. Two slices of bread is also an example of two servings. One small roll plus one-half cup of peas plus one small potato is an example of three servings. One cup of rice is also an example of three servings.

What are healthy ways to eat starches?

- Buy whole grain breads and cereals.

- Eat fewer fried and high-fat starches such as regular tortilla chips and potato chips, french fries, pastries, or biscuits. Try pretzels, fat-free popcorn, baked tortilla chips or potato chips, baked potatoes, or low-fat muffins.

- Use low-fat or fat-free plain yogurt or fat-free sour cream instead of regular sour cream on a baked potato.

- Use mustard instead of mayonnaise on a sandwich.

- Use low-fat or fat-free substitutes such as low-fat mayonnaise or light margarine on bread, rolls, or toast.

- Eat cereal with fat-free (skim) or low-fat (1%) milk.

Vegetables

Vegetables provide vitamins, minerals, and fiber. They are low in carbohydrate. Examples of vegetables are lettuce, broccoli, vegetable juice, spinach, peppers, carrots, green beans, tomatoes, celery, chilies, greens, and cabbage.

Examples of one serving of a vegetable include one-half cup of cooked carrots or one-half cup of cooked green beans or one cup of salad. One-half cup of cooked carrots plus one cup of salad is an example of two servings. One-half cup of vegetable juice plus one half cup of cooked green beans is another example of two servings. One cup of cooked green beans plus one small tomato is an example of three servings. One-half cup of broccoli plus one cup of tomato sauce is another example of three servings.

What are healthy ways to eat vegetables?

- Eat raw and cooked vegetables with little or no fat, sauces, or dressings.

- Try low-fat or fat-free salad dressing on raw vegetables or salads.

- Steam vegetables using water or low-fat broth.
- Mix in some chopped onion or garlic.
- Use a little vinegar or some lemon or lime juice.
- Add a small piece of lean ham or smoked turkey instead of fat to vegetables when cooking.
- Sprinkle with herbs and spices.
- If you do use a small amount of fat, use canola oil, olive oil, or soft margarines (liquid or tub types) instead of fat from meat, butter, or shortening.

Fruits

Fruits provide carbohydrate, vitamins, minerals, and fiber. Examples of fruit include apples, fruit juice, strawberries, dried fruit, grapefruit, bananas, raisins, oranges, watermelon, peaches, mango, guava, papaya, berries, and canned fruit.

Examples of one serving of fruit include one small apple or one-half cup of juice or one-half grapefruit. One banana is an example of two servings of a fruit. One-half cup of orange juice plus one and one-quarter cups of whole strawberries is another example of two servings of a fruit.

What are healthy ways to eat fruits?

- Eat fruits raw or cooked, as juice with no sugar added, canned in their own juice, or dried.
- Buy smaller pieces of fruit.
- Choose pieces of fruit more often than fruit juice. Whole fruit is more filling and has more fiber.
- Save high-sugar and high-fat fruit desserts such as peach cobbler or cherry pie for special occasions.

Milk

Milk provides carbohydrate, protein, calcium, vitamins, and minerals. Examples of one serving of milk include one cup of fat-free or low-fat yogurt or one cup of fat-free (skim) or low-fat (1%) milk.

What are healthy ways to have milk?

- Drink fat-free (skim) or low-fat (1%) milk.

- Eat low-fat or fat-free fruit yogurt sweetened with a low-calorie sweetener.

- Use low-fat plain yogurt as a substitute for sour cream.

Meat and Meat Substitutes

The meat and meat substitutes group includes meat, poultry, eggs, cheese, fish, and tofu. Eat small amounts of some of these foods each day. Meat and meat substitutes provide protein, vitamins, and minerals. Examples of meat and meat substitutes include chicken, beef, fish, canned tuna or other fish, eggs, peanut butter, tofu, cottage cheese, cheese, pork, lamb, and turkey.

Examples of a one-ounce serving of meat and meat substitutes include one egg or two tablespoons of peanut butter. Examples of a two-ounce serving include one slice (one ounce) of turkey plus one slice (one ounce) of low fat cheese. Examples of three-ounce servings include three ounces of cooked lean meat, chicken, or fish. Three ounces of meat (after cooking) is about the size of a deck of cards.

What are healthy ways to eat meat or meat substitutes?

- Buy cuts of beef, pork, ham, and lamb that have only a little fat on them. Trim off the extra fat.

- Eat chicken or turkey without the skin.

- Cook meat or meat substitutes in low-fat ways: broil, grill, stir-fry, roast, steam, stew, or microwave.

- To add more flavor, use vinegars, lemon juice, soy sauce, salsa, ketchup, barbecue sauce, herbs, and spices.

- Cook eggs using a non-stick pan or with cooking spray.

- Limit the amounts of nuts, peanut butter, and fried foods that you eat. They are high in fat.

- Check food labels. Choose low-fat or fat-free cheese.

Fats and Sweets

Limit the amount of fats and sweets you eat. Fats and sweets are not as nutritious as other foods. Fats have a lot of calories. Sweets can be high in carbohydrate and fat. Some contain saturated fats, trans fats, and cholesterol that increase your risk of heart disease.

Limiting these foods will help you lose weight and keep your blood glucose and blood fats under control.

Examples of fats include salad dressing, oil, cream cheese, butter, margarine, mayonnaise, avocado, olives, and bacon. Examples of sweets include cake, ice cream, pie, syrup, cookies, and doughnuts.

Examples of one serving of sweets include one 3-inch cookie or one plain cake doughnut or one tablespoon of maple syrup. Examples of one serving of fat include one strip of bacon or one teaspoon of oil. One tablespoon of regular salad dressing is an example of two servings of fat. Another example of two servings of fat is two tablespoons of reduced-fat salad dressing plus one tablespoon of reduced-fat mayonnaise.

How can I satisfy my sweet tooth?

It's okay to have sweets once in a while. Try having sugar-free popsicles, diet soda, fat-free ice cream or frozen yogurt, or sugar-free hot cocoa mix.

Other tips include sharing desserts in restaurants, ordering small or child-size servings of ice cream or frozen yogurt, or dividing home-made desserts into small servings and wrapping each individually. Freeze extra servings.

Remember, fat-free and low-sugar foods still have calories. Talk with your diabetes teacher about how to fit sweets into your meal plan.

Alcoholic Drinks

Alcoholic drinks have calories but no nutrients. If you have alcoholic drinks on an empty stomach, they can make your blood glucose level go too low. Alcoholic drinks also can raise your blood fats. If you want to have alcoholic drinks, talk with your doctor or diabetes teacher about how much to have.

Your Meal Plan

Plan your meals and snacks for one day. Work with your diabetes teacher if you need help. An organized chart separating what and how much you will eat for breakfast, lunch, dinner, and snacks might help.

Measuring Your Food

To make sure your food servings are the right size, you can use measuring cups, measuring spoons, and a food scale. Or you can use the

This much	is the same as

3 ounces
1 serving of meat, chicken, turkey, or fish

1 cup
1 serving of
- cooked vegetables
- salads
- casseroles or stews, such as chili with beans
- milk

1/2 cup
1 serving of
- fruit or fruit juice
- starchy vegetables, such as potatoes or corn
- pinto beans and other dried beans
- rice or noodles
- cereal

1 ounce
1 serving of
- snack food
- cheese (1 slice)

1 tablespoon
1 serving of
- salad dressing
- cream cheese

1 teaspoon
1 serving of
- margarine or butter
- oil
- mayonnaise

Figure 11.2. Guide to Sensible Serving Sizes.

guide shown in Figure 11.2. Also, the Nutrition Facts label on food packages tells you how much of that food is in one serving.

When You're Sick

Take care of yourself when you're sick. Being sick can make your blood glucose go too high. Here are some tips on what to do:

- Check your blood glucose level every four hours. Write down the results.

- Keep taking your diabetes medicine. You need it even if you can't keep food down.

- Drink at least one cup (8 ounces) of water or other calorie-free, caffeine-free liquid every hour while you're awake.

- If you can't eat your usual food, try drinking juice or eating crackers, popsicles, or soup.

- If you can't eat at all, drink clear liquids such as ginger ale. Eat or drink something with sugar in it if you have trouble keeping food down, because you still need calories. If you can't eat enough, you increase your risk of low blood glucose (hypoglycemia).

- In people with type 1 diabetes, when blood glucose is very high, the body produces ketones. Ketones can make you very sick. Test your urine for ketones if your blood glucose is over 240 or you can't keep food or liquids down.

Call your health care provider right away under these conditions:

- your blood glucose has been over 240 for longer than a day
- you have moderate to large amounts of ketones in your urine
- you feel sleepier than usual
- you have trouble breathing
- you can't think clearly
- you throw up more than once
- you've had diarrhea for more than six hours

101

Chapter 12

Tips for Healthy Meal Planning

Chapter Contents

Section 12.1—Recipe and Meal Planning Guide 104

Section 12.2—How Does Fiber Affect Blood Glucose
　　　　　　　Levels? 108

Section 12.3—Calorie Counting vs. Exchanges in Meal
　　　　　　　Planning 109

Section 12.4—Carbohydrate Counting 111

Section 12.5—Is the Glycemic Index a Helpful Tool? 118

Section 12.6—Diabetes and Alcohol 119

Section 12.7—Tips for Using Less Salt 122

Section 12.8—Ordering Fast-Food Wisely 124

Section 12.9—Buffet Table Tips for People with Diabetes 126

Section 12.1

Recipe and Meal Planning Guide

"Recipe and Meal Planner Guide," National Diabetes
Education Program (http://ndep.nih.gov), October 2004.

Follow these steps to healthy eating and a healthy lifestyle to control and manage diabetes:

- Begin with a healthy eating plan. Healthy eating means eating more grains, fruits, and vegetables, and less meat, sweets, and fats every day. "Let the food be the medicine and medicine be the food" (Hippocrates).

- Be physically active every day to help prevent weight gain and improve blood sugar control.

- Check the sugar in your blood and take your medication every day if needed.

How to Create a Healthy Meal Plan

To create a healthy meal plan you should do the following:

- Eat a variety of foods as recommended in the Diabetes Food Pyramid to get a balanced intake of the nutrients your body needs—carbohydrates, proteins, fats, vitamins, and minerals.

- Make changes gradually because it takes time to accomplish lasting goals.

- Reduce the amount of fat you eat by choosing fewer high-fat foods and cooking with less fat.

- Eat more fiber by eating at least five servings of fruits and vegetables every day.

- Eat fewer foods that are high in sugar like fruit juices, fruit-flavored drinks, sodas, and tea or coffee sweetened with sugar.

- Use less salt in cooking and at the table. Eat fewer foods that are high in salt, like canned and packaged soups, pickles, and processed meats.

- Eat smaller portions and never skip meals.
- Learn about the right serving sizes for you.
- Learn how to read food labels.
- Limit use of alcohol.

What is the Diabetes Food Pyramid?

The Diabetes Food Pyramid is a general guide of what and how much to eat each day. It is similar to the Food Pyramid you see on many food packages. The pyramid is divided into six groups. You should eat more foods from the largest group at the base of the pyramid and less from the smaller groups at the top of the pyramid. The number of servings needed every day is not the same for everyone, so a range of servings is given to ensure you get the foods you need for good health. The food groups and suggested servings per day are listed below, beginning with the food group at the base of the pyramid.

- Grains, beans, and starchy vegetables (good source of B vitamins and fiber): 6 or more servings/day
- Fruits (contain vitamins C, A, potassium, folate, and fiber): 3–4 servings/day
- Vegetables (provide vitamins A, C, folate, and fiber): 3–5 servings/day
- Milk (source of calcium, protein, and vitamins A and D): 2–3 servings/day
- Meats and others (good source of iron, zinc, B vitamins, and protein): 2–3 servings/day
- Fats, sweets, and alcohol: The foods at the tip of the pyramid should be eaten in small amounts. Fats and oils should be limited because they are high in calories. Sweets are high in sugar and should only be eaten once in a while.

What is the right number of servings for you?

The Diabetes Food Pyramid gives a range of servings for each group, but it is only a guide. If you have diabetes, a dietitian can design a specific meal plan for you.

Remember that the number of servings listed is for the entire day. Since food raises blood sugar levels, it is best to space servings throughout the day. For example, four servings of fruit might be divided between three meals and one snack.

What is a serving size in the Food Pyramid?

Each of the following represents one serving from each of the food groups in the Diabetes Food Pyramid:

- **Grains, beans, and starchy vegetables:** 1 slice of bread; ½ small bagel, English muffin, or bun; ½ cup cooked cereal, pasta, rice; ¾ cup ready-to-eat cereal; ½ cup cooked dried beans, corn, peas

- **Vegetable group:** 1 cup raw vegetable; ½ cup vegetable juice

- **Fruit group:** 1 medium-size fresh fruit; ½ cup canned fruit; ½ cup fruit juice

- **Milk group:** 1 cup (8 ounces) milk or yogurt

- **Meat group:** 2–3 ounces cooked lean meat, skinless poultry, or fish; 1 egg; 2 tablespoons peanut butter; 2–3 ounces cheese

- **Fats, sweets, and alcohol:** 1 teaspoon butter, margarine, or mayonnaise; 1 tablespoon cream cheese or salad dressing; 1 tablespoon cream cheese; ½ cup ice cream

Many dishes are made up of several types of foods. Therefore, they do not fit in one specific group. Here are some examples (recipes can be found online at http://ndep.nih.gov/diabetes/MealPlanner/en_recipes.htm).

- Spanish omelet: 1 grains/beans/starchy vegetables; 1 meat, ½ fat

- Beef or turkey stew: 1 grains/beans/starchy vegetables; 1 vegetable; 1 meat; 1 fat

- Caribbean red snapper: 1 meat; 1½ fat

- Two-cheese pizza: 2 grains/beans/starchy vegetables; 1 meat; 1½ fat

- Eggplant lasagna: 1 vegetable; 1 meat; 1 fat

- Rice with chicken, Spanish style: 1½ grains/beans/starchy vegetables; 1 vegetable; 1 meat; 1 fat

- Seafood stew: 2 meat; ½ fat

These are just examples. If you have diabetes, consult a registered dietitian to help you make your own meal plan. Your meal plan will be based on many factors, including your weight goal, height, age, and physical activity. The following Sample Meal Plan, shown in Table 12.1, includes three meals and two snacks, with suggested servings.

Table 12.1. Sample Meal Plan for a Day

Meal	Food Pyramid	Group Servings	Suggested Menu
Breakfast	Fruit	1	Fresh orange, 1 medium
	Grains/Beans/Starchy Veg.	2	Baked plantain, 1 medium
	Milk	1	Milk, 1% low fat, 1 cup
	Fat	1	Oil, 1 teaspoon
Lunch	Meat	1	Two-Cheese Pizza*
	Grains/Beans/Starchy Veg.	2	2 slices
	Fat	1	
	Fruit	1	Melon, 1 cup/cubes
	Vegetable	1	Mixed green salad
Afternoon Snack	Fruit	1	Apple, 1 medium
	Meat	1	Peanut butter, 2 tablespoons
	Grains/Beans/Starchy Veg.	1	Whole wheat crackers, 5
Dinner	Grains/Beans/Starchy Veg.	1	Rice with Chicken Spanish Style*
	Meat	1	1 cup
	Vegetable	1	
	Fat	1	
	Fruit	1	Pineapple rings, ½ cup
	Vegetable	1	Spinach, 1 cup raw
	Fat	1	Vinaigrette, 1 tablespoon
Evening Snack	Milk	1	Yogurt, low fat, 1 cup
	Grains/Beans/Starchy Veg.	1	Bread sticks, 2

*Recipes can be found online at http://ndep.nih.gov/diabetes/MealPlanner/en _recipes.htm.

Section 12.2

How Does Fiber Affect Blood Glucose Levels?

Fiber is a type of carbohydrate (just like sugars and starches) but since it is not broken down by the human body, it does not contribute any calories. Yet, on a food label, fiber is listed under total carbohydrate. So this gets kind of confusing for people who have diabetes. Carbohydrate is the one nutrient that has the biggest impact on blood glucose. So, does fiber have any effect on your blood glucose?

The answer is that fiber does not raise blood glucose levels. Because it is not broken down by the body, the fiber in an apple or a slice of whole grain bread has no effect on blood glucose levels because it isn't digested. The grams of fiber can actually be subtracted from the total grams of carb you are eating if you are using carbohydrate counting for meal planning.

So, fiber is a good thing for people with diabetes. Of course, most of the foods that contain fiber (fruits, vegetables, whole grain breads, cereals, and pastas) also contain other types of non-fiber carbohydrate (sugar, starch) that must be accounted for in your meal plan.

The average person should eat between 20–35 grams of fiber each day. Most Americans eat about half that amount. A study in the *New England Journal of Medicine* showed that people with diabetes who ate 50 grams of fiber a day—particularly soluble fiber—were able to control their blood glucose better than those who ate far less.

So if fiber does not give us any calories, why exactly should you eat it? There are two types of fiber: insoluble and soluble. Insoluble fiber keeps your digestive tract working well. Whole wheat bran is an example of this type of fiber. Soluble fiber can help lower your cholesterol level and improve blood glucose control if eaten in large amounts. Oatmeal is an example of this type of fiber.

Another benefit of fiber is that it adds bulk to help make you feel full. Given these benefits, fiber is important to include in the daily diet for people with diabetes, as well as those who don't have diabetes. You can add fiber by eating whole grain products, fruits, vegetables, and legumes. Leave the skin on fruits and vegetables, as it is high in fiber. Eat whole grain breads and crackers. And be sure to increase your fiber intake generally, and remember to drink 6–8 glasses of water per day to avoid constipation.

Section 12.3

Calorie Counting vs. Exchanges in Meal Planning

Counting calories alone is not a very effective way to manage your diabetes because calories that come from carbohydrate will have a larger and quicker effect raising your blood glucose than calories that come from protein or fat. So if you eat an average-sized meal, but it is all carbohydrate, your blood glucose may rise to an unhealthy level. On the other hand, for many people with diabetes—particularly older people with type 2 diabetes—weight loss is a very important goal to help keep their blood sugars under control. So calories do matter.

Both exchange meal planning and newer meal planning tools like carbohydrate counting and fat gram counting can help you monitor calories while controlling blood glucose.

Many people who have had diabetes for a decade or longer were taught exchange meal planning to manage their diabetes. This system divides all food into six categories—starch, fruit, milk, vegetable, meat, and fat groups. A defined serving or "exchange" of each food item in one of these categories has the same calories, grams of fat, protein, and carbohydrate in it as every other food item in that category. So, under the "fruit choices" in the exchange system, for example, ½ cup of applesauce and a small banana each equals one "fruit exchange" that has 60 calories, 15 grams of carbohydrate, and no protein or fat.

In the exchange meal planning system, your healthcare team works with you to develop a meal plan that distributes a number of exchanges from each of the six food categories through each of three meals and two or three snacks each day. The meal plan is developed based on the patient's diabetes treatment plan and goals. If weight loss is a goal, for example, the patient will have fewer exchanges to spend at each meal, so that total calories are kept at a level to enable the patient to lose weight. Patients then use food lists to figure out how to "spend" those exchanges at each meal.

This system has been fairly complicated for many patients to use successfully, though many people who have used this system for years are very happy with it.

More recently—and particularly with the growing use of prepackaged foods—the focus has shifted to carbohydrate counting and fat gram counting for meal planning. Because carbohydrate has the biggest effect on blood glucose, clinicians believe that if the patient is allocated a number of grams of carbohydrate to eat at each meal, they can keep their blood glucose under control with much less mathematical gymnastics. Similarly, some patients who need to lose weight may focus on counting grams of fat, because each gram of fat in a food has 9 calories in it (versus carbohydrate or protein, which have only 4 calories per gram). Because fat grams and carbohydrate grams per serving are listed on all packaged foods, this becomes a much easier way for people to manage their meals for good blood glucose control.

The bottom line: talk with your healthcare team about what your diabetes treatment goals are, and with a dietitian who has experience in diabetes about what type of meal planning methods are available that will be easiest for you to use to achieve those treatment goals.

Section 12.4

Carbohydrate Counting

There are several different ways people with diabetes can manage their food intake to keep their blood sugars as close to normal as possible. One such method is carbohydrate counting. Carbohydrate counting is a method of calculating the grams of carbohydrate you eat at meals and snacks. The reason you focus on counting grams of carbohydrate is because carbohydrates tend to have the greatest effect on your blood sugar.

When you understand how to count grams of carbohydrates, you can have a wider choice of foods in your meal plan. It is easier to fit in combination foods such as soups and frozen dinners because you look at the grams of carbohydrate listed on the package, rather than trying to calculate how that particular food fits into the more traditional exchange meal plan. Also, some people find they can control their blood sugars more precisely.

Carbohydrate counting can be used by anyone with diabetes—not just people taking insulin. This method can assure that the right amount of carbohydrate is eaten at each meal and snack. Now that foods are more clearly labeled, it is easy to find the carbohydrate content of packaged foods.

This method is also useful for people who are using more aggressive methods of adjusting insulin to control their diabetes. The amount of meal and snack carbohydrate is adjusted based on the pre-meal blood sugar reading. Depending on the reading, more or less carbohydrate may be eaten. Likewise, insulin may be adjusted based on what the person wants to eat. For example, if you want to eat a much larger meal, this approach can guide you to determine how much extra insulin to take.

The following is an explanation of how to use carbohydrate meal planning. Feel free to discuss them with your nurse educator, dietitian, or physician at your next visit.

111

Tools of the Trade

In order to count carbohydrates, you must begin by knowing your meal plan and the average carbohydrate values of the food groups. If you don't have some form of a meal plan developed by your health care team, you will be unable to figure out how many grams of carbohydrate you are supposed to eat at each meal and snack. Start by making sure you know the average amount of carbohydrates per serving in each food group. Good resources for exchange systems are Joslin's Menu Planning—Simple! (http://www.joslin.org/2802.asp), Joslin's Guide to Diabetes (http://www.joslin.org/815_2817.asp) (which also contains a chapter discussing meal planning, including carbohydrate counting) or the American Diabetes Association's *Exchange Lists for Meal Planning*. It is also helpful if you also have a carbohydrate counting reference book. We suggest: *The Complete Book of Food Counts* by Corinne Netzer, *The Diabetes Carbohydrate and Fat Gram Guide* by Lea Holzmeister, *Calories and Carbohydrates* by Barbara Kraus, *Carbohydrate Guide to Brand Names and Basic Foods* by Barbara Kraus, *The Carbohydrate Addict's Gram Counter* by Richard Heller, and *The Restaurant Lovers' Fat Gram Counter* by Kalia Doner. Measuring equipment, such as a food scale, measuring cups and spoons, is essential. Probably the most frequently used tool will be food labels.

Step 1: Know Your Meal Plan

Indicate on the Chart 12.1 the number of servings from each food group planned as part of your meal plan. The last row will be completed in Step 2.

Step 2: Know Your Carbohydrates

Most of the carbohydrates we eat comes from three food groups: starch, fruit, and milk. Vegetables also contain some carbohydrates, but foods in the meat and fat groups contain very little carbohydrates. This list shows the average amount of carbohydrates in each food group per serving:

- Starch: 15 carbohydrate grams
- Fruit: 15 carbohydrate grams
- Milk: 12 carbohydrate grams

- Vegetable: 5 carbohydrate grams
- Meat: 0 carbohydrate grams
- Fat: 0 carbohydrate grams

To make things easy, many people begin carbohydrate counting by rounding the carbohydrate values of milk up to 15. In other words, one serving of starch, fruit, or milk all contain 15 grams of carbohydrates or one carbohydrate serving. Three servings of vegetable also contain 15 grams. One or two servings of vegetables do not need to be counted. Each meal and snack will contain a total number of grams of carbohydrates.

Complete the following to test your understanding:

- 1 slices of bread = _____ grams of carbohydrates
- 1 whole banana (9" size) = _____ grams of carbohydrates
- 1 cup oatmeal with 1 cup milk = _____ grams of carbohydrates

Look back at your meal plan in Step 1. Total up the number of grams of carbohydrate for each meal and snack and write the totals in the last row. It is more important to know your carbohydrate allowance for each meal and snack than it is to know your total for the day. The amount of carbohydrates eaten at each meal should remain consistent (unless you learn to adjust your insulin for a change in the amount of carbohydrates eaten).

Chart 12.1.

Food Groups	Breakfast	Snack	Lunch	Snack	Dinner	Snack
Starch						
Fruit						
Vegetable						
Milk						
Protein						
Fat						
Carbohydrates						

Step 3 : Using Carbohydrate Counting in Meal Planning

Here is an example to show how carbohydrate counting can make meal planning easier. Let's say your dinner meal plan contains five carbohydrate servings or 75 grams of carbohydrates. (This is based on a meal plan of three starch servings, four protein, one vegetable, one fruit, one milk, and three fat.) The label on a frozen dinner of beef enchiladas says it contains 62 grams of carbohydrate. Instead of calculating how many exchanges that converts to, just figure out how many more grams of carbohydrates you need to meet your 75 gram total. Add about 15 more grams of carbohydrates (one serving of fruit or milk, for example) and you have almost matched your total.

Try another example. If you want to have chili for lunch, what else can you have with it? The label on the chili says it contains 29 grams of carbohydrate per 1 cup serving.

Portion Control: A Key to Successful Meal Planning

The amount of food you eat is closely related to blood sugar control. If you eat more food than is recommended on your meal plan, your blood sugar goes up. Although foods containing carbohydrate have the most impact on blood sugars, the calories from all foods will affect blood sugar. The only way you can tell if you are eating the right amount is to measure your foods carefully.

Measuring Hints

- Practice, practice, practice. Don't rely on measuring once and then just "guesstimating." Pull out the scales at least once a week to check yourself and reinforce your skills.

- Use a glass which you know only holds 4 or 8 ounces to better control your portion. You can also place a piece of tape on the outside of a glass to mark a 4 or 8 ounce line so you will be able to measure easily.

- A bread serving is based on a one-ounce slice of bread. Many single bread servings may weigh more than one ounce, and therefore have more impact on blood sugar. Check the weight or the label of such things as light breads, bagels, or rolls.

- To be more precise, know the weight of fruit servings for portion control.

- Check your cereal portion using measuring cups. The cereal label will give you a more precise nutrition information such as calories, carbohydrate, and fat grams than the food group averages.

Test Your Memory

How much of each of these foods can you have for a 15 gram carbohydrates (or 1 fruit or 1 bread) serving?

- Cherries
- Raisins
- Grapefruit juice
- Rice
- Vanilla Wafers
- Lentils/dried beans

Fitting Sugar in Your Meal Plan

It is commonly thought that people with diabetes should avoid all forms of sugar. Most people with diabetes can eat foods containing sugar as long as the total amount of carbohydrate for that meal or snack is consistent and sugar foods are added within the context of healthy eating. Many research studies have shown that meals which contain sugar do not make the blood sugar rise higher than meals of equal carbohydrate levels which do not contain sugar. However, if the sugar-containing meal contains more carbohydrates, the blood sugar levels will go up.

Which will have the greater effect on blood sugar?

- 1 tsp sugar
- ½ cup potatoes

The potatoes will contribute about 15 grams of carbohydrates, while a level teaspoon of sugar will only give 4 grams of carbohydrates. Therefore, the potatoes will have about three times the effect on blood sugar as compared to the table sugar.

Meal Planning Practice

Using the foods listed in Table 12.2, plan two breakfast meals containing approximately 45 grams of carbohydrate. Notice that there

115

are some foods on this list you might think would not be "allowed" on your meal plan. But again, any of these foods can be used as long as you limit the amount of carbohydrates you eat at a given meal to what is indicated on your individualized meal plan. (In the example below, this means you can choose whatever foods you want as long as the total carbohydrate equals no more than 45 grams).

Table 12.2. Meal Planning

Food	Amount	Carbohydrate Grams
1% fat milk	1 cup	12
Bran Chex	2/3 cup	23
Frosted Flakes	3/4 cup	26
Raisin Bran	3/4 cup	28
bread/toast	1 slice	15
sugar, white table	1 teaspoon	4
pancakes—4 inches	2	15
low-fat granola	1/2 cup	30
yogurt, fruited	1 cup	40
yogurt, fruit with NutraSweet fruit juice	1 cup	19
fruit juice	1/2 cup	15
banana	1/2	15
pancake syrup	2 tablespoons	30
light pancake sugar free syrup	2 tablespoons	4

Sample Breakfast

- Fruit yogurt (with NutraSweet): 19 carbohydrate grams
- Cinnamon-sugar toast—1 slice with 1 teaspoon sugar and 1 teaspoon margarine: 19 carbohydrate grams
- Milk, ½ cup: 6 carbohydrate grams
- Carbohydrate total = 44 carbohydrate grams

Does this mean I can eat cake and not worry about it?

No! A slice of white cake with chocolate icing (1/12 of a cake or 80 gram weight) will give you about 300 calories, 45 grams of carbohydrates, and 12 grams of fat. That is three starch servings and over two fat servings. Before you have a slice of cake, ask yourself the following questions: Will that small piece of cake be satisfying or will I still be hungry? How it will fit into my meal plan? Do I have 300 calories to "spend" on this? Are there other choices I could make which would contribute less fat? A 1/12 slice of angel food cake has less than 1 gram of fat and only 30 carbohydrates. This may be a better choice.

Controlling All Carbohydrates

It is important to realize that sugar is not the only carbohydrate that you have to "control." The body will convert all carbohydrates to glucose—so eating extra servings of rice, pasta, bread, fruit, or other carbohydrates foods will make the blood sugar rise. Just because something doesn't have sugar in it doesn't mean you can eat as much as you want. Your meal plan is designed so that the carbohydrate content of your meals remains as consistent as possible from day to day.

A Word of Caution

Although sugar does not cause the blood sugar to rise any higher than other carbohydrates, it should be eaten along with other healthy foods. If you choose to drink a 12 ounce can of a sugar-sweetened soft drink, that would use up about 45 grams carbohydrates—and you wouldn't have gotten any nutrition (protein, vitamins, or minerals). What a waste of calories!

High sugar foods are more concentrated in carbohydrates. Therefore the volume would be smaller than a low sugar food. What is your eating style? Are you able to control your portion size—or are you likely to overeat? High sugar foods might not be a good choice if they will just tempt you to eat more. If you would rather eat larger portions, select low sugar choices. Look at the differences in portion size you get for equal amounts of carbohydrate in these cereals.

- 1/4 cup Granola
- 1/3 cup Frosted Flakes
- 3/4 cup Cornflakes
- 1 cup Cheerios
- 1 1/4 cup Puffed Wheat

In addition, many sugar-containing foods also contain a lot of fat. Foods such as cookies, pastries, ice cream, and cakes should be avoided largely because of the fat content and because they don't contribute much nutritional value. If you do want a "sweet"—make a low-fat choice, such as low-fat frozen yogurt, gingersnaps, fig bars, or graham crackers and substitute it for another carbohydrate on your meal plan.

Talk with your diabetes dietitian educator to select the best "sweet" choices for your meal plan. If you have not met with a dietitian in the past year or if you do not have a personal meal plan, scheduling an appointment with a dietitian would help you to incorporate these guidelines in the best way for you and your diabetes control.

Section 12.5

Is the Glycemic Index a Helpful Tool?

"What Is the Glycemic Index and Is It a Helpful Tool?"
copyright © 2007 by Joslin Diabetes Center. All rights reserved.
Reprinted with permission from Joslin's website: www.joslin.org.

The glycemic index indicates the after-meal response your body has to a particular food compared to a standard amount of glucose. If that sounds complicated—it is. Many factors come into play, including your age and activity level, the amount of fiber and fat in the particular food, how refined (processed) the food is, what else was eaten with the food, what the composition of the food is in terms of carb, protein, and fat, how the food was cooked, and how quickly your body digests the food (which varies from person to person).

In general, fiber-rich foods are often the same foods that are thought to be low glycemic foods and seem to have less effect on blood glucose. Sucrose (table sugar) also has a lower effect on blood glucose than some starches, such as potatoes. There are lists of such "high" and "low" glycemic index foods.

Health professionals agree that the more complex a meal plan is, the less likely people are to follow it. The glycemic index is a fairly complex meal planning tool, and the fact that people's blood glucose can react differently to so-called "low" and "high" glycemic index foods has limited the usefulness of the index in teaching patients with diabetes how to manage their food intake to keep their blood glucose under control. However, the glycemic index may be used as an additional tool together with a patient's current meal planning system. Registered dietitians often encourage patients to determine their own individual glycemic index of foods based on how their blood glucose responds to the various meals and snacks they tend to eat.

Most dietitians and other healthcare professionals working with patients prefer to talk in terms of the number of grams of carbohydrate in a food, rather than the "glycemic index" of a food. Carbohydrate has the greatest effect on blood glucose, so in general two foods that have the same number of grams of carbohydrate in them will have a similar effect on your blood glucose level. Your dietitian works with you to determine—based on your weight, how active you are, and other factors—how many grams of carbohydrate you can eat at each meal and snack to keep your blood glucose under control. This type of meal planning is simpler to use, offers greater flexibility, and enables many people to manage their diabetes successfully.

Section 12.6

Diabetes and Alcohol

How to Stay Safe When You Drink Alcohol: An Ounce of Prevention

You need to take certain added precautions when you plan on having a drink or two:

- Always eat something when you drink. Have a well-balanced meal before you drink and snack while you are out drinking. You need glucose from food, since your liver will stop producing it once you drink alcohol.

- Carefully check the alcohol level of what you're drinking. Make sure that mixed drinks are accurately measured, and be sure to account for added calories and carbohydrates in fruit juices, sodas, and other mixers. Check the proof of distilled spirits and the alcohol level of beer and wines.

- Don't exercise before drinking. Exercise lowers blood glucose levels, and drinking will reduce them even further. Dancing counts as exercise, so think about skipping the drinks if you are hitting the dance floor.

- Be prepared for hypoglycemia. Make sure you have a high carbohydrate snack available in case your blood glucose levels dip below 65 (3.61 mmol/l) to 70 mg/dl (3.89 mmol/l). Glucagon will not help treat alcohol-induced hypoglycemia.

- Monitor, monitor, monitor. The best precaution against alcohol-induced hypoglycemia is to bring along your blood glucose monitor and check your levels frequently.

Pick Your Drinking Buddies Wisely

Make sure at least one friend or trusted companion knows that you have diabetes and is aware of what should be done in case of a hypoglycemic attack. And make sure they remain sober enough to do so. This is extremely important, because hypoglycemia can resemble intoxication, and others may assume you are drunk rather than suffering from a dangerous diabetic complication. Your friend should be able to recognize the symptoms of hypoglycemia (that is, confusion, dizziness, shaking, paleness, etc.) and to get you a snack high in carbohydrates or glucose tablets or gel if symptoms occur. They should also be prepared to seek immediate medical attention if you lose consciousness or start vomiting.

After the Party

When you go to sleep after a few evening drinks, blood sugar levels may crash in the middle of the night. As a safety precaution, have a snack before bed. You should also set the alarm to wake you up after a few hours of sleep, so you can test your blood glucose and eat something if required.

When to Just Say No

Under certain circumstances, alcohol and diabetes don't mix:

- If you suffer from neuropathy, drinking can make it worse. Heavy or prolonged alcohol use can cause nerve damage (in people with and without diabetes), and even moderate drinking can aggravate existing diabetic neuropathy.

- If you have high triglyceride levels (over 200 mg/dl or 11.11 mmol/l), you should also abstain. Alcohol impairs the ability of the liver to clear fat from the blood and increases triglyceride production.

- If you have chronic hypertension, limit or eliminate your alcohol intake. People with diabetes are already at risk for high blood pressure, and alcohol has been shown to raise blood pressure levels even further. Chronic high blood pressure can contribute to a host of diabetic complications, including kidney failure, heart disease, and retinopathy.

- A number of diabetes medications and other prescription and over-the-counter drugs should not be taken with alcohol. Check the label, and ask your pharmacist and/or physician if you are unsure.

- If you are practicing tight control, you may do better to forgo the drinks altogether. Tight control and the impaired judgment that comes with intoxication is a recipe for disaster. In addition, since tight control means you are fairly close to normal glucose levels, hypoglycemia may occur more quickly.

And of course, never drink if you are planning to test your blood glucose, drive any type of vehicle (automobile, boat, snowmobile, even dog sled), or if you are pregnant or trying to become pregnant.

There are other medical conditions that may contraindicate the use of alcohol, such as liver disease, peptic ulcer, gastritis, and pancreatitis. Check with your healthcare provider if you think your medical history may have an influence on your alcohol intake.

Section 12.7

Tips for Using Less Salt

Excerpted from "A Healthier You,"
U.S. Department of Health and Human Services, 2005.

Nearly all of us eat too much salt (sodium). On average, the more salt a person eats, the higher his or her blood pressure is. Most salt we eat comes from processed foods, not necessarily from the salt shaker. Some people are surprised by this, and that is why we are going to talk about the Nutrition Facts label—you'll see "salt" listed as sodium there. For our purposes, we can use the terms "salt" and "sodium" interchangeably.

Eating less salt is an important way to reduce the risk of high blood pressure, which may in turn reduce the risk of heart disease, stroke, congestive heart failure, and kidney damage.

In addition to eating less salt, other lifestyle changes may prevent or delay getting high blood pressure and may help lower high blood pressure. These lifestyle changes include eating more potassium-rich foods, losing excess weight, being more physically active, and eating a healthy diet.

Eating Less Salt

- When you're choosing packaged foods, look at the sodium content on the Nutrition Facts label. Use the percent Daily Value (% DV) to help limit your sodium intake. 5% DV or less is low and 20% DV or more is high. You don't want to exceed a total of 100% DV for sodium in a day. Some people (people with high blood pressure, African-Americans/blacks, and people who are middle-aged or older) should get even less—about half as much.

- Compare sodium content for similar foods. This can really make a difference. By comparing brands of similar foods, you can save over hundreds of milligrams of sodium. Use the Nutrition Facts label on the food package to select food brands that are lower in sodium.

- Use the claims on the front of the food package to quickly identify foods that contain less salt or that are a good source of potassium, a nutrient you want to get more of in your daily diet. Example s include "low in sodium," "very low sodium," and "high in potassium."

- When you're preparing food at home, use herbs and spices to add flavor to your foods so you don't depend too heavily on salt. Don't salt foods before or during cooking—and limit salt use at the table.

- When you're eating out, ask that your meal be prepared without added salt or ask the server to identify foods on the menu that are made without added salt.

Tips for Using Herbs and Spices Instead of Salt

- **Basil:** Use in soups, salads, vegetables, fish, and meats.
- **Cinnamon:** Use in salads, vegetables, breads, and snacks.
- **Chili Powder:** Use in soups, salads, vegetables, and fish.
- **Cloves:** Use in soups, salads, and vegetables.
- **Dill Weed and Dill Seed:** Use in fish, soups, salads, and vegetables.
- **Ginger:** Use in soups, salads, vegetables, and meats.
- **Marjoram:** Use in soups, salads, vegetables, beef, fish, and chicken.
- **Nutmeg:** Use in vegetables, meats, and snacks.
- **Oregano:** Use in soups, salads, vegetables, meats, and chicken.
- **Parsley:** Use in salads, vegetables, fish, and meats.
- **Rosemary:** Use in salads, vegetables, fish, and meats.
- **Sage:** Use in soups, salads, vegetables, meats, and chicken.
- **Thyme:** Use in salads, vegetables, fish, and chicken.

Note: To start, use small amounts of these herbs and spices to see whether you like them.

Section 12.8

Ordering Fast-Food Wisely

"Ordering Fast-Food Wisely," © Michigan Diabetes Research and
Training Center (www.med.umich.edu/mdrtc). Reprinted with permission.

About 46% of the average American's food budget is spent on eating out. Unfortunately, it's not always easy to eat a nutritious and balanced meal away from home. Fast-food restaurants are probably the biggest challenge. You can still have a healthy, relatively low-calorie meal that can fit into your diabetes meal plan, if you know how to order.

Fast-foods are generally very low in fiber and complex carbohydrates, but are high in fat, salt, and sugar. Fat has twice as many calories as an equal amount of carbohydrate or protein, so most fast-foods are very "calorie dense." It doesn't take very much food to add up to too many calories. Fast-food dinners such as fried chicken or a fish sandwich and fries get about half their calories from fat. Such a meal could easily top the 1000 calorie mark—over half the total suggested daily calories for most adults.

The easiest answer to the fast-food dilemma is to keep such foods to a minimum. But fast-foods are here to stay and, admittedly, they're tasty, inexpensive, and fast. Here are some suggestions for how to deal with them:

- When you eat a fast-food meal, try to balance this with healthier foods for the remaining meals of the day. Choose fresh vegetables and fruit, whole grain breads, and low-fat dairy products at your other meals.

- Don't assume that anything you get from a salad bar is low in calories and fat. A plate of prepared salads such as potato and macaroni salads, coleslaw, or salad greens covered with bacon bits, croutons, cheeses, and heavy dressings could be more calories and fat than a burger, fries, and shake.

- Many fast-food restaurants offer broiled chicken, which is much lower in fat and calories than fried. For example, save 400 calories and 35 grams of fat by ordering a grilled chicken sandwich instead of a deluxe burger. But whether you order broiled or fried chicken, don't eat the skin, which is where most of the fat lies. Also, when ordering something fried, choose larger pieces rather than tidbits, which have more greasy batter.

- Shakes and colas are high in sugar and have little or no nutritive value. Skim milk, fruit juice, or even glasses of ice water or diet soda are healthier alternatives.

- Go easy on the condiments. Big Mac sauce, tartar sauce, and mayonnaise add more than 100 calories each. Most barbecue sauces add 60 calories. Try ketchup and mustard or order your sandwich plain.

- Many fast-food breakfasts are little more than grease on a bun. A croissant may contain as much as four and a half pats of butter or fat. If you're in a hurry, you're much better off having a quick breakfast of toast or a bagel.

- Fast-food portions are intended for large appetites. In fact, fast-food advertisers emphasize "BIG," "JUMBO," and "SUPER" portions. Order smaller versions when you can. Choose fast-food restaurants with salad bars, and have a salad of fresh fruit and vegetables on the side if you want more food.

- Get information on the calorie/nutrient values of fast-foods so you know just what you're eating. Almost every fast-food restaurant has this information available.

Section 12.9

Buffet Table Tips for People with Diabetes

National Diabetes Education Program, November 2005.

Barbecues, picnics, and family reunions are gatherings to enjoy and treasure. If you have diabetes, these events can pose special challenges. How can you stick with your meal plan, yet join in the celebration and have some fun? You can do it. If you choose wisely and watch how much you eat, you can have a delicious meal and feel good too. So, grab your plate and head for the buffet table.

Look for the high fiber, low-fat dishes. Great choices are beans, peas, and lentils, and dark green vegetables such as broccoli, cabbage, spinach, and kale. Go for the green bean, three-bean, black bean, and black-eyed pea dishes or pasta salads mixed with summer vegetables. Choose whole grain foods such as brown rice, couscous, whole wheat bread, and pasta. Everyone benefits from eating these foods, not just people with diabetes.

Watch out for dishes loaded with mayonnaise, sour cream, and butter. Choose veggies that are light on salad dressing, cheese, or cream sauce. If you can, make your own dressing with a little olive oil and vinegar.

Vegetables and grains should fill up most of your plate, but leave room for some lean meat, poultry, or fish. Be sure to choose grilled chicken—and remove the skin—instead of the fried variety. If you're going to make a sandwich, use whole wheat bread with mustard or salsa, rather than mayonnaise.

What's for dessert? Summer means terrific fruits. It's hard to beat a fresh peach, fruit salad, cantaloupe, or watermelon. Fruit is an excellent source of fiber, vitamins, and minerals, and has zero fat. Everyone, including people with diabetes, should eat three to four servings of fruit a day. Pies, cakes, and cookies are high in fat and cholesterol. If you can't resist, have a small serving.

It's best to drink water, unsweetened tea, or diet soda. Add a wedge of lemon for flavor. If you choose to drink alcoholic beverages, limit your intake to no more than one drink a day for women, two for men, and drink only with a meal.

Chapter 13

Physical Activity Guidelines for People with Diabetes

What I Need to Know about Physical Activity and Diabetes

How can I take care of my diabetes?

Diabetes means that your blood glucose (also called blood sugar) is too high. Your body uses glucose for energy. But having too much glucose in your blood can hurt you. When you take care of your diabetes, you'll feel better. You'll reduce your risk for problems with your kidneys, eyes, nerves, feet and legs, and teeth. You'll also lower your risk for a heart attack or a stroke. You can take care of your diabetes by being physically active, following a healthy meal plan, and taking medicines (if prescribed by your doctor).

What can a physically active lifestyle do for me?

Research has shown that physical activity can help with the following:

• lower your blood glucose and your blood pressure

"What I Need to Know about Physical Activity and Diabetes," National Diabetes Information Clearinghouse, National Institute of Diabetes and Digestive and Kidney Diseases, NIH Pub. 04-5180, June 2004. Text under the heading "Frequently Asked Questions about Diabetes and Exercise," is from the National Center for Chronic Disease Prevention and Health Promotion, Centers for Disease Control and Prevention, June 2006.

- lower your bad cholesterol and raise your good cholesterol
- improve your body's ability to use insulin
- lower your risk for heart disease and stroke
- keep your heart and bones strong
- keep your joints flexible
- lower your risk of falling
- help you lose weight
- reduce your body fat
- give you more energy
- reduce your stress

Physical activity also plays an important part in preventing type 2 diabetes. A major government study, the Diabetes Prevention Program (DPP), showed that a healthy diet and a moderate exercise program resulting in a five to seven percent weight loss can delay and possibly prevent type 2 diabetes.

What kinds of physical activity can help me?

Four kinds of activity can help. You can try being extra active every day, doing aerobic exercise, doing strength training, and stretching.

Be extra active every day: Being extra active can increase the number of calories you burn. There are many ways to be extra active:

- Walk around while you talk on the phone.
- Play with the kids.
- Take the dog for a walk.
- Get up to change the TV channel instead of using the remote control.
- Work in the garden or rake leaves.
- Clean the house.
- Wash the car.
- Stretch out your chores. For example, make two trips to take the laundry downstairs instead of one.

- Park at the far end of the shopping center lot and walk to the store.

- At the grocery store, walk down every aisle.

- At work, walk over to see a co-worker instead of calling or e-mailing.

- Take the stairs instead of the elevator.

- Stretch or walk around instead of taking a coffee break and eating.

- During your lunch break, walk to the post office or do other errands.

Do aerobic exercise: Aerobic exercise is activity that requires the use of large muscles and makes your heart beat faster. You will also breathe harder during aerobic exercise. Doing aerobic exercise for 30 minutes a day, most days of the week, provides many benefits. You can even split up those 30 minutes into several parts. For example, you can take three brisk 10-minute walks, one after each meal.

If you haven't exercised lately, see your doctor first to make sure it's OK for you to increase your level of physical activity. Talk with your doctor about how to warm up and stretch before exercise and how to cool down after exercise. Then start slowly with five to ten minutes a day. Add a little more time each week, aiming for 150 to 200 minutes per week. Try these activities:

- walking briskly
- hiking
- climbing stairs
- swimming or taking a water-aerobics class
- dancing
- riding a bicycle outdoors or a stationary bicycle indoors
- taking an aerobics class
- playing basketball, volleyball, or other sports
- in-line skating, ice skating, or skate boarding
- playing tennis
- cross-country skiing

Do strength training: Doing exercises with hand weights, elastic bands, or weight machines two or three times a week builds muscle.

When you have more muscle and less fat, you'll burn more calories because muscle burns more calories than fat, even between exercise sessions. Strength training can help make daily chores easier, improving your balance and coordination, as well as your bones' health. You can do strength training at home, at a fitness center, or in a class. Your health care team can tell you more about strength training and what kind is best for you.

Stretch: Stretching increases your flexibility, lowers stress, and helps prevent muscle soreness after other types of exercise. Your health care team can tell you what kind of stretching is best for you.

Can I exercise any time I want?

Ask your health care team about the best time of day for you to exercise. Consider your daily schedule, your meal plan, and your diabetes medications in deciding when to exercise.

If you exercise when your blood glucose is above 300, your level can go even higher. It's best not to exercise until your blood glucose is lower. Also, exercise is not recommended if your fasting blood glucose is above 250 and you have ketones in your urine.

Are there any types of physical activity I shouldn't do?

If you have diabetes complications, some exercises can make your problems worse. For example, activities that increase the pressure in the blood vessels of your eyes, such as lifting heavy weights, can make diabetic eye problems worse. If nerve damage from diabetes has made your feet numb, your doctor may suggest that you try swimming instead of walking for aerobic exercise.

Numbness means that you may not feel any pain from sores or blisters on your feet and so may not notice them. Then they can get worse and lead to more serious problems. Make sure you exercise in cotton socks and comfortable, well-fitting shoes that are designed for the activity you are doing. After you exercise, check your feet for cuts, sores, bumps, or redness. Call your doctor if any foot problems develop.

Can physical activity cause low blood glucose?

Physical activity can cause hypoglycemia (low blood glucose) in people who take insulin or certain diabetes pills, including sulfonylureas and meglitinides. Ask your health care team whether your diabetes pills can cause hypoglycemia. Some types of diabetes pills do not.

Hypoglycemia can happen while you exercise, right afterward, or even up to a day later. It can make you feel shaky, weak, confused, irritable, hungry, or tired. You may sweat a lot or get a headache. If your blood glucose drops too low, you could pass out or have a seizure.

However, you should still be physically active. These steps can help you be prepared for hypoglycemia:

Before Exercise

- Be careful about exercising if you have skipped a recent meal. Check your blood glucose. If it's below 100, have a small snack.

- If you take insulin, ask your health care team whether you should change your dosage before you exercise.

During Exercise

- Wear your medical identification or other ID.

- Always carry food or glucose tablets so that you'll be ready to treat hypoglycemia.

- If you'll be exercising for more than an hour, check your blood glucose at regular intervals. You may need snacks before you finish.

After Exercise

- Check to see how exercise affected your blood glucose level.

Treating hypoglycemia: If your blood glucose is 70 or lower, have one of the following right away:

- 2 or 3 glucose tablets
- ½ cup (4 ounces) of any fruit juice
- ½ cup (4 ounces) of a regular (not diet) soft drink
- 1 cup (8 ounces) of milk
- 5 or 6 pieces of hard candy
- 1 or 2 teaspoons of sugar or honey

After 15 minutes, check your blood glucose again. If it's still too low, have another serving. Repeat until your blood glucose is 70 or higher. If it will be an hour or more before your next meal, have a snack as well.

131

What should I do first?

Check with your doctor. Always talk with your doctor before you start a new physical activity program. Ask about your medications—prescription and over the counter—and whether you should change the amount you take before you exercise. If you have heart disease, kidney disease, eye problems, or foot problems, ask which types of physical activity are safe for you.

Decide exactly what you'll do and set some goals. Make the following choices:

- the type of physical activity you want to do
- the clothes and items you'll need to get ready
- the days and times you'll add activity
- the length of each session
- your warm up and cool down plan for each session
- alternatives, such as where you'll walk if the weather is bad
- your measures of progress

Find an exercise buddy: Many people find that they are more likely to do something active if a friend joins them. If you and a friend plan to walk together, for example, you may be more likely to do it.

Keep track of your physical activity: Write down when you exercise and for how long in your blood glucose record book. You'll be able to track your progress and to see how physical activity affects your blood glucose.

Decide how you'll reward yourself: Do something nice for yourself when you reach your activity goals. For example, treat yourself to a movie or buy a new plant for the garden.

What can I do to make sure I stay active?

One of the keys to staying on track is finding some activities you like to do. If you keep finding excuses not to exercise, think about why. Are your goals realistic? Do you need a change in activity? Would another time be more convenient? Keep trying until you find a routine that works for you. Once you make physical activity a habit, you'll wonder how you lived without it.

Frequently Asked Questions about Exercise and Diabetes

Why is it important for people with diabetes to be physically active?

Physical activity can help you control your blood glucose, weight, and blood pressure, as well as raise your "good" cholesterol and lower your "bad" cholesterol. It can also help prevent heart and blood flow problems, reducing your risk of heart disease and nerve damage, which are often problems for people with diabetes.

How much and how often should people with diabetes exercise?

Experts recommend moderate-intensity physical activity for at least 30 minutes on five or more days of the week. Some examples of moderate-intensity physical activity are walking briskly, mowing the lawn, dancing, swimming, or bicycling.

If you are not accustomed to physical activity, you may want to start with a little exercise, and work your way up. As you become stronger, you can add a few extra minutes to your physical activity. Do some physical activity every day. It's better to walk 10 or 20 minutes each day than one hour once a week.

Talk to your health care provider about a safe exercise plan. He or she may check your heart and your feet to be sure you have no special problems. If you have high blood pressure, eye, or foot problems, you may need to avoid some kinds of exercise.

What are some good types of physical activity for people with diabetes?

Walking vigorously, hiking, climbing stairs, swimming, aerobics, dancing, bicycling, skating, skiing, tennis, basketball, volleyball, or other sports are just some examples of physical activity that will work your large muscles, increase your heart rate, and make you breathe harder—important goals for fitness.

In addition, strength training exercises with hand weights, elastic bands, or weight machines can help you build muscle. Stretching helps to make you flexible and prevent soreness after other types of exercise.

Do physical activities you really like. The more fun you have, the more likely you will do it each day. It can be helpful to exercise with a family member or friend.

133

Are there any safety considerations for people with diabetes when they exercise?

Exercise is very important for people with diabetes to stay healthy, but there are a few things to watch out for.

You should avoid some kinds of physical activity if you have certain diabetes complications. Exercise involving heavy weights may be bad for people with blood pressure, blood vessel, or eye problems. Diabetes-related nerve damage can make it hard to tell if you've injured your feet during exercise, which can lead to more serious problems. If you do have diabetes complications, your health care provider can tell you which kinds of physical activity would be best for you. Fortunately, there are many different ways to get exercise.

Physical activity can lower your blood glucose too much, causing hypoglycemia, especially in people who take insulin or certain oral medications. Hypoglycemia can happen at the time you're exercising, just afterward, or even up to a day later. You can get shaky, weak, confused, irritable, anxious, hungry, tired, or sweaty. You can get a headache, or even lose consciousness.

To help prevent hypoglycemia during physical activity, check your blood glucose before you exercise. If it's below 100, have a small snack. In addition, bring food or glucose tablets with you when you exercise just in case. It is not good for people with diabetes to skip meals at all, but especially not prior to exercise. After you exercise, check to see how it has affected your blood glucose level. If you take insulin, ask your health care provider if there is a preferable time of day for you to exercise, or whether you should change your dosage before physical activity, before beginning an exercise regimen.

On the other hand, you should not exercise when your blood glucose is very high because your level could go even higher. Do not exercise if your blood glucose is above 300, or your fasting blood glucose is above 250 and you have ketones in your urine.

When you exercise, wear cotton socks and athletic shoes that fit well and are comfortable. After you exercise, check your feet for sores, blisters, irritation, cuts, or other injuries.

Drink plenty of fluids during physical activity, since your blood glucose can be affected by dehydration.

Chapter 14

Take Care of Your Feet and Skin

What are diabetes problems?

Too much glucose in the blood for a long time can cause diabetes problems. This high blood glucose, also called blood sugar, can damage many parts of the body, such as the heart, blood vessels, eyes, and kidneys. Heart and blood vessel disease can lead to heart attacks and strokes. You can do a lot to prevent or slow down diabetes problems.

This chapter is about feet and skin problems caused by diabetes. You will learn the things you can do each day and during each year to stay healthy and prevent diabetes problems.

What should I do each day to stay healthy with diabetes?

- Follow the healthy eating plan that you and your doctor or dietitian have worked out.

- Be active a total of 30 minutes most days. Ask your doctor what activities are best for you.

- Take your medicines as directed.

- Check your blood glucose every day. Each time you check your blood glucose, write the number in your record book.

"Prevent Diabetes Problems: Keep Your Feet and Skin Healthy," National Diabetes Information Clearinghouse, National Institute of Diabetes and Digestive and Kidney Diseases, NIH Pub. No. 07-4282, February 2007.

- Check your feet every day for cuts, blisters, sores, swelling, redness, or sore toenails.

- Brush and floss your teeth every day.

- Control your blood pressure and cholesterol.

- Don't smoke.

How can diabetes hurt my feet?

High blood glucose from diabetes causes two problems that can hurt your feet:

- **Nerve damage:** One problem is damage to nerves in your legs and feet. With damaged nerves, you might not feel pain, heat, or cold in your legs and feet. A sore or cut on your foot may get worse because you do not know it is there. This lack of feeling is caused by nerve damage, also called diabetic neuropathy. Nerve damage can lead to a sore or an infection.

- **Poor blood flow:** The second problem happens when not enough blood flows to your legs and feet. Poor blood flow makes it hard for a sore or infection to heal. This problem is called peripheral vascular disease, also called PVD. Smoking when you have diabetes makes blood flow problems much worse.

These two problems can work together to cause a foot problem. For example, you get a blister from shoes that do not fit. You do not feel the pain from the blister because you have nerve damage in your foot. Next, the blister gets infected. If blood glucose is high, the extra glucose feeds the germs. Germs grow and the infection gets worse. Poor blood flow to your legs and feet can slow down healing. Once in a while a bad infection never heals. The infection might cause gangrene. If a person has gangrene, the skin and tissue around the sore die. The area becomes black and smelly.

To keep gangrene from spreading, a doctor may have to do surgery to cut off a toe, foot, or part of a leg. Cutting off a body part is called an amputation.

What can I do to take care of my feet?

- Wash your feet in warm water every day. Make sure the water is not too hot by testing the temperature with your elbow. Do not soak your feet. Dry your feet well, especially between your toes.

136

- Look at your feet every day to check for cuts, sores, blisters, redness, calluses, or other problems. Checking every day is even more important if you have nerve damage or poor blood flow. If you cannot bend over or pull your feet up to check them, use a mirror. If you cannot see well, ask someone else to check your feet.

- If your skin is dry, rub lotion on your feet after you wash and dry them. Do not put lotion between your toes.

- File corns and calluses gently with an emery board or pumice stone. Do this after your bath or shower.

- Cut your toenails once a week or when needed. Cut toenails when they are soft from washing. Cut them to the shape of the toe and not too short. File the edges with an emery board.

- Always wear slippers or shoes to protect your feet from injuries.

- Always wear socks or stockings to avoid blisters. Do not wear socks or knee-high stockings that are too tight below your knee.

- Wear shoes that fit well. Shop for shoes at the end of the day when your feet are bigger. Break in shoes slowly. Wear them one to two hours each day for the first few weeks.

- Before putting your shoes on, feel the insides to make sure they have no sharp edges or objects that might injure your feet.

How can my doctor help me take care of my feet?

- Tell your doctor right away about any foot problems.

- Ask your doctor to look at your feet at each diabetes checkup. To make sure your doctor checks your feet, take off your shoes and socks before your doctor comes into the room.

- Ask your doctor to check how well the nerves in your feet sense feeling.

- Ask your doctor to check how well blood is flowing to your legs and feet.

- Ask your doctor to show you the best way to trim your toenails. Ask what lotion or cream to use on your legs and feet.

137

• If you cannot cut your toenails or you have a foot problem, ask your doctor to send you to a foot doctor. A doctor who cares for feet is called a podiatrist.

What are common diabetes foot problems?

Anyone can have corns, blisters, and athlete's foot. If you have diabetes and your blood glucose stays high, these foot problems can lead to infections.

Corns and calluses are thick layers of skin caused by too much rubbing or pressure on the same spot. Corns and calluses can become infected.

Blisters can form if shoes always rub the same spot. Wearing shoes that do not fit or wearing shoes without socks can cause blisters. Blisters can become infected.

Ingrown toenails happen when an edge of the nail grows into the skin. The skin can get red and infected. Ingrown toenails can happen if you cut into the corners of your toenails when you trim them. If toenail edges are sharp, smooth them with an emery board. You can also get an ingrown toenail if your shoes are too tight.

A bunion forms when your big toe slants toward the small toes and the place between the bones near the base of your big toe grows big. This spot can get red, sore, and infected. Bunions can form on one or both feet. Pointed shoes may cause bunions. Bunions often run in the family. Surgery can remove bunions.

Plantar warts are caused by a virus. The warts usually form on the bottoms of the feet.

Hammertoes form when a foot muscle gets weak. The weakness may be from diabetic nerve damage. The weakened muscle makes the tendons in the foot shorter and makes the toes curl under the feet. You may get sores on the bottoms of your feet and on the tops of your toes. The feet can change their shape. Hammertoes can cause problems with walking and finding shoes that fit well. Hammertoes can run in the family. Wearing shoes that are too short can also cause hammertoes.

Dry and cracked skin can happen because the nerves in your legs and feet do not get the message to keep your skin soft and moist. Dry skin can become cracked and allow germs to enter. If your blood glucose is high, it feeds the germs and makes the infection worse.

Athlete's foot is a fungus that causes itchiness, redness, and cracking of the skin. The cracks between the toes allow germs to get under the skin. If your blood glucose is high, it feeds the germs and makes

138

the infection worse. The infection can spread to the toenails and make them thick, yellow, and hard to cut.

Tell your doctor about any foot problem as soon as you see it.

How can special shoes help my feet?

Special shoes can be made to fit softly around your sore feet or feet that have changed shape. These special shoes help protect your feet. Medicare and other health insurance programs may pay for special shoes. Talk with your doctor about how and where to get them.

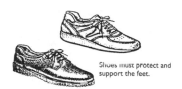
Shoes must protect and support the feet.

Shoes must accommodate foot deformities.

Shoe shape must match foot shape.

Figure 14.1. *Properly fitted athletic or walking shoes are recommended for daily wear. If off-the-shelf shoes are used, make sure that there is room to accommodate any deformities. High risk patients may require depth-inlay shoes or custom-molded inserts (orthoses), depending on the degree of foot deformity and history of ulceration. (Source: Feet Can Last a Lifetime: A Health Care Provider's Guide to Preventing Diabetes Foot Problems," National Diabetes Education Program, November 2000.*

How can diabetes hurt my skin?

Diabetes can hurt your skin in two ways:

- If your blood glucose is high, your body loses fluid. With less fluid in your body, your skin can get dry. Dry skin can be itchy, causing you to scratch and make it sore. Also, dry skin can crack. Cracks allow germs to enter and cause infection. If your blood glucose is high, it feeds germs and makes infections worse. Skin can get dry on your legs, feet, elbows, and other places on your body.

- Nerve damage can decrease the amount you sweat. Sweating helps keep your skin soft and moist. Decreased sweating in your feet and legs can cause dry skin.

What can I do to take care of my skin?

- After you wash with a mild soap, make sure you rinse and dry yourself well. Check places where water can hide, such as under the arms, under the breasts, between the legs, and between the toes.

- Keep your skin moist by using a lotion or cream after you wash. Ask your doctor to suggest one.

- Drink lots of fluids, such as water, to keep your skin moist and healthy.

- Wear all-cotton underwear. Cotton allows air to move around your body better.

- Check your skin after you wash. Make sure you have no dry, red, or sore spots that might lead to an infection.

- Tell your doctor about any skin problems.

Chapter 15

Take Care of Your Teeth and Gums

This chapter is about the tooth and gum problems caused by diabetes. You will learn what you can do each day and during each year to stay healthy and prevent diabetes problems.

How can diabetes hurt my teeth and gums?

Tooth and gum problems can happen to anyone. A sticky film full of germs, called plaque (plak), builds up on your teeth. High blood glucose helps germs, also called bacteria, grow. Then you can get red, sore, and swollen gums that bleed when you brush your teeth.

People with diabetes can have tooth and gum problems more often if their blood glucose stays high. High blood glucose can make tooth and gum problems worse. You can even lose your teeth.

Smoking makes it more likely for you to get a bad case of gum disease, especially if you have diabetes and are age 45 or older.

Red, sore, and bleeding gums are the first sign of gum disease. These problems can lead to periodontitis. Periodontitis is an infection in the gums and the bone that holds the teeth in place. If the infection gets worse, your gums may pull away from your teeth, making your teeth look long.

Call your dentist if you think you have problems with your teeth or gums.

"Prevent Diabetes Problems: Keep Your Teeth and Gums Healthy," National Diabetes Information Clearinghouse, National Institute of Diabetes and Digestive and Kidney Diseases, NIH Pub. No. 07-4280, February 2007.

How do I know if I have damage to my teeth and gums?

If you have one or more of these problems, you may have tooth and gum damage from diabetes:

- red, sore, swollen gums
- bleeding gums
- gums pulling away from your teeth so your teeth look long
- loose or sensitive teeth
- bad breath
- a bite that feels different
- dentures—false teeth—that do not fit well

How can I keep my teeth and gums healthy?

- Keep your blood glucose as close to normal as possible.
- Use dental floss at least once a day. Flossing helps prevent the buildup of plaque on your teeth. Plaque can harden and grow under your gums and cause problems. Using a sawing motion, gently

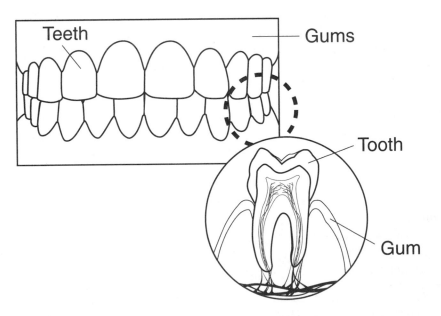

Figure 15.1. High blood glucose can cause tooth and gum problems.

bring the floss between the teeth, scraping from bottom to top several times.

- Brush your teeth after each meal and snack. Use a soft tooth-brush. Turn the bristles against the gum line and brush gently. Use small, circular motions. Brush the front, back, and top of each tooth.

- If you wear false teeth, keep them clean.

- Ask the person who cleans your teeth to show you the best way to brush and floss your teeth and gums. Ask this person about the best toothbrush and toothpaste to use.

- Call your dentist right away if you have problems with your teeth and gums.

- Call your dentist if you have red, sore, or bleeding gums; gums that are pulling away from your teeth; a sore tooth that could be infected; or soreness from your dentures.

- Get your teeth and gums cleaned and checked by your dentist twice a year.

- If your dentist tells you about a problem, take care of it right away.

- Be sure your dentist knows that you have diabetes.

- If you smoke, talk to your doctor about ways to quit smoking.

How can my dentist take care of my teeth and gums?

Your dentist can help you take care of your teeth and gums by cleaning and checking your teeth and gums twice a year, helping you learn the best way to brush and floss your teeth and gums, telling you if you have problems with your teeth or gums and what to do about them, and making sure your false teeth fit well.

Plan ahead: You may be taking a diabetes medicine that can cause low blood glucose, also called hypoglycemia. Talk to your doctor and dentist before the visit about the best way to take care of your blood glucose during the dental work. You may need to bring some diabetes medicine and food with you to the dentist's office.

If your mouth is sore after the dental work, you might not be able to eat or chew for several hours or days. For guidance on how to adjust your normal routine while your mouth is healing, ask your doctor what foods and drinks you should have, how you should change your diabetes medicines, and how often you should check your blood glucose.

Chapter 16

Taking Care of Your Diabetes during Challenging Times

Diabetes is part of your life. It's very important to take care of it when you're sick, when you're at school or work, when you travel, or when you're pregnant or thinking about having a baby. Here are some tips to help you take care of your diabetes at these times.

When You're Sick

Take good care of yourself when you have a cold, the flu, an infection, or other illnesses. Being sick can raise your blood glucose. When you're sick, do the following:

- Check your blood glucose every four hours. Write down the results.

- Keep taking your diabetes medicines. Even if you can't keep food down, you still need your diabetes medicine. Ask your doctor or diabetes educator whether to change the amount of diabetes medicine you take.

- Drink at least a cup (8 ounces) of water or other calorie-free, caffeine-free liquid every hour while you're awake.

- If you can't eat your usual food, try drinking juice or eating crackers, popsicles, or soup.

From "Your Guide to Diabetes: Type 1 and Type 2," National Diabetes Information Clearinghouse, National Institute of Diabetes and Digestive and Kidney Diseases, NIH Pub. 07-4016, October 2006.

- If you can't eat at all, drink clear liquids such as ginger ale. Eat or drink something with sugar in it if you have trouble keeping food down.

- Test your urine for ketones if your blood glucose is over 240 or you can't keep food or liquids down

Call your health care provider right away in these circumstances:

- your blood glucose has been over 240 for longer than a day

- you have moderate to large amounts of ketones in your urine

- you feel sleepier than usual

- you have trouble breathing

- you can't think clearly

- you throw up more than once

- you've had diarrhea for more than six hours

Action Steps

If you use insulin: Take your insulin, even if you've been throwing up. Ask your doctor about how to adjust your insulin dose, based on your blood glucose test results.

If you don't use insulin: Take your diabetes medicines, even if you've been throwing up.

When You're at School or Work

Take care of your diabetes when you're at school or at work:

- Follow your meal plan.

- Take your medicine and check your blood glucose as usual.

- Tell your teachers, friends, or close co-workers about the signs of hypoglycemia. You may need their help if your blood glucose drops too low.

- Keep snacks nearby and carry some with you at all times to treat hypoglycemia.

- Tell your company nurse or school nurse that you have diabetes.

When You're Away from Home

Taking care of your diabetes, even on vacation, is very important. Here are some tips:

- Follow your meal plan as much as possible when you eat out. Always carry a snack with you in case you have to wait to be served.

- Limit your drinking of beer, wine, or other alcoholic beverages. Ask your diabetes educator how much alcohol you can safely drink. Eat something when you drink.

- If you're taking a long trip by car, check your blood glucose before driving. Stop and check your blood glucose every two hours. Always carry snacks like fruit, crackers, juice, or soda in the car in case your blood glucose drops too low.

- Ask ahead of time for a diabetes meal if you're traveling by plane. Most airlines serve special meals for people with health needs. Carry food (like crackers or fruit) with you in case meals are late.

- Carry your diabetes medicines and your blood testing supplies with you. Never put them in your checked luggage.

- Ask your health care team how to adjust your medicines, especially your insulin, if you're traveling across time zones.

- Take comfortable, well-fitting shoes on vacation. You'll probably be walking more than usual, so you should take extra care of your feet.

- If you're going to be away for a long time, ask your doctor for a written prescription for your diabetes medicine and the name of a doctor in the place you're going to visit.

- Don't count on buying extra supplies when you're traveling, especially if you're going to another country. Different countries use different kinds of diabetes medicines.

Action Steps

If you use insulin: Here are some tips for when you travel:

- take a special insulated bag to carry your insulin to keep it from freezing or getting too hot

147

- bring extra supplies for taking insulin and testing your blood glucose in case of loss or breakage

- ask your doctor for a letter saying that you have diabetes and need to carry supplies for taking insulin and testing blood glucose

When You're Planning a Pregnancy

Planning ahead is very important if you want to have a baby. High blood glucose can be harmful to both a mother and her unborn baby. Even before you become pregnant, your blood glucose should be close to the normal range. Keeping blood glucose near normal before and during pregnancy helps protect both mother and baby.

Your insulin needs may change when you're pregnant. Your doctor may want you to take more insulin and check your blood glucose more often. If you take diabetes pills, you'll take insulin instead when you're pregnant.

If you plan to have a baby, do the following:

- Work with your health care team to get your blood glucose as close to the normal range as possible.

- See a doctor who has experience in taking care of pregnant women with diabetes.

- Have your eyes and kidneys checked. Pregnancy can make eye and kidney problems worse.

- Don't smoke, drink alcohol, or use harmful drugs.

- Follow the meal plan you get from your dietitian or diabetes educator to make sure you and your unborn baby have a healthy diet.

- If you're already pregnant, see your doctor right away. It's not too late to bring your blood glucose close to normal so that you'll stay healthy during the rest of your pregnancy.

Chapter 17

Adjusting to Life with Diabetes

Chapter Contents

Section 17.1—Feelings about Diabetes 150

Section 17.2—Getting Your Diabetes Ready for Winter 152

Section 17.3—Diabetes-Friendly Tips for Handling the
Summer Heat 154

Section 17.4—Driving when You Have Diabetes 156

Section 17.5—Traveling with Diabetes 159

Section 17.6—Diabetes and Work 162

Section 17.7—Growing Older and Staying Healthy with
Diabetes 165

Section 17.1

Feelings about Diabetes

"Feelings about Diabetes," © Michigan Diabetes Research and Training Center (www.med.umich.edu/mdrtc). Reprinted with permission.

Diabetes can affect your whole self—not just your body. It can affect your feelings about yourself and how you get along with others. An important step in learning to live with diabetes is to become aware of how you are feeling. Each person has different feelings about having diabetes. When you first found out that you had diabetes, it might have been hard to believe. You may have been frightened or wondered "why me?" These are very real feelings that many people have when they first find out that they have diabetes. As you live with diabetes, you may find that your feelings change. Some common feelings are listed below. As you read the list, you may become aware that you've had some of these feelings.

- **Denial:** Some people find it hard to believe they have diabetes. They may also believe that they do not really have to take care of their diabetes. This is called denial.

- **Anger:** When people feel angry about having diabetes, they may wonder, "Why me?" They may act angry at family, friends, or health care professionals. In fact, they are angry about having diabetes.

- **Depression:** Sometimes when people are angry about having diabetes, they keep their feelings bottled up inside. As time goes on, they begin to feel very sad and blue—even hopeless.

- **Acceptance:** Gradually people adjust or adapt to having diabetes. They still wish that they didn't have diabetes, but they are able to handle it.

These feelings do not always happen in this order. Most people find that these feelings come and go. Also, you may have two or more of these feelings at one time or you may have none of these feelings. You may have had some of these same feelings when you had other problems in your life. Think about how you handled your feelings then. The way you handled your feelings in the past can help you to find ways to deal with your feelings now. Many people find that it helps to talk about their feelings. Family, friends, and health care professionals can help by listening. Most of the time, other people want to be helpful. It's up to you to let them know the best way they can help you. Many areas have support groups especially for people with diabetes and their families. These are groups of people who talk about what it's like to have diabetes and ways to handle problems. Your health care team can tell you about one in your area.

Other sources of support for you and your feelings about diabetes are available. Sometimes it helps to talk with someone who is not a friend or family member. It may help to talk to a minister, rabbi, or priest; a mental health counselor; or a social worker.

You may find that you are feeling sad, down, or depressed. If you feel depressed tell your physician. There are treatments for depression that are very effective. Learning to live with diabetes takes a long time. For most people, it is a lifelong journey. The first step is to learn to recognize how you are feeling. Think about how your feelings are affecting the way you cope with other stresses, get along with family and friends and take care of your diabetes. Most journeys are easier if you have some help along the way. Find someone to talk with and support you. Take one step and one day at a time and you'll reach your goal.

Section 17.2

Getting Your Diabetes Ready for Winter

"Getting Your Diabetes Ready for Winter," © Michigan Diabetes
Research and Training Center (http://www.med.umich.edu/mdrtc).
Reprinted with permission.

If you live in a northern climate, you know all about getting ready
for winter. You make sure that the storm windows are in, the furnace
is working, your car has snow tires and antifreeze and you get out
your gloves and warm coat. But did you know that winter affects your
diabetes as well?

A recent study showed that A1C levels (a measure of long-term
blood glucose levels) are higher in the winter. In all climates, levels
were highest from February through April, and were lowest in August
through September. The people who had the greatest rise were
those who lived in moderate climates, where the winter temperatures
ranged between 32 and 40 degrees. People who lived in the coldest
parts of the country had less of an effect, perhaps because it is so cold
that they spend very little time outside.

Scientists don't really know for sure why this happens. It was not
related to how people manage their diabetes. Because heart attacks and
strokes also are more common during the winter months, it is thought
that cold may cause the blood pressure and heart rate to go up. This
same response may also cause blood glucose levels to go up as well.

In this very large study, the average increase in A1C was 0.22%.
This means that if the A1C reading was 7.0% in the fall, it would go
up to 7.22% by the end of the winter. Although this does not seem like
a very big increase, it might help explain why you notice your blood
glucose readings are higher even though you are working just as hard.
So, what can you do to get your diabetes ready for winter?

- Ask your provider for an A1C check before winter begins so you
  know where you stand.

- Do more of the things that help to lower your blood glucose levels, such as watch your food intake and be active physically. It is
  easy to eat an extra snack or two in winter when you spend long

evenings in the house. If you like to exercise outside, make a plan for an indoor activity—walk in the mall, dance in your living room, put in an exercise video, use a treadmill, and go to the gym.

- Use caution about exercising in very cold weather. Because heart attacks and strokes also are more likely in winter, talk with your health care provider about what is safe for you. Shoveling snow is probably best left to others.

- Your skin needs extra care in the winter as well. Cold weather and forced air heat can be very drying. Using lotion will help to keep your skin from becoming dry and cracked. Cracked places in your skin give bacteria an easy way to enter and can cause an infection. This is especially true for your feet and legs.

- Keeping your feet warm can be hard to do if the blood flow to your legs and feet has been affected by diabetes. Well-fitting, waterproof boots, and mostly cotton or wool socks will help keep your feet warm and dry when you are outdoors. If you have lost some of the feeling in your feet due to nerve damage, hot water bottles or heating pads are not recommended because they can cause burns.

- It seems like everyone you meet in the winter has a cold or the flu. Protect yourself by getting a flu shot. If you haven't had a pneumonia shot, remind your health care provider that people with diabetes need this injection at least once in their lifetimes. Since most of us don't get through the winter without catching one bug or another, talk with your diabetes educator about how to handle your diabetes care during an illness.

- Some people find that they feel sad and blue in the winter. If these feelings are severe, this is called SAD (seasonal affective disorder). If you find that your feelings keep you from doing the things that you enjoy or are affecting how you care for your diabetes, talk with your provider. There is help available.

- Even if you don't have SAD, but find that you feel blue from time to time in the winter, don't ignore those feelings. Think of something you enjoy that would help you to feel better. Sometimes calling a friend for a few minutes is enough to lighten your mood. It may seem easier to stay inside, but you may find that even a brief outing may help your mood.

- The days are getting shorter and winter is here. While you are getting your house, car, and clothes ready for winter, don't forget about your diabetes as well.

153

Section 17.3

Diabetes-Friendly Tips for Handling the Summer Heat

The heat being experienced in many parts of the nation these days is tough enough for the average healthy person, but for the estimated 21 million Americans with diabetes, special precautions may be required.

"People with chronic diseases like diabetes as well as people taking certain medications, including heart disease medications and diuretics, which are often used to treat complications of diabetes, are at increased risk of experiencing difficulties in the heat, even though they may not be aware of it," says Catherine Carver, M.S., A.N.P., C.D.E, Director of Educational Services at Joslin Clinic.

Carver and her colleagues at Joslin Clinic offer the following tips for people with diabetes during these steamy summer days:

- Keep hydrated. Dehydration, or the loss of body fluids, can happen on these very hot summer days whether you have diabetes or not. If you have diabetes, dehydration also can occur when blood glucose is not under control. When blood glucose is elevated, this can lead to an increase in the body's excretion of urine. To prevent dehydration drink plenty of caffeine-free fluids such as water, seltzer, or sugar-free iced tea and lemonade. Limit your intake of alcohol.

- Watch for signs of heat exhaustion, especially if you are working or exercising outdoors. People with diabetes and other chronic diseases like heart disease are more susceptible to overheating. Symptoms include: feeling dizzy or fainting; sweating excessively; muscle cramps; skin that is cold or clammy; headaches; rapid heartbeat, and/or nausea. If you experience any of these symptoms, move to a cooler environment, drink fluids like water, juice or sports drinks (based on your healthcare provider's instructions), and seek medical attention.

- Exercise in a cool place such as an air-conditioned gym, or early in the morning or later in the evening when temperatures may be more moderate.

- Check blood glucose levels at least four times per day, and more often if you are not feeling well. Remember that heat can cause blood glucose levels to fluctuate. Carry plenty of water and snacks.

- Store your blood glucose meter, strips, and insulin in a cool, dry place. Do not store insulin in extreme temperatures. Never store insulin in the freezer, in direct sunlight, in the car, or the car's glove compartment. Examine your vials of insulin. Clear insulin (Regular, Humalog, Novolog, Apidra, Lantus, Levemir) should remain clear. NPH insulin should not have any clumping or "frosting" on the vials.

Additional Tips for Insulin Pump Users

- For insulin pump users, excessive perspiration can be a problem in hot weather or during strenuous activities. This can loosen the adhesive securing the infusion set, the part of the device that attaches to your body. If perspiration is a problem, try using a spray of antiperspirant on the insertion site after your usual skin-preparation routine. Others have success with skin-barrier preparations such as Mastisol, Skin-Tac H, or a compound tincture of benzoin applied to the skin.

- The pump housing provides some insulation from the heat. If you are concerned about heat, you can use a protective pouch with a small, cold gel pack placed inside the pouch as a way to protect your insulin from the effects of heat. If you are spending an extended amount of time in the sun, cover the pump with a towel to protect it from prolonged direct sunlight. Disconnecting your pump for up to an hour is another option, but if it is disconnected for a longer time, you will need to adjust your insulin infusion rate accordingly to allow for the missed doses.

If you have diabetes and have any questions about coping with heat or other extreme weather conditions, consult with your medical team.

Section 17.4

Driving when You Have Diabetes

U.S. Department of Transportation, National Highway
Traffic Safety Administration, DOT HS 809 684, November 2003.

- For most people, driving represents freedom, control, and competence. Driving enables most people to get to the places they want or need to go. For many people, driving is important economically—some drive as part of their job or to get to and from work.

- Driving is a complex skill. Our ability to drive safely can be affected by changes in our physical, emotional, and mental condition. This section is designed to give you the information you need to talk to your health care team about driving and diabetes.

How can having diabetes affect my driving?

- In the short term, diabetes can make your blood glucose (sugar) levels too high or too low. As a result, diabetes can make you feel sleepy or dizzy, feel confused, have blurred vision, or lose consciousness or have a seizure.

- In the long run, diabetes can lead to problems that affect driving. Diabetes may cause nerve damage in your hands, legs and feet, or eyes. In some cases, diabetes can cause blindness or lead to amputation.

Can I still drive with diabetes?

- Yes, people with diabetes are able to drive unless they are limited by certain complications of diabetes. These include severe low blood glucose levels or vision problems. If you are experiencing diabetes-related complications, you should work closely with your diabetes health care team to find out if diabetes affects your ability to drive. If it does, discuss if there are actions you can take to continue to drive safely.

What can I do to ensure that I can drive safely with diabetes?

- Insulin and some oral medications can cause blood glucose levels to become dangerously low (hypoglycemia). Do not drive if your blood glucose level is too low. If you do, you might not be able to make good choices, focus on your driving, or control your car. Your health care team can help you determine when you should check your blood glucose level before driving and how often you should check while driving.

- Make sure you always carry your blood glucose meter and plenty of snacks (including a quick-acting source of glucose) with you. Pull over as soon as you feel any of the signs of a low blood glucose level. Check your blood glucose.

- If your glucose level is low, eat a snack that contains a fast-acting sugar such as juice, soda with sugar (not diet), hard candy, or glucose tablets. Wait 15 minutes, and then check your blood glucose again. Treat again as needed. Once your glucose level has risen to your target range, eat a more substantial snack or meal containing protein. Do not continue driving until your blood glucose level has improved.

- Most people with diabetes experience warning signs of a low blood glucose level. However, if you experience hypoglycemia without advance warning, you should not drive. Talk to your health care team about how glycemic awareness training might help you sense the beginning stages of hypoglycemia.

- In extreme situations, high blood glucose levels (hyperglycemia) also may affect driving. Talk to your health care team if you have a history of very high glucose levels to determine at what point such levels might affect your ability to be a safe driver.

- The key to preventing diabetes-related eye problems is good control of blood glucose levels, good blood pressure control, and good eye care. A yearly exam with an eye care professional is essential.

- If you are experiencing long-term complications of diabetes such as vision or sensation problems, or if you have had an amputation, your diabetes health care team can refer you to a driving specialist. This specialist can give you on and off-road tests to see if, and how, your diabetes is affecting your driving. The specialist also may offer training to improve your driving skills.

- Improving your driving skills could help keep you and others around you safe. To find a specialist near you, call the Association of Driver Rehabilitation Specialists at 800-290-2344 or go to their website at www.aded.net. You also can call hospitals and rehabilitation facilities to find an occupational therapist who can help with the driving skills assessment.

What if I have to cut back or give up driving?

- You can keep your independence even if you have to cut back or give up on your driving. It may take planning ahead on your part, but planning will help get you to the places you need to go and to the people you want to see.

  Consider rides with family and friends; taxi cabs; shuttle buses or vans; public buses, trains and subways; and walking. Also, senior centers and religious and other local service groups often offer transportation services for older adults in your community.

Who can I call for help with transportation?

- Call the ElderCare Locator at 800-677-1116 and ask for the phone number of your local Office on Aging, or go to their website at http://www.nhtsa.dot.gov/exit.cfm?Link=http://www.eldercare.gov.

- Contact your regional transit authority to find out which bus or train to take.

- Call Easter Seals Project ACTION (Accessible Community Transportation In Our Nation) at 800-659-6428 or go to their website http://www.nhtsa.dot.gov/exit.cfm?Link=http://www.projectaction.org.

Wear Your Safety Belt

- Always wear your safety belt when you are driving or riding in a car. Make sure that every person who is riding with you also is buckled up. Wear your safety belt even if your car has air bags.

Section 17.5

Traveling with Diabetes

"Have Diabetes. Will Travel,"
National Diabetes Education Program, June 2006.

Heading out of town? Leaving your troubles behind? Off on an important business trip? Whenever you travel, your diabetes comes along with you. And while having diabetes shouldn't stop you from traveling in style, you will have to do some careful planning. Here are some helpful diabetes travel tips from the National Diabetes Education Program.

Plan Ahead

- Get all your immunizations. Find out what's required for where you're going, and make sure you get the right shots, on time.

- Control your **ABCs**: **A**1C, **B**lood pressure, and **C**holesterol. See your health care provider for a check-up four to six weeks before your trip to make sure your ABCs are under control and in a healthy range before you leave.

- Ask your health care provider for a prescription and a letter explaining your diabetes medications, supplies, and any allergies. Carry this with you at all times on your trip. The prescription should be for insulin or diabetes medications and could help in case of an emergency.

- Wear identification that explains you have diabetes. The identification should be written in the languages of the places you are visiting.

- Plan for time zone changes. Make sure you'll always know when to take your diabetes medicine, no matter where you are. Remember: eastward travel means a shorter day. If you inject insulin, less may be needed. Westward travel means a longer day, so more insulin may be needed.

- Find out how long the flight will be and whether meals will be served. However, you should always carry enough food to cover

159

the entire flight time in case of delays or unexpected schedule changes.

Pack Properly

- Take twice the amount of diabetes medication and supplies that you'd normally need. Better safe than sorry.

- Keep your insulin cool by packing it in an insulated bag with refrigerated gel packs.

- Keep snacks, glucose gel, or tablets with you in case your blood glucose drops.

- If you use insulin, make sure you also pack a glucagon emergency kit.

- Make sure you keep your medical insurance card and emergency phone numbers handy.

- Don't forget to pack a first aid kit with all the essentials.

If You Are Flying

- Plan to carry all your diabetes supplies in your carry-on luggage. Don't risk a lost suitcase.

- Have all syringes and insulin delivery systems (including vials of insulin) clearly marked with the pharmaceutical preprinted label that identifies the medications. The FAA recommends that patients travel with their original pharmacy labeled packaging.

- Keep your diabetes medications and emergency snacks with you at your seat—don't store them in an overhead bin.

- If the airline offers a meal for your flight call ahead for a diabetic, low fat, or low cholesterol meal.

- Wait until your food is about to be served before you take your insulin. Otherwise, a delay in the meal could lead to low blood glucose.

- If no food is offered on your flight, bring a meal on board yourself.

- If you plan on using the restroom for insulin injections, ask for an aisle seat for easier access.

- Don't be shy about telling the flight attendant that you have diabetes—especially if you are traveling alone.

- When drawing up your dose of insulin don't inject air into the bottle (the air on your plane will probably be pressurized).

- Because prescription laws may be very different in other countries, write for a list of International Diabetes Federation groups: IDF, 1 rue Defaeqz, B-1000, Belgium or visit www.idf.org. You may also want to get a list of English-speaking foreign doctors in case of an emergency. Contact the American Consulate, American Express, or local medical schools for a list of doctors.

- Insulin in foreign countries comes in different strengths. If you purchase insulin in a foreign country, be sure to use the right syringe for the strength. An incorrect syringe may cause you to take too much or too little insulin.

On a Road Trip

- Don't leave your medications in the trunk, glove compartment, or near a window—they might overheat. If possible, carry a cooler in the car to keep medications cool.

- Bring extra food with you in the car in case you can't find a restaurant.

General Traveling Tips

- Stay comfortable and reduce your risk for blood clots by moving around every hour or two.

- Always tell at least one person traveling with you about your diabetes.

- Protect your feet. Never go barefoot in the shower or pool.

- Check your blood glucose often. Changes in diet, activity, and time zones can affect your blood glucose in unexpected ways.

You may not be able to leave your diabetes behind, but you can control it and have a relaxing, safe trip. To learn more about controlling your diabetes, visit the National Diabetes Education Program at http://www.ndep.nih.gov.

Section 17.6

Diabetes and Work

Excerpted from "Questions and Answers About Diabetes in the
Workplace and the Americans with Disabilities Act (ADA)," U.S. Equal
Employment Opportunity Commission, October 29, 2003.

The Americans with Disabilities Act (ADA) is a federal law that
prohibits discrimination against individuals with disabilities. Title I
of the ADA covers employment by private employers with 15 or more
employees as well as state and local government employers. The Rehabilitation Act provides similar protections related to federal employment. In addition, most states have their own laws prohibiting
employment discrimination on the basis of disability. Some of these
state laws may apply to smaller employers and provide protections
in addition to those available under the ADA.

The U.S. Equal Employment Opportunity Commission (EEOC) en-
forces the employment provisions of the ADA. This guide explains
how the ADA might apply to job applicants and employees with diabetes.

People with Diabetes at Work

Individuals with diabetes successfully perform all types of jobs from
heading major corporations to protecting public safety. Yet, many employers still automatically exclude them from certain positions based
on myths, fears, or stereotypes. For example, some employers wrongly
assume that anyone with diabetes will be unable to perform a particular job (for example, one that requires driving) or will need to use a
lot of sick leave. The reality is that, because many individuals with diabetes work with few or no restrictions, their employers do not know
that they have diabetes. Some employees, however, tell their employers that they have diabetes because they need a "reasonable accommodation" (a change or adjustment in the workplace to better manage
and control their condition). Most of the accommodations requested
by employees with diabetes—such as regular work schedules, meal

162

breaks, a place to test their blood sugar levels, or a rest area—do not cost employers anything to provide.

When is diabetes a disability under the ADA?

Diabetes is a disability when it substantially limits one or more of a person's major life activities. Major life activities are basic activities that an average person can perform with little or no difficulty, such as eating or caring for oneself. Diabetes also is a disability when it causes side effects or complications that substantially limit a major life activity. Even if diabetes is not currently substantially limiting because it is controlled by diet, exercise, oral medication, and/or insulin, and there are no serious side effects, the condition may be a disability because it was substantially limiting in the past (before it was diagnosed and adequately treated). Finally, diabetes is a disability when it does not significantly affect a person's everyday activities, but the employer treats the individual as if it does. For example, an employer may assume that a person is totally unable to work because he has diabetes. Under the ADA, the determination of whether an individual has a disability is made on a case-by-case basis.

May an employer ask job applicants for medical information?

The ADA limits the medical information that an employer can seek from a job applicant. During the application stage, an employer may not ask questions about an applicant's medical condition or require an applicant to take a medical examination before it makes a conditional job offer. This means that an employer cannot ask questions about whether an applicant has diabetes or questions about an applicant's use of insulin or other prescription drugs.

After making a job offer, an employer may ask questions about an applicant's health (including asking whether the applicant has diabetes) and may require a medical examination as long as it treats all applicants the same.

May an employer ask any follow-up questions if an applicant reveals that she has diabetes?

If an applicant voluntarily tells an employer that she has diabetes, an employer only may ask two questions: whether she needs a reasonable accommodation and what type of accommodation.

What types of reasonable accommodations may employees with diabetes need?

Some employees may need one or more of the following accommodations:

- A private area to test blood sugar levels or to take insulin

- A place to rest until blood sugar levels become normal

- Breaks to eat or drink, take medication, or test blood sugar levels

- Leave for treatment, recuperation, or training on managing diabetes

- Modified work schedule or shift change

- Allowing a person with diabetic neuropathy (a nerve disorder caused by diabetes) to use a stool.

Although these are some examples of the types of accommodations commonly requested by employees with diabetes, other employees may need different changes or adjustments. Employers should ask the particular employee requesting an accommodation because of his diabetes what he needs that will help him do his job. There also are extensive public and private resources to help employers identify reasonable accommodations. For example, the website for the Job Accommodation Network (http://janweb.icdi.wvu.edu/media/diabetes.html) provides information about many types of accommodations for employees with diabetes.

How does an employee with diabetes request a reasonable accommodation?

There are no "magic words" that a person has to use when requesting a reasonable accommodation. A person simply has to tell the employer that she needs an adjustment or change at work because of her diabetes.

A request for a reasonable accommodation also can come from a family member, friend, health professional, or other representative on behalf of a person with diabetes. If the employer does not already know that an employee has diabetes, the employer can ask the employee for verification from a health care professional.

Does an employer have to grant every request for a reasonable accommodation?

No. An employer does not have to provide a reasonable accommodation if doing so will be an undue hardship. Undue hardship means that providing the reasonable accommodation would result in significant difficulty or expense. If a requested accommodation is too difficult or expensive, an employer still would be required to determine whether there is another easier or less costly accommodation that would meet the employee's needs.

Section 17.7

Growing Older and Staying Healthy with Diabetes

Chances are that you or someone you know has diabetes. One out of every five people over age 60 has diabetes. It is a complicated disease to manage, but for older adults with many other health issues, it can be overwhelming.

Diabetes care is necessarily left in the hands of the person with diabetes, who "self-manages" by monitoring blood glucose, taking medications and/or insulin, following diet plans, and getting more physical activity. Goals for diabetes care for older adults and the plan for how to achieve them should take into account their unique challenges. We don't treat a 10-year-old child with diabetes as we would a 40 year-old adult, and we should not treat an 80-year-old the same way either.

Our overall goal is for older adults with diabetes to have the best quality of life possible. And that can't happen if they are having trouble following through with care instructions due to undiagnosed depression, memory problems, or other medical conditions.

Who Is Old?

There is something to be said for the saying "You are as young as you feel." Medicare sets 65 as the age for eligibility, but that by no means answers the question: "Who is old?" Many people with diabetes over age 65 are managing quite well—they eat in moderation, are physically active, and have a positive outlook on life.

But then there are some older adults who may have just been diagnosed and are having trouble coping with the required changes in routine. Or, they may have had diabetes for years, but they've had a stroke or heart attack or lost significant vision, and their blood glucose control has suddenly deteriorated. With major changes such as these, their diabetes management goals need to be reassessed.

Unique Challenges

Several conditions occur more commonly in older adults with diabetes. A major reason why some older adults have a difficult time is that they are experiencing "cognitive dysfunction," abnormalities in brain function that make it hard to problem-solve, plan and organize, and be attentive. Depression is also highly prevalent in older patients, as are vision and hearing impairments, leading to difficulty coping with daily activities. Diabetes should be seen in the context of these and other medical conditions.

We are good at identifying vision and hearing impairments and screening for cardiovascular problems. But cognitive dysfunction and depression often go undiagnosed. Our recently published research shows that one-third of our patients in the Joslin Geriatrics Clinic have cognitive problems associated with poor diabetes control.

People with diabetes are about twice as likely to be depressed than those without diabetes. In our study of patients older than 70, we also found that more than one-third have symptoms of depression. Once identified, we can treat cognitive dysfunction or depression, which can improve quality of life and probably diabetes control as well.

Family members are most likely to see subtle changes of cognitive dysfunction or depression in their loved ones. Signs that an older adult with diabetes should be screened for these conditions include:

- blood glucose control that is suddenly worse;
- subtle changes in mental status, that is, more forgetful about monitoring or taking medications; making more mistakes;

- sudden difficulty coping, or acting more stressed;
- less socially active or showing other signs of depression, such as sadness or hopelessness or isolation from friends and family.

Many Meds

Another important aspect to caring for older adults with diabetes is to re-evaluate their medications. For example, for those on insulin, there are now once-a-day insulins. Insulin pens with pre-measured amounts can help those who face difficulties because of arthritis, impaired vision, or cognitive problems. Oral medications may need to be changed or monitored more closely for side effects (such as risk of hypoglycemia) that particularly affect older adults.

Drug interactions are a big problem for anyone on multiple medicines. It is important to bring a list of all one's medications to every medical visit. It is common to find that one medicine causes a side effect, which is being treated by another medication. It becomes a chain effect. But it might be possible to find an alternative to the medication that started the chain, making other medications unnecessary.

Simplify, Simplify, Simplify

Goals for diabetes care aim to keep blood glucose levels as near normal as possible to avoid diabetes complications that can develop over time—eye, kidney and nerve disease, heart attacks, and stroke. Blood glucose control is important no matter what one's age. But for older adults, quality of life and safety become most important.

One side effect that occurs in the quest to maintain tight control of blood glucose is hypoglycemia—glucose levels falling too low. This is much more dangerous in the elderly. They may be more severely affected and become confused, delirious, dizzy, or weak. A frail person using a cane or a walker who is even mildly hypoglycemic may get dizzy and fall, ending up in a nursing home.

We try to simplify the care plan so that an elderly person with diabetes can follow the plan without feeling stressed. Our goal is to achieve the best diabetes control possible without any episodes of hypoglycemia. Keeping quality of life in mind, the short-term goal of avoiding these episodes becomes more important than a long-term goal of reducing the risk of complications, for which an occasional episode of hypoglycemia is expected.

The Best Possible Life

An overall objective in the care of older adults is to maintain good quality of life and functional independence. We've seen people with diabetes who had to go to a nursing home because they couldn't manage injections of insulin four times a day or were having too many low blood glucose reactions that could not be managed at home. It was not the disease that put them there—it was the treatment. We can avoid this from happening. By keeping their unique needs in mind and treating them differently, we can keep older adults healthier and happier longer.

Part Three

Medical Interventions for Diabetes Management

Chapter 18

Managing Diabetes Is Your Responsibility

Chapter Contents

Section 18.1—Keep Your Diabetes under Control 172

Section 18.2—Frequently Asked Questions about
                      Diabetes Examinations and Tests 177

Section 18.3—Diabetes Management Numbers At-a-Glance ... 180

Section 18.1

Keep Your Diabetes under Control

Excerpted from "Prevent Diabetes Problems: Keep Your Diabetes Under Control," National Diabetes Information Clearinghouse, National Institute of Diabetes and Digestive and Kidney Diseases, NIH Pub. No. 07-4349, January 2007.

What are diabetes problems?

Too much glucose in the blood for a long time can cause diabetes problems. This high blood glucose, also called blood sugar, can damage many parts of the body, such as the heart, blood vessels, eyes, and kidneys. Heart and blood vessel disease can lead to heart attacks and strokes. You can do a lot to prevent or slow down diabetes problems.

What should my blood glucose numbers be?

Keeping your blood glucose on target can prevent or delay diabetes problems. The information below shows target blood glucose levels for most people with diabetes.

- Before meals: 90 to 130

- One to two hours after the start of a meal: less than 180

Talk with your health care provider about what your blood glucose numbers should be and record them.

Talk with your health care provider about when you need to check your blood glucose using a blood glucose meter. You will do the checks yourself. Your health care provider can teach you how to use your meter.

Keep track of your blood glucose checks. Make copies for yourself or ask your health care provider for a blood glucose record book. Your blood glucose check results will help you and your health care provider make a plan for keeping your blood glucose under control. Always bring your record book to your doctor visits so you can talk about reaching your glucose goals.

How can I find out what my average blood glucose is?

Ask your health care provider for the A1C test. This blood test shows the average amount of glucose in your blood during the past two to three months. Have this test done at least twice a year. If your A1C result is not on target, your health care provider may do this test more often to see if your result is improving as your treatment changes. Your A1C result plus your blood glucose meter results can show whether your blood glucose is under control.

Aim for a result below seven percent. If your A1C test result is below seven percent, then your blood glucose is in a desirable range and your diabetes treatment plan is working. The lower your A1C is, the lower your chance of having health problems.

If your result is more than eight percent, you may need a change in your diabetes plan. Your health care team can help you decide what part of your plan to change. You may need to change your meal plan, your diabetes medicines, or your physical activity plan.

Table 18.1. What Your A1C Result Means

My A1C Result	My Average Blood Glucose
6%	135
7%	170
8%	205
9%	240
10%	275
11%	310
12%	345

What should my blood pressure be?

Normal blood pressure will help prevent damage to your eyes, kidneys, heart, and blood vessels. Blood pressure is written with two numbers separated by a slash. For example, 120/70 is said as "120 over 70." The first number should be below 130 and the second number should be below 80. Keep your blood pressure as close to these numbers as you can. If you already have kidney disease, ask your doctor what numbers are best for you.

Meal planning, medicines, and physical activity can help you reach your blood pressure target.

What should my cholesterol be?

Normal cholesterol and blood fat levels will help prevent heart disease and stroke, the biggest health problems for people with diabetes. Keeping cholesterol levels under control can also help with blood flow. Have your blood fat levels checked at least once a year. Meal planning, physical activity, and medicines can help you reach your blood fat targets:

Table 18.2. Target Blood Fat Levels for People With Diabetes

Total cholesterol	below 200
LDL cholesterol	below 100
HDL cholesterol	above 40 (men)
	above 50 (women)
Triglycerides	below 150

What does smoking have to do with diabetes problems?

Smoking and diabetes are a dangerous combination. Smoking raises your risk for diabetes problems. If you quit smoking, you'll lower your risk for heart attack, stroke, nerve disease, and kidney disease. Your cholesterol and your blood pressure levels may improve. Your blood circulation will also improve.

If you smoke, ask your health care provider for help in quitting.

What else can I do to prevent diabetes problems?

You can do many things to prevent diabetes problems. For example, to keep your feet healthy, check them each day. Ask your health care team whether you should take a low-dose aspirin every day to lower your risk for heart disease. To keep your eyes healthy, visit an eye care professional once a year for a complete eye examination that includes using drops in your eyes to dilate the pupils.

Make sure your doctor checks your urine for protein every year. At least once a year, your blood creatinine level should be checked. Also once a year, your health care provider should do a complete foot exam.

What things should I check for good diabetes care?

Taking care of diabetes is a team effort between you and your health care team—doctor, diabetes nurse educator, diabetes dietitian educator, pharmacist, and others. You are the most important member of the team.

Take charge of your diabetes by learning what to do for good diabetes care.

You can prevent or slow down diabetes problems by reaching your blood glucose, blood pressure, and cholesterol goals most of the time.

Things to Do Every Day for Good Diabetes Care

- Follow the healthy eating plan that you and your doctor or dietitian have worked out.

- Be active a total of 30 minutes most days. Ask your doctor what activities are best for you.

- Take your medicines as directed.

- Check your blood glucose every day. Each time you check your blood glucose, write the number in your record book.

- Check your feet every day for cuts, blisters, sores, swelling, redness, or sore toenails.

- Brush and floss your teeth every day.

- Control your blood pressure and cholesterol.

- Don't smoke.

Things for Your Health Care Provider to Look at Every Time You Have a Checkup

- Your blood glucose records:
  - Show your records to your health care provider.
  - Tell your health care provider if you often have low blood glucose or high blood glucose.

- Your weight:
  - Talk with your health care provider about how much you should weigh.
  - Talk about ways to reach your goal that will work for you.

175

- Your blood pressure:
  - The goal for most people with diabetes is less than 130/80.
  - Ask your health care provider about ways to reach your goal.
- Your diabetes medicines plan:
  - Talk to your health care provider about any problems you have had with your diabetes medicines.
- Your feet
  - Ask your health care provider to check your feet for sores.
- Your plan for physical activity
  - Talk with your health care provider about what you do to stay active.
- Your meal plan
  - Talk about what you eat, how much you eat, and when you eat.
- Your feelings
  - Ask your health care provider about ways to handle stress.
  - If you are feeling sad or unable to cope with problems, ask about how to get help.
- Your smoking
  - If you smoke, talk with your health care provider about how you can quit.

Things for You or Your Health Care Provider to Do at Least Once or Twice a Year

These test results will help you plan how to prevent heart attack and stroke.

- A1C test: Have this blood test at least twice a year. Your result will tell you what your average blood glucose level was for the past two to three months.
- Blood lipid (fats) lab tests: Get a blood test to check your:
  - total cholesterol: aim for below 200;
  - LDL: aim for below 100;

- HDL: men: aim for above 40; women: aim for above 50;
- triglycerides: aim for below 150.

- Kidney function tests: Once a year, get a urine test to check for protein. At least once a year, get a blood test to check for creatinine. The results will tell you how well your kidneys are working.

- Dilated eye exam: See an eye care professional once a year for a complete eye exam.

- Dental exam: See your dentist twice a year for a cleaning and checkup.

- Foot exam: Ask your health care provider to check your feet to make sure your foot nerves and your blood circulation are OK.

- Flu shot: Get a flu shot each year.

- Pneumonia vaccine: Get one; if you're over 64 and your shot was more than five years ago, get one more.

Section 18.2

Frequently Asked Questions about Diabetes Examinations and Tests

Excerpted from "Frequently Asked Questions: Staying Healthy with Diabetes," National Center for Chronic Disease Prevention and Health Promotion, Centers for Disease Control and Prevention, June 2006.

How does maintaining healthy blood glucose levels help people with diabetes stay healthy?

Research studies in the United States and other countries have shown that controlling blood glucose benefits people with either type 1 or type 2 diabetes. In general, for every 1% reduction in results of A1C blood tests (for example, from 8.0% to 7.0%), the risk of developing eye, kidney, and nerve disease is reduced by 40%.

How does maintaining a healthy body weight help people with diabetes stay healthy?

Most people newly diagnosed with type 2 diabetes are overweight. Excess weight, particularly in the abdomen, makes it difficult for cells to respond to insulin, resulting in high blood glucose. Often, people with type 2 diabetes are able to lower their blood glucose by losing weight and increasing physical activity. Losing weight also helps lower the risk for other health problems which especially affect people with diabetes, such as cardiovascular disease.

How does maintaining a healthy blood pressure level help people with diabetes stay healthy?

About 73% of adults with diabetes have high blood pressure or use prescription medications to reduce high blood pressure. Maintaining normal blood pressure—less than 130/80 millimeters of mercury (mm Hg) helps to prevent damage to the eyes, kidneys, heart, and blood vessels. Blood pressure measurements are written like a fraction, with the two numbers separated by a slash. The first number represents the pressure in your blood vessels when your heart beats (systolic pressure); the second number represents the pressure in the vessels when your heart is at rest (diastolic pressure).

In general, for every 10 mm Hg reduction in systolic blood pressure (the first number in the fraction), the risk for any complication related to diabetes is reduced by 12%. Maintaining normal blood pressure control can reduce the risk of eye, kidney, and nerve disease (microvascular disease) by approximately 33%, and the risk of heart disease and stroke (cardiovascular disease) by approximately 33% to 50%. Healthy eating, medications, and physical activity can help you bring high blood pressure down.

How does maintaining healthy cholesterol levels help people with diabetes stay healthy?

Several things, including having diabetes, can make your blood cholesterol level too high. When cholesterol is too high, the insides of large blood vessels become narrowed, even clogged, which can lead to heart disease and stroke, the biggest health problems for people with diabetes. Maintaining normal cholesterol levels will help prevent these diseases, and can help prevent circulation problems, also an issue for people with diabetes. Have your cholesterol checked at least once a year. Total cholesterol should be under 200; LDL ("bad" cholesterol) should be under 100; HDL ("good" cholesterol) should be above 40 in men and above 50 in women; and triglycerides should be under 150. Healthy eating, medications, and physical activity can help you reach your cholesterol targets. Keeping cholesterol levels under control can reduce the risk of cardiovascular complications of diabetes by 20% to 50%.

How does exercise help people with diabetes stay healthy?

Physical activity can help you control your blood glucose, weight, and blood pressure, as well as raise your "good" cholesterol and lower your "bad" cholesterol. It can also help prevent heart and blood flow problems.

Experts recommend moderate-intensity physical activity for at least 30 minutes on five or more days of the week. Talk to your health care provider about a safe exercise plan. He or she may check your heart and your feet to be sure you have no special problems. If you have high blood pressure, eye, or foot problems, you may need to avoid some kinds of exercise.

How does quitting smoking help people with diabetes stay healthy?

Smoking puts people with diabetes at particular risk. Smoking raises your blood glucose, cholesterol, and blood pressure, all of which people with diabetes need to be especially concerned about. When you have diabetes and use tobacco, the risk of heart and blood vessel problems is even greater. If you quit smoking, you'll lower your risk for heart attack, stroke, nerve disease, kidney disease, and oral disease.

Why is it important for people with diabetes to get an annual flu shot?

Diabetes can make the immune system more vulnerable to severe cases of the flu. People with diabetes who come down with the flu may become very sick and may die. You can help keep yourself from getting the flu by getting a flu shot every year. Everyone with diabetes—even pregnant women—should get a yearly flu shot. The best time to get one is between October and mid-November, before the flu season begins.

Section 18.3

Diabetes Management Numbers At-a-Glance

From the National Diabetes Education Program (NDEP), February 2007. NDEP is jointly sponsored by the National Institutes of Health and the Centers for Disease Control and Prevention with the support of more than 200 partner organizations. For more information, visit http://www.ndep.nih.gov.

Criteria for Diagnosis of Pre-Diabetes

- Impaired fasting glucose: 100–125 mg/dl (IFG) (Fasting plasma glucose) and/or

- Impaired glucose tolerance 140–199 mg/dl (IGT) (2-hr post 75g glucose challenge)

Criteria for Diagnosis of Diabetes

- Random plasma glucose more than 200 mg/dl* with symptoms (polyuria, polydipsia, and unexplained weight loss) and/or

- Fasting plasma glucose more than 126 mg/dl* and/or

- 2-hr plasma glucose more than 200 mg/dl* post 75g glucose challenge

*Repeat to confirm on subsequent day.

Treatment Goals for the ABCs of Diabetes

A1C Less Than 7%

- Preprandial plasma glucose 90–130 mg/dl
- Peak postprandial plasma glucose less than 180 mg/dl (usually 1 to 2 hr after the start of a meal)

Blood Pressure (mmHg)

- Systolic less than 130
- Diastolic less than 80

Cholesterol—Lipid Profile (mg/dl)

- LDL Cholesterol less than 100
- HDL Cholesterol Men more than 40; Women more than 50
- Triglycerides less than 150

Individualize Treatment Goals

For example, consider the following:

- A1C goal as close to normal (less than 6%) as possible without significant hypoglycemia.
- Less stringent A1C goal for people with severe or frequent hypoglycemia or if other factors exist (for example, limited life expectancy).
- Lower blood pressure goals for people with nephropathy.

Diabetes Management Schedule

People with diabetes should receive medical care from a physician-coordinated team of health care professionals. Referrals to these team members should be made as appropriate.

At each regular diabetes visit:

- Measure weight and blood pressure.
- Inspect feet.
- Review self-monitoring glucose record.
- Review/adjust medications to control glucose, lipids, and blood pressure—include regular use of aspirin for CVD prevention.
- Review self-management skills, dietary needs, and physical activity.
- Assess for depression or other mood disorder.
- Counsel on smoking cessation and alcohol use.

Quarterly

- Obtain A1C in patients whose therapy has changed or who are not meeting glycemic goals (twice a year if at goal with stable glycemia).

Annually

- Obtain fasting lipid profile (every two years if at goal).
- Obtain serum creatinine and estimate glomerular filtration rate.
- Perform urine test for albumin-to-creatinine ratio in patients with type 1 diabetes more than 5 years and in all patients with type 2 diabetes.
- Refer for dilated eye exam (if normal, an eye care specialist may advise an exam every two to three years).
- Perform comprehensive foot exam.
- Refer for dental/oral exam at least once a year.
- Administer influenza vaccination.
- Review need for other preventive care or treatment.

Lifetime

- Administer pneumococcal vaccination (repeat if over 64 or immunocompromised and last vaccination was more than five years ago).

Chapter 19

Tests Used to Monitor Diabetes

Chapter Contents

Section 19.1—Glucose Tolerance Testing 184

Section 19.2—The ABCs of A1C Testing 191

Section 19.3—Ketone Testing 194

Section 19.4—Blood Urea Nitrogen (BUN) 196

Section 19.5—Creatinine 199

Section 19.6—Microalbumin and Microalbumin/
Creatinine Ratio 203

Section 19.7—Glomerular Filtration Rate (GFR) 207

Section 19.1

Glucose Tolerance Testing

"Glucose: The Test Sample, The Test, Common Questions," © 2007 American Association for Clinical Chemistry. Reprinted with permission. For additional information about clinical lab testing, visit the Lab Tests Online website at www.labtestsonline.org.

What is being tested?

Glucose is a simple sugar that serves as the main source of energy for the body. The carbohydrates we eat are broken down into glucose (and a few other simple sugars), absorbed by the small intestine, and circulated throughout the body. Most of the body's cells require glucose for energy production; brain and nervous system cells not only rely on glucose for energy, they can only function when glucose levels in the blood remain above a certain level.

The body's use of glucose hinges on the availability of insulin, a hormone produced by the pancreas. Insulin acts as a traffic director, transporting glucose into the body's cells, directing the body to store excess glucose as glycogen (for short-term storage), and as triglycerides in adipose (fat) cells. We cannot live without glucose or insulin, and they must be in balance.

Normally, blood glucose levels rise slightly after a meal, and insulin is secreted to lower them, with the amount of insulin released matched up with the size and content of the meal. If blood glucose levels drop too low, such as might occur in between meals or after a strenuous workout, glucagon (another pancreatic hormone) is secreted to tell the liver to turn some glycogen back into glucose, raising the blood glucose levels. If the glucose/insulin feedback mechanism is working properly, the amount of glucose in the blood remains fairly stable. If the balance is disrupted and glucose levels in the blood rise, then the body tries to restore the balance, both by increasing insulin production and by excreting glucose in the urine.

Severe, acute hyperglycemia or hypoglycemia can be life-threatening, causing organ failure, brain damage, coma, and, in extreme cases, death. Chronically high blood glucose levels can cause progressive damage to body organs such as the kidneys, eyes, heart and blood vessels, and nerves. Chronic hypoglycemia can lead to brain and nerve damage.

Some women may develop hyperglycemia during pregnancy and this may lead to gestational diabetes. If untreated, this can cause these mothers to give birth to large babies who may have low glucose levels. Women who have had gestational diabetes may or may not go on to develop diabetes.

How is the sample collected for testing?

A blood sample is obtained by inserting a needle into a vein in the arm or a drop of blood is taken by pricking your skin with a small, pointed lancet. Sometimes, a random urine sample is collected.

Is any test preparation needed to ensure the quality of the sample?

It is generally recommended that you fast before having a blood glucose test.

How is it used?

The blood glucose test is ordered to measure the amount of glucose in the blood right at the time of sample collection. It is used to detect both hyperglycemia and hypoglycemia and to help diagnose diabetes. Blood glucose may be measured on a fasting basis (collected after an 8 to 10 hour fast), randomly (anytime), post prandial (after a meal), and/or as part of an oral glucose tolerance test (OGTT/GTT). An OGTT is a series of blood glucose tests. A fasting glucose is collected; then the patient drinks a standard amount of a glucose solution to "challenge" their system. This is followed by one or more additional glucose tests performed at specific intervals to track glucose levels over time. The OGTT may be ordered to help diagnose diabetes and as a follow-up test to an elevated blood glucose.

The American Diabetes Association recommends either the fasting glucose or the OGTT to diagnose diabetes but says that testing should be done twice, at different times, in order to confirm a diagnosis of diabetes.

Most pregnant women are screened for gestational diabetes, a temporary form of hyperglycemia, between their 24th and 28th week of pregnancy using a version of the OGTT, a 1-hour glucose challenge. If either fasting glucose or a random glucose is above the values used to diagnose diabetes in those who are not pregnant, the woman is considered to have gestational diabetes and neither the screening nor the glucose tolerance test is needed. If the 1-hour level is higher than the defined value, a longer OGTT is performed to clarify the patient's status.

Diabetics must monitor their own blood glucose levels, often several times a day, to determine how far above or below normal their glucose is and to determine what oral medications or insulin(s) they may need. This is usually done by placing a drop of blood from a skin prick onto a glucose strip and then inserting the strip into a glucose meter, a small machine that provides a digital readout of the blood glucose level.

In those with suspected hypoglycemia, glucose levels are used as part of the "Whipple triad" to confirm a diagnosis.

The urine glucose is seldom ordered by itself. At one time, it was used to monitor diabetics, but it has been largely replaced by the more sensitive and "real time" blood glucose. The urine glucose is, however, one of the substances measured when a urinalysis is performed. A urinalysis may be done routinely as part of a physical, when a doctor suspects that a patient may have a urinary tract infection, or for a variety of other reasons. The doctor may follow an elevated urine glucose test with blood glucose testing.

When is it ordered?

Blood glucose testing can be used to screen healthy, asymptomatic individuals for diabetes and pre-diabetes because diabetes is a common disease that begins with few symptoms. Screening for glucose may occur during public health fairs or as part of workplace health programs. It may also be ordered when a patient has a routine physical exam. Screening is especially important for people at high risk of developing diabetes, such as those with a family history of diabetes, those who are overweight, and those who are more than 40 to 45 years old.

The glucose test may also be ordered to help diagnose diabetes when someone has symptoms of hyperglycemia (such as increased thirst, increased urination, fatigue, blurred vision, and slow-healing infections) or symptoms of hypoglycemia (such as sweating, hunger, trembling, anxiety, confusion, and blurred vision).

Blood glucose testing is also done in emergency settings to determine if low or high glucose is contributing to symptoms such as fainting and unconsciousness. If a patient has pre-diabetes (characterized by fasting or OGTT levels that are higher than normal but lower than those defined as diabetic), the doctor will order a glucose test at regular intervals to monitor the patient's status. With known diabetics, doctors will order glucose levels in conjunction with other tests such as hemoglobin A1C to monitor glucose control over a period of time. Occasionally, a blood glucose level may be ordered along with insulin and C-peptide to monitor insulin production.

Diabetics may be required to self-check their glucose, once or several times a day, to monitor glucose levels and to determine treatment options as prescribed by their doctor.

Pregnant women are usually screened for gestational diabetes late in their pregnancies, unless they have early symptoms or previously have had gestational diabetes. When a woman has gestational diabetes, her doctor will usually order glucose levels throughout the rest of her pregnancy and after delivery to monitor her condition.

What does the test result mean?

High levels of glucose most frequently indicate diabetes, but many other diseases and conditions can also cause elevated glucose. The information in Table 19.1 summarizes the meaning of the test results. These are based on the clinical practice recommendations of the American Diabetes Association.

Some of the other diseases and conditions that can result in elevated glucose levels include the following:

- Acromegaly
- Acute stress (response to trauma, heart attack, and stroke for instance)
- Chronic renal failure
- Cushing syndrome
- Drugs, including: corticosteroids, tricyclic antidepressants, diuretics, epinephrine, estrogens (birth control pills and hormone replacement), lithium, phenytoin (Dilantin), salicylates
- Excessive food intake
- Hyperthyroidism
- Pancreatic cancer
- Pancreatitis

Low to non-detectible urine glucose results are considered normal. Anything that raises blood glucose levels also has the potential

Table 19.1. Glucose Test Result Meanings

Fasting Blood Glucose

From 70 to 99 mg/dL (3.9 to 5.5 mmol/L)	Normal glucose tolerance
From 100 to 125 mg/dL (5.6 to 6.9 mmol/L)	Impaired fasting glucose (pre-diabetes)
126 mg/dL (7.0 mmol/L) and aboveon more than one testing occasion	Diabetes

Oral Glucose Tolerance Test (OGTT) (except pregnancy)
(2 hours after a 75-gram glucose drink)

Less than 140 mg/dL (7.8 mmol/L)	Normal glucose tolerance
From 140 to 200 mg/dL (7.8 to 11.1 mmol/L)	Impaired glucose tolerance (pre-diabetes)
Over 200 mg/dL (11.1 mmol/L) on more than one testing occasion	Diabetes

Gestational Diabetes Screening: Glucose Challenge Test
(1 hour after a 50-gram glucose drink)

Less than 140[1] mg/dL (7.8 mmol/L)	Normal glucose tolerance
140[1] mg/dL (7.8 mmol/L) and over	Abnormal, needs OGTT (see below)

Gestational Diabetes Diagnostic: OGTT
(100-gram glucose drink)

Fasting[2]	95 mg/dL (5.3 mmol/L)
1 hour after glucose load[2]	180 mg/dL (10.0 mmol/L)
2 hours after glucose load[2]	155 mg/dL (8.6 mmol/L)
3 hours after glucose load[2,3]	140 mg/dL (7.8 mmol/L)

1. Some use a cutoff of >130 mg/dL (7.2 mmol/L) because that identifies 90% of women with gestational diabetes, compared to 80% identified using the threshold of >140 mg/dL (7.8 mmol/L).

2. If two or more values are above the criteria, gestational diabetes is diagnosed.

3. A 75-gram glucose load may be used, although this method is not as well validated as the 100-gram OGTT; the 3-hour sample is not drawn if 75 grams is used.

to elevate urine glucose levels. Increased urine glucose levels may be seen with medications, such as estrogens and chloral hydrate, and with some forms of renal disease.

Moderately increased levels may be seen with pre-diabetes. This condition, if left un-addressed, often leads to type 2 diabetes.

Low glucose levels (hypoglycemia) are also seen with the following:

- Adrenal insufficiency
- Drinking alcohol
- Drugs, such as acetaminophen and anabolic steroids
- Extensive liver disease
- Hypopituitarism
- Hypothyroidism
- Insulin overdose
- Insulinomas (insulin-producing pancreatic tumors)
- Starvation

Is there anything else I should know?

Hypoglycemia is characterized by a drop in blood glucose to a level where first it causes nervous system symptoms (sweating, palpitations, hunger, trembling, and anxiety), then begins to affect the brain (causing confusion, hallucinations, blurred vision, and sometimes even coma and death). An actual diagnosis of hypoglycemia requires satisfying the "Whipple triad." These three criteria include:

- Documented low glucose levels (less than 40 mg/dL (2.2 mmol/L) often tested along with insulin levels and sometimes with C-Peptide levels);
- Symptoms of hypoglycemia;
- Reversal of the symptoms when blood glucose levels are returned to normal.

Primary hypoglycemia is rare and often diagnosed in infancy. People may have symptoms of hypoglycemia without really having low blood sugar. In such cases, dietary changes such as eating frequent small meals and several snacks a day and choosing complex carbohydrates over simple sugars may be enough to ease symptoms. Those with fasting hypoglycemia may require IV (intravenous) glucose if dietary measures are insufficient.

Can I test myself at home for blood glucose levels?

If you are not diabetic or pre-diabetic, there is usually no reason to test glucose levels at home. Screening done as part of your regular physical should be sufficient.

If you have been diagnosed with diabetes, however, your doctor or diabetes educator will recommend a home glucose monitor (glucometer, or one of the newer methods that uses very tiny amounts of blood or tests the interstitial fluid—the fluid between your cells—for glucose). You will be given guidelines for how high or low your blood sugar should be at different times of the day. By checking your glucose regularly, you can see if the diet and medication schedule you are following is working properly.

Can I test my urine glucose instead of my blood?

Not in most cases. Glucose will usually only show up in the urine if it is at sufficiently high levels in the blood so that the body is "dumping" the excess into the urine, or if there is some degree of kidney damage and the glucose is leaking out into the urine. Urine glucose, however, is sometimes used as a rough indicator of high glucose levels and the urine indicator strip (dipstick) that measures the glucose is occasionally useful for tracking the presence of protein and ketones in the urine.

What are the usual treatments for diabetes?

For type 2 diabetes, which is the most common type of diabetes, losing excess weight, eating a healthy diet that is high in fiber and restricted in carbohydrates, and getting regular amounts of exercise may be enough to lower your blood glucose levels. In many cases however, oral medications that increase the body's secretion of and sensitivity to insulin are necessary to achieve the desired glucose level. With type 1 diabetes (and with type 2 diabetes that does not respond well enough to oral medications), insulin injections several times a day are necessary.

How can a diabetic educator help me?

If you are diabetic, a diabetic educator (often a nurse with specialized training) can make sure that you know how to:

- Plan meals (a dietitian can help with this also). Diet is extremely important in minimizing swings in blood glucose levels.

- Recognize and know how to treat both high and low blood sugar.

- Test and record your self-check glucose values.

- Adjust your medications.

- Administer insulin (which types in which combinations to meet your needs).

- Handle medications when you get ill.

- Monitor your feet, skin, and eyes to catch problems early.

- Buy diabetic supplies and store them properly.

Section 19.2

The ABCs of A1C Testing

"The ABCs of A1C Testing . . . The Best Test of Blood Sugar Control for People with Diabetes," an undated fact sheet produced by the U.S. Department of Veterans' Affairs; available online at http://www1.va.gov/diabetes/docs/ABCs_of_A1C_Testing.doc; accessed in August 2007.

What is the A1C test?

The A1C test (also called H-b-A-one-c) is a simple lab test that shows the average amount of sugar (also called glucose) that has been in a person's blood over the last three months.

The A1C test shows if a person's blood sugar is close to normal or too high. It is the best test for a health care provider to tell if a person's blood sugar is under control.

What does this test measure?

Sugar in the bloodstream can become attached to the hemoglobin (the part of the cell that carries oxygen) in red blood cells. This process is called glycosylation (pronounced gli-kos-a-lay'-shen). Once the sugar is attached, it stays there for the life of the red blood cell, which is about 120 days. The higher the level of blood sugar, the more sugar attaches to red blood cells. The A1C test measures the amount of sugar sticking to the red blood cells. Results are given in percentages.

Why do more people need to know about this test?

The findings of a major diabetes study, the Diabetes Control and Complications Trial (DCCT), have shown just how important the A1C test is. The study showed that lowering the A1C number can delay or prevent the development of serious eye, kidney, and nerve disease in people with diabetes. The study also showed that lowering A1C levels by any amount improves a person's chances of staying healthy.

When should this test be done?

All people with diabetes should have an A1C test at least twice a year. People with diabetes should get the test more often if their blood sugar stays too high or if their health care provider makes any change in their treatment plan.

How is the A1C test done?

This test is usually done in a health care provider's office. To do the test, a small sample of blood is taken. The blood sample is sent to a laboratory for testing, and the laboratory sends the results to the patient's health care provider.

Where does self-monitoring of blood glucose fit in?

Self-monitoring of blood glucose is also very important. A finger-stick test using a blood glucose meter measures the actual level of sugar in the blood at the time of the test. The meter reading is reported in milligrams per deciliter (mg/dl).

Self-monitoring of blood glucose helps people with diabetes see how food, physical activity, and diabetes medicine affect their blood sugar. The readings from these tests can help people with diabetes manage their disease day by day or even hour by hour. The readings can also tell them when their blood sugar is too low or too high, so they can work with their health care provider to change their treatment plan.

All people with diabetes need regular A1C tests. Most people with diabetes also need to self-monitor their blood glucose to get a complete picture of blood sugar control. Self-monitoring blood glucose gives a snapshot of control at the time of the test, while the A1C test gives the big picture of control over the past three months. Together, these tests tell a patient and his or her health care provider whether the patient's blood sugar is under control.

What does an A1C test result mean?

The A1C goal for people with diabetes is less than seven percent. The DCCT findings showed that people with diabetes who keep their A1C levels close to seven percent have a much better chance of delaying or preventing diabetes problems that affect the eyes, kidneys, and nerves than people with A1C levels eight percent or higher. A change in treatment is almost always needed if a person's A1C is over eight percent. But, if people with diabetes can lower their A1C number by any amount, they will improve their chances of staying healthy.

How does the A1C relate to readings from self-monitoring of blood glucose?

People with high daily blood sugar readings most of the time will usually have a high A1C test result. To maintain an A1C level less than seven percent means that the blood sugar should rarely go above 150 mg/dl on any self-monitoring blood glucose test performed before meals during the previous three months. The blood sugar also should not drop below 60-70 mg/dl, or low blood sugar occurs.

How can people with diabetes keep their A1C at less than seven percent?

Staying in control of diabetes over a prolonged period of time requires following a recommended meal plan, sticking to a physical activity program, taking prescribed diabetes medicines, self-monitoring of blood glucose if recommended, and consulting a health care provider often. When a patient has a high A1C test result, a health care provider can work with the patient to identify what is causing high blood sugar by examining the patient's record of self-monitoring blood glucose. Common causes of high blood sugar include eating too much food or eating the wrong foods, lack of physical activity, stress, a need to change medicines, and infection or illness. By finding the source of the problem, a health care provider can decide if and how to change a patient's treatment plan to meet the A1C goal of less than seven percent.

193

How can people with diabetes use their A1C test results?

When people with diabetes know the results from their A1C test, they can take an active role in their diabetes management. A high A1C is one that is greater than eight percent. People with diabetes who have a test result that is greater than eight percent need to work with their health care provider to change their treatment plan.

An A1C test result that is close to normal is one that is less than seven percent. When people with diabetes have a test result that is less than seven percent, their treatment plan is probably working and it is likely that their blood sugar is under good control.

Section 19.3

Ketone Testing

What are ketones?

Ketones are produced when the body burns fat for energy or fuel. They are also produced when you lose weight or there is not enough insulin to help your body use sugar for energy. Without enough insulin, glucose builds up in the blood. Since the body is unable to use glucose for energy, it breaks down fat instead. When this occurs, ketones form in the blood and spill into the urine. These ketones can make you very sick.

How can I test for ketones?

You can test to see if your body is making any ketones by doing a simple urine test. There are several products available for ketone testing and they can be purchased, without a prescription, at your pharmacy. Common product names include: Ketostix, Chemstrip K, and Acetest. The test result can be negative, or show small, moderate, or large quantities of ketones.

When should I test for ketones?

- Anytime your blood glucose is over 250 mg/dl for two tests in a row.

- When you are ill. Often illness, infections, or injuries will cause sudden high blood glucose and this is an especially important time to check for ketones.

- When you are planning to exercise and the blood glucose is over 250 mg/dl.

- If you are pregnant, you should test for ketones each morning before breakfast and any time the blood glucose is over 250 mg/dl.

If ketones are positive, what does this mean?

There are situations when you might have ketones without the blood glucose being too high. Positive ketones are not a problem when blood glucose levels are within range and you are trying to lose weight.

It is a problem if blood glucose levels are high and left untreated. Untreated high blood glucose with positive ketones can lead to a life-threatening condition called diabetic ketoacidosis (DKA).

What should I do if the ketone test is positive?

Call your diabetes educator or physician, as you may need additional insulin. Drink plenty of water and fluids containing no calories to "wash out" the ketones. Continue testing your blood glucose every three to four hours, testing for ketones if the blood glucose is over 250 mg/dl. Do not exercise if your blood glucose is over 250 mg/dl and ketones are present.

Section 19.4

Blood Urea Nitrogen (BUN)

What is being tested?

This test measures the amount of urea nitrogen in the blood. Nitrogen, in the form of ammonia, is produced in the liver when protein is broken into its component parts (amino acids) and metabolized. The nitrogen combines with other molecules in the liver to form the waste product urea. The urea is then released into the bloodstream and carried to the kidneys, where it is filtered out of the blood and excreted in the urine. Since this is an ongoing process, there is usually a small but stable amount of urea nitrogen in the blood.

Most diseases or conditions that affect the kidneys or liver have the potential to affect the amount of urea present in the blood. If increased amounts of urea are produced by the liver or decreased amounts are excreted by the kidneys, then urea concentrations will rise. If significant liver damage or disease inhibits the production of urea, then BUN concentrations may fall.

How is the sample collected for testing?

A blood sample is drawn from a vein in the arm.

How is it used?

The BUN test is primarily used, along with the creatinine test, to evaluate kidney function under a wide range of circumstances and to monitor patients with acute or chronic kidney dysfunction or failure. It also may be used to evaluate a person's general health status when ordered as part of a basic metabolic panel (BMP) or comprehensive metabolic panel (CMP).

When is it ordered?

BUN is part of both the BMP and CMP, groups of tests that are widely used:

- when someone has non-specific complaints;
- as part of a routine testing panel;
- to check how the kidneys are functioning before starting to take certain drug therapies;
- when an acutely ill person comes to the emergency room and/or is admitted to the hospital; or
- during a hospital stay.

BUN is often ordered with creatinine:

- when kidney problems are suspected;
- at regular intervals to monitor kidney function in patients with chronic diseases such as diabetes, congestive heart failure, and myocardial infarction (heart attack);
- at regular intervals to monitor kidney function and treatment in patients with known kidney disease;
- prior to and during certain drug treatments to monitor kidney function; or
- at regular intervals to monitor the effectiveness of dialysis.

What does the test result mean?

Increased BUN levels suggest impaired kidney function. This may be due to acute or chronic kidney disease, damage, or failure. It may also be due to a condition that results in decreased blood flow to the kidneys, such as congestive heart failure, shock, stress, recent heart attack, or severe burns, to conditions that cause obstruction of urine flow, or to dehydration.

BUN concentrations may be elevated when there is excessive protein catabolism (breakdown), significantly increased protein in the diet, or gastrointestinal bleeding (because of the proteins present in the blood).

Low BUN levels are not common and are not usually a cause for concern. They may be seen in severe liver disease, malnutrition, and

197

sometimes when a patient is overhydrated (too much fluid volume), but the BUN test is not usually used to diagnose or monitor these conditions.

Both decreased and increased BUN concentrations may be seen during a normal pregnancy.

If one kidney is fully functional, BUN concentrations may be normal even when significant dysfunction is present in the other kidney.

NOTE: The result of your test is measured by your doctor against a reference range for the test to determine whether the result is "normal" (it is within the range of numbers), high (it is above the high end of the range), or low (it is below the low end of the range). Because there can be many variables that affect the determination of the reference range, the reference range for this test is specific to the lab where your test sample is analyzed. For this reason, the lab is required to report your results with an accompanying reference range. Typically, your doctor will have sufficient familiarity with the lab and your medical history to interpret the results appropriately.

While there is no such thing as a "standard" reference range for BUN, most labs will report a similar, though maybe not exactly the same, set of numbers as that included in medical textbooks or found elsewhere online. For this reason, it is recommend that you talk with your doctor about your lab results.

Is there anything else I should know?

BUN levels can increase with the amount of protein in your diet. High-protein diets may cause abnormally high BUN levels while very low-protein diets can cause an abnormally low BUN.

What other tests are used with BUN to check how my kidneys are functioning?

BUN and creatinine are the primary tests used to check how well the kidneys are able to filter waste products from your blood. Your doctor may also order electrolyte tests such as sodium and potassium or calcium to help understand how your kidneys are functioning.

How does BUN change with age?

BUN levels increase with age. BUN levels in very young babies are about 2/3 of the levels found in healthy young adults, while levels in adults over 60 years of age are slightly higher than younger adults. Levels are also slightly higher in men than women.

What is a BUN/Creatinine ratio?

Occasionally, a doctor will look at the ratio between a person's BUN and blood creatinine to help them determine what is causing these concentrations to be higher than normal. The ratio of BUN to creatinine is usually between 10:1 and 20:1. An increased ratio may be due to a condition that causes a decrease in the flow of blood to the kidneys, such as congestive heart failure or dehydration. It may also be seen with increased protein, from gastrointestinal bleeding, or increased protein in the diet. The ratio may be decreased with liver disease (due to decrease in the formation of urea) and malnutrition.

Section 19.5

Creatinine

What is being tested?

This test measures the amount of creatinine in your blood and/or urine. Creatinine is a waste product produced in your muscles from the breakdown of a compound called creatine. Creatine is part of the cycle that produces energy needed to contract your muscles and it as well as creatinine are produced at a relatively constant rate. Almost all creatinine is excreted by the kidneys, so blood levels are a good measure of how well your kidneys are working. The quantity produced depends on the size of the person and their muscle mass. For this reason, creatinine concentrations will be slightly higher in men than in women and children.

How is the sample collected for testing?

A blood sample is drawn from a vein in the arm. You may be asked to collect a complete 24-hour urine sample in addition to having your blood drawn. Your doctor or the laboratory will give you a large container and instructions for properly collecting this sample. Typically, you start collecting urine after you wake up in the morning and empty your bladder and save all of the urine produced until the same time the following day.

How is it used?

The creatinine blood test is usually ordered along with a BUN (blood urea nitrogen) test to assess kidney function. Both are frequently ordered as part of a basic or comprehensive metabolic panel (BMP or CMP), groups of tests that are performed to evaluate the function of the body's major organs. BMP or CMP tests are ordered on healthy people during routine physical exams and on acutely or chronically ill patients in the emergency room and/or hospital. If the creatinine and BUN tests are found to be abnormal or if the patient has an underlying disease, such as diabetes, that is known to affect the kidneys, then these two tests may be used to monitor the progress of kidney dysfunction and the effectiveness of treatment. Blood creatinine and BUN tests may also be ordered to evaluate kidney function prior to some procedures, such as a computed tomography (CT) scan, that may require the use of drugs that can damage the kidneys.

A combination of blood and urine creatinine levels may be used to calculate a creatinine clearance. This measures how effectively your kidneys are filtering small molecules like creatinine out of your blood. Urine creatinine may also be used with a variety of other urine tests as a sort of correction factor. Since it is produced and removed at a relatively constant rate, the amount of urine creatinine can be compared to the amount of the other substance (such as protein) being measured.

Serum creatinine measurements (along with your age, weight, and gender) also are used to calculate the estimated glomerular filtration rate (EGFR), which is used as a screening test to look for evidence of kidney damage.

When is it ordered?

Creatinine may be ordered routinely as part of a comprehensive or basic metabolic panel, when someone has non-specific health complaints, is acutely ill, and/or when a doctor suspects kidney dysfunction. The creatinine blood test may be ordered, along with the BUN test, at regular intervals when the patient has a known kidney disorder or has a disease that may affect kidney function or be exacerbated by dysfunction. Both may be ordered when a CT scan is planned, prior to and during certain drug therapies, and before and after dialysis to monitor the effectiveness of treatments.

What does the test result mean?

Increased creatinine levels in the blood suggest diseases or conditions that affect kidney function. These can include:

- damage to or swelling of blood vessels in the kidneys (glomerulonephritis) caused by, for example, infection or autoimmune diseases;

- bacterial infection of the kidneys (pyelonephritis);

- death of cells in the kidneys' small tubes (acute tubular necrosis) caused, for example, by drugs or toxins;

- prostate disease, kidney stone, or other causes of urinary tract obstruction; or

- reduced blood flow to the kidney due to shock, dehydration, congestive heart failure, atherosclerosis, or complications of diabetes.

Creatinine can also increase temporarily as a result of muscle injury.

Low levels of creatinine are not common and are not usually a cause for concern. They can be seen with conditions that result in decreased muscle mass.

Creatinine levels are generally slightly lower during pregnancy.

NOTE: The result of your creatinine test is measured by your doctor against a reference range for the test to determine whether the result is "normal" (it is within the range of numbers), high (it is above the high end of the range), or low (it is below the low end of the range). Because there can be many variables that affect the determination of the reference range, the reference range for this test is specific to the lab where your test sample is analyzed. For this reason, the lab is required to report your results with an accompanying reference range. Typically, your doctor will have sufficient familiarity with the lab and your medical history to interpret the results appropriately.

While there is no such thing as a "standard" reference range for creatinine, most labs will report a similar, though maybe not exactly the same, set of numbers as that included in medical textbooks or found elsewhere online. For this reason, it is recommend that you talk with your doctor about your lab results.

Is there anything else I should know?

Drugs such as aminoglycosides (gentamicin) can cause kidney damage and so creatinine is monitored. Other drugs, such as cephalosporins (cefoxitin), may increase creatinine concentration without reflecting kidney damage.

Will exercise affect my creatinine levels?

In general, moderate exercise will not affect your creatinine levels. As you continue to exercise and build muscle mass, your creatinine levels may increase slightly, but not to abnormal levels.

How does diet affect creatinine levels?

In general, creatinine levels will not vary with a normal diet. Creatinine levels may be 10%–30% higher in people who eat a diet that is very high in meat.

What is creatine? If I take creatine, will my creatinine levels go up?

Creatine is a compound that is made primarily in the liver and then transported to your muscles, where it is used as an energy source for muscle activity. Once in the muscle, some of the creatine is spontaneously converted to creatinine. The amount of both creatine and creatinine depend on muscle mass, so men usually have higher levels than women. Creatine is now available as a dietary supplement. If you take creatine, your creatinine levels may be higher than when you do not take the supplement. You should tell your doctor about all of the dietary supplements you are taking to help her evaluate your lab results.

Do creatinine levels change with age?

Creatinine levels relate to both muscle mass and to kidney function. As you age, your muscle mass decreases but your kidneys tend to function less effectively. The net result is not much change in creatinine levels in the blood as you get older.

What is a BUN/Creatinine ratio?

Occasionally, a doctor will look at the ratio between a person's BUN and blood creatinine to help them determine what is causing these concentrations to be higher than normal. The ratio of BUN to creatinine is usually between 10:1 and 20:1. An increased ratio may be due to a condition that causes a decrease in the flow of blood to the kidneys, such as congestive heart failure or dehydration. It may also be seen with increased protein, from gastrointestinal bleeding, or increased protein in the diet. The ratio may be decreased with liver disease (due to decrease in the formation of urea) and malnutrition.

Section 19.6

Microalbumin and Microalbumin/Creatinine Ratio

What is being tested?

The microalbumin test is an early indicator of kidney failure. It measures the tiny amounts of albumin that the body begins to release into the urine several years before significant kidney damage becomes apparent. Albumin is a protein that is produced in the liver. It is present in high concentrations in the blood, but when the kidneys are functioning properly, virtually no albumin is allowed to leak through into the urine. If a person's kidneys become damaged or diseased, however, they begin to lose their ability to filter proteins out of the urine. This is frequently seen in chronic diseases, such as diabetes and hypertension, with increasing amounts of protein in the urine reflecting increasing kidney failure.

Since the albumin molecule is small, it is one of the first proteins to be detected in the urine with kidney damage. Patients who have consistently detectible amounts of albumin in their urine (microalbuminuria) have an increased risk of developing progressive kidney failure and cardiovascular disease in the future. Because the amount of albumin in the urine varies throughout the day, the most accurate microalbumin measurement is the 24-hour urine test. This test, which requires the collection of all urine over a 24-hour period, is cumbersome and relies on patient compliance. In the case of young children, it can be difficult or impossible to conduct without the use of a catheter. Since not collecting all of the urine will affect the accuracy of the 24-hour test, doctors have begun to order timed (4-hour or overnight) or random (spot) microalbumin tests as an alternative.

Although timed urine samples are not as reliable as 24-hour samples, they can be corrected using creatinine measurement. Creatinine, a byproduct of muscle metabolism, is normally excreted into the urine on a consistent basis. Its level in the urine is relatively stable. Since the concentration (or dilution) of urine varies throughout the day, this property of creatinine allows its measurement to be used as a corrective factor in random urine samples. When a creatinine measurement is performed along with a random microalbumin, the resulting microalbumin/creatinine ratio approaches the accuracy of the 24-hour microalbumin test without the extended collection hassle.

How is the sample collected for testing?

You will be asked to collect either a random sample of urine while you are at the doctor's office or laboratory, a timed urine sample (such as four hours or overnight), or you may be requested to collect a complete 24-hour urine sample. Your doctor or the laboratory will give you a container and instructions for properly collecting a timed or 24-hour urine sample.

How is it used?

The random microalbumin test or microalbumin/creatinine ratio is frequently ordered as a screening test on patients with chronic conditions, such as diabetes and hypertension, that put them at an increased risk of developing kidney failure. Studies have shown that identifying the very early stages of kidney disease (microalbuminuria) helps patients and doctors adjust treatment. With better control of diabetes and hypertension, the progression of diabetic kidney disease can be slowed or prevented.

A timed microalbumin test (four hour or overnight) may be ordered as an alternative screening tool. If significant amounts of microalbumin are detected with these screening tests, they may be confirmed with a 24-hour microalbumin test.

When is it ordered?

The National Kidney Foundation recommends that type 2 diabetics under the age of 70 and type 1 diabetics over the age of 12 be screened annually for microalbuminuria. In addition, microalbumin may be ordered when a person is first diagnosed with type 2 diabetes. According to the American Diabetes Association, in type 1 diabetes, annual testing should begin five years after diagnosis.

Patients with hypertension may be tested at regular intervals, with the frequency determined by their doctor.

What does the test result mean?

NOTE: A standard reference range is not available for this test. Because reference values are dependent on many factors, including patient age, gender, sample population, and test method, numeric test results have different meanings in different labs. Your lab report should include the specific reference range for your test. Lab Tests Online strongly recommends that you discuss your test results with your doctor.

Moderately increased microalbumin levels in urine indicate that a person is in one of the very early phases of developing kidney disease. Very high levels are an indication that kidney disease is present in a more severe form. Normal levels are an indication that kidney function is normal.

Is there anything else I should know?

Recently, studies have shown that in type 2 diabetics, an abnormal microalbumin result indicates an increased risk of developing cardiovascular disease (CVD).

What is the difference between albumin, prealbumin, and microalbumin tests?

The prealbumin test measures a protein that reflects your nutritional status, particularly before and after surgery, or if you are hospitalized or taking nutritional supplements. Albumin testing is more often used to test for liver or kidney disease or to learn if your body is not absorbing enough amino acids. Albumin can also be used to monitor nutritional status. However, prealbumin changes more quickly, making it more useful for detecting changes in short-term nutritional status than albumin. The microalbumin test measures very small levels of albumin in your urine and may indicate whether you are at risk for developing kidney disease.

Is microalbumin just smaller molecules of albumin?

Microalbumin tests for a small amount of albumin, not smaller molecules.

What is the test finding in my urine?

If you are diabetic, each year your doctor will test a sample of your urine to see if your kidneys are leaking albumin, even in small amounts. It is good news if your kidneys are not leaking even small amounts of albumin.

Are there other reasons for having increased microalbumin levels in urine?

Yes, microalbuminuria is not specific for diabetes. It may also be associated with hypertension (high blood pressure), some lipid abnormalities, and several immune disorders. Elevated results may also be caused by vigorous exercise, blood in the urine, urinary tract infection, dehydration, and some drugs.

Section 19.7

Glomerular Filtration Rate (GFR)

"Understanding GFR: A Guide for Patients,"
National Kidney Disease Education Program, December 2005.

What is glomerular filtration rate?

Your glomerular filtration rate (GFR) is a measure of how well your kidneys are filtering wastes from your blood. Your GFR has been estimated from a routine measurement of creatinine in your blood.

Creatinine is a waste product formed by the normal breakdown of muscle cells. Healthy kidneys take creatinine out of the blood and put it into the urine to leave the body. When kidneys are not working well, creatinine builds up in the blood.

What does my GFR number mean?

As you get older, the average GFR number drops. However, a low GFR with a value below 60 suggests some kidney damage has occurred. This means that your kidneys are not working at full strength.

How important is my GFR number?

Your doctor will use your GFR number as one clue to how well your kidneys are working. Your doctor will also look at other factors, including protein (albumin) in your urine, diabetes, and high blood pressure.

Depending on these factors, your doctor may decide that you have chronic kidney disease. If you have chronic kidney disease, controlling your diabetes or high blood pressure can help prevent more damage to your kidneys and other problems like heart attacks and strokes.

What do my kidneys do?

Healthy kidneys filter your blood. They remove waste and extra water, which become urine. The wastes in your blood come from the normal breakdown of active tissues and from food you eat. After your body has taken what it needs from the food, waste is sent to the blood. If your kidneys do not remove these wastes, the wastes build up in the blood and damage your body.

Chapter 20

Self-Monitoring of Blood Glucose

When people with diabetes can control their blood sugar (glucose), they are more likely to stay healthy. People with diabetes use two kinds of management devices: glucose meters and other diabetes management tests. Glucose meters help people with diabetes check their blood sugar at home, school, work, and play. Other blood and urine tests reveal trends in diabetes management and help identify diabetes complications.

The process of monitoring one's own blood glucose with a glucose meter is often referred to as self-monitoring of blood glucose or "SMBG."

Portable glucose meters are small battery-operated devices.

To test for glucose with a typical glucose meter, place a small sample of blood on a disposable "test strip" and place the strip in the meter. The test strips are coated with chemicals (glucose oxidase, dehydrogenase, or hexokinase) that combine with glucose in blood. The meter measures how much glucose is present. Meters do this in different ways. Some measure the amount of electricity that can pass through the sample. Others measure how much light reflects from it. The meter displays the glucose level as a number. Several new models can record and store a number of test results. Some models can connect to personal computers to store test results or print them out.

Excerpted from "Glucose Meters and Diabetes Management," U.S. Food and Drug Administration, June 2005. The complete text of this document, with links to additional information, is available online at http://www.fda.gov/diabetes/glucose.html.

Choosing a Glucose Meter

At least 25 different meters are commercially available. They differ in several ways including the amount of blood needed for each test, testing speed, overall size, ability to store test results in memory, cost of the meter, and cost of the test strips used.

To search the U.S. Food and Drug Administration (FDA)'s 510(k) database for glucose meters available over-the-counter (without a prescription), visit http://www.fda.gov/search/databases/html and click on the link under "Medical Devices."

Newer meters often have features that make them easier to use than older models. Some meters allow you to get blood from places other than your fingertip. Some new models have automatic timing, error codes and signals, or barcode readers to help with calibration. Some meters have a large display screen or spoken instructions for people with visual impairments.

Using Your Glucose Meter

Diabetes care should be designed for each individual patient. Some patients may need to test (monitor) more often than others do. How often you use your glucose meter should be based on the recommendation of your health care provider. Self-monitoring of blood glucose (SMBG) is recommended for all people with diabetes, but especially for those who take insulin. The role of SMBG has not been defined for people with stable type 2 diabetes treated only with diet.

As a general rule, the American Diabetes Association (ADA) recommends that most patients with type 1 diabetes test glucose three or more times per day. Pregnant women taking insulin for gestational diabetes should test two times per day. ADA does not specify how often people with type 2 diabetes should test their glucose, but testing often helps control.

Often, self-monitoring plans direct you to test your blood sugar before meals, two hours after meals, at bedtime, at 3 A.M., and anytime you experience signs or symptoms. You should test more often when you change medications, when you have unusual stress or illness, or in other unusual circumstances.

Learning to Use Your Glucose Meter

Not all glucose meters work the same way. Since you need to know how to use your glucose meter and interpret its results, you should get training from a diabetes educator. The educator should watch you test your glucose to make sure you can use your motor correctly. This training is better if it is part of an overall diabetes education program.

Instructions for Using Glucose Meters

The following are the general instructions for using a glucose meter:

1. Wash hands with soap and warm water and dry completely or clean the area with alcohol and dry completely.

2. Prick the fingertip with a lancet.

3. Hold the hand down and hold the finger until a small drop of blood appears; catch the blood with the test strip.

4. Follow the instructions for inserting the test strip and using the SMBG meter.

5. Record the test result.

The Food and Drug Administration (FDA) requires that glucose meters and the strips used with them have instructions for use. You should read carefully the instructions for both the meter and its test strips. Meter instructions are found in the user manual. Keep this manual to help you solve any problems that may arise. Many meters use "error codes" when there is a problem with the meter, the test strip, or the blood sample on the strip. You will need the manual to interpret these error codes and fix the problem.

You can get information about your meter and test strips from several different sources. Your user manual should include a toll free number in case you have questions or problems. If you have a problem and can't get a response from this number, contact your healthcare provider or a local emergency room for advice. Also, the manufacturer of your meter should have a website. Check this website regularly to see if it lists any issues with the function of your meter.

New devices are for sale such as laser lancets and meters that can test blood taken from "alternative sites" of the body other than fingertips. Since new devices are used in new ways and often have new use restrictions, you must review the instructions carefully.

Important Features of Glucose Meters

There are several features of glucose meters that you need to understand so you can use your meter and understand its results. These features are often different for different meters. You should understand the features of your own meter.

Measurement range: Most glucose meters are able to read glucose levels over a broad range of values from as low as 0 to as high as 600 mg/dL. Since the range is different among meters, interpret very high or low values carefully. Glucose readings are not linear over their entire range. If you get an extremely high or low reading from your meter, you should first confirm it with another reading. You should also consider checking your meter's calibration.

Whole blood glucose vs. plasma glucose: Glucose levels in plasma (one of the components of blood) are generally 10–15% higher than glucose measurements in whole blood (and even more after eating). This is important because home blood glucose meters measure the glucose in whole blood while most lab tests measure the glucose in plasma. There are many meters on the market now that give results as "plasma equivalent." This allows patients to easily compare their glucose measurements in a lab test and at home. Remember, this is just the way that the measurement is presented to you. All portable blood glucose meters measure the amount of glucose in whole blood. The meters that give "plasma equivalent" readings have a built in algorithm that translates the whole blood measurement to make it seem like the result that would be obtained on a plasma sample. It is important for you and your healthcare provider to know whether your meter gives its results as "whole blood equivalent" or "plasma equivalent."

Cleaning: Some meters need regular cleaning to be accurate. Clean your meter with soap and water, using only a dampened soft cloth to avoid damage to sensitive parts. Do not use alcohol (unless recommended in the instructions), cleansers with ammonia, glass cleaners, or abrasive cleaners. Some meters do not require regular cleaning but contain electronic alerts indicating when you should clean them. Other meters can be cleaned only by the manufacturer.

Display of high and low glucose values: Part of learning how to operate a meter is understanding what the meter results mean. Be sure you know how high and low glucose concentrations are displayed on your meter.

Factors That Affect Glucose Meter Performance

The accuracy of your test results depends partly on the quality of your meter and test strips and your training. Other factors can also make a difference in the accuracy of your results.

Hematocrit. Hematocrit is the amount of red blood cells in the blood. Patients with higher hematocrit values will usually test lower for blood glucose than patients with normal hematocrit. Patients with lower hematocrit values will test higher. If you know that you have abnormal hematocrit values you should discuss its possible effect on glucose testing (and HbA1C testing) with your health care provider. Anemia and sickle cell anemia are two conditions that affect hematocrit values.

Other substances: Many other substances may interfere with your testing process. These include uric acid (a natural substance in the body that can be more concentrated in some people with diabetes), glutathione (an "anti-oxidant" also called "GSH"), and ascorbic acid (vitamin C). You should check the package insert for each meter to find what substances might affect its testing accuracy, and discuss your concerns with your health care provider.

Altitude, temperature, and humidity: Altitude, room temperature, and humidity can cause unpredictable effects on glucose results. Check the meter and test strip package insert for information on these issues. Store and handle the meter and test strips according to the instructions.

Third-party test strips: Third-party or "generic glucose reagent strips" are test strips developed as a less expensive option than the strips that the manufacturer intended the meter to be used with. They are typically developed by copying the original strips. Although these strips may work on the meter listed on the package, they could look like strips used for other meters. Be sure the test strip you use is compatible with your glucose meter.

Sometimes manufacturers change their meters and their test strips. These changes are not always communicated to the third-party strip manufacturers. This can make third-party strips incompatible with your meter without your knowledge. Differences can involve the amount, type or concentration of the chemicals (called "reagents") on the test strip, or the actual size and shape of the strip itself. Meters are sensitive to these features of test strips and may not work well or consistently if they are not correct for a meter. If you are unsure whether or not a certain test strip will work with you meter, contact the manufacturer of your glucose meter.

Making Sure Your Meter Works Properly

You should perform quality-control checks to make sure that your home glucose testing is accurate and reliable. Several things can reduce the accuracy of your meter reading even if it appears to still work. For instance, the meter may have been dropped or its electrical components may have worn out. Humidity or heat may damage test strips. It is even possible that your testing technique may have changed slightly. Quality control checks should be done on a regular basis according to the meter manufacturer's instructions. There are two kinds of quality control checks:

Check using test quality control solutions or electronic controls: Test quality control solutions and electronic controls are both used to check the operation of your meter. Test quality control solutions check the accuracy of the meter and test strip. They may also give an indication of how well you use your system. Electronic controls only check that the meter is working properly.

Test quality control solutions have known glucose values. Essentially, when you run a quality control test, you substitute the test solution for blood. The difference is that you know what the result should be.

To test your meter with a quality control solution, follow the instructions that accompany the solution. These will guide you to place a certain amount of solution on your test strip and run it through your meter. The meter will give you a reading for the amount of glucose in the sample. Compare this number to the number listed on the test quality control solution. If the results of your test match the values given in the quality control solution labeling, you can be assured the entire system (meter and test strip) is working properly. If results are not correct, the system may not be accurate—contact the manufacturer for advice.

Manufacturers sometimes include quality control solution with their meter. However, most often you must order it separately from a manufacturer or pharmacy.

Some glucose meters also use electronic controls to make sure the meter is working properly. With this method, you place a cartridge or a special "control" test strip in the meter and a signal will appear to indicate if the meter is working.

Take your meter with you to the health care provider's office: This way you can test your glucose while your health care provider watches your technique to make sure you are using the meter correctly. Your healthcare provider will also take a sample of blood and evaluate it using a routine laboratory method. If values obtained on the glucose meter match the laboratory method, you and your healthcare provider will see that your meter is working well and that you are using good technique. If results do not match the laboratory method results, then results you get from your meter may be inaccurate and you should discuss the issue with your healthcare provider and contact the manufacturer if necessary.

New Technologies: Alternative Site Testing

Some glucose meters allow testing blood from alternative sites, such as the upper arm, forearm, base of the thumb, and thigh.

Sampling blood from alternative sites may be desirable, but it may have some limitations. Blood in the fingertips show changes in glucose levels more quickly than blood in other parts of the body. This means that alternative site test results may be different from fingertip test results not because of the meter's ability to test accurately, but because the actual glucose concentration can be different. FDA believes that further research is needed to better understand these differences in test values and their possible impact on the health of people with diabetes.

Glucose concentrations change rapidly after a meal, insulin, or exercise. Glucose levels at the alternative site appear to change more slowly than in the fingertips. Because of this concern, FDA has now requested that manufacturers either show their device is not affected by differences between alternative site and fingertip blood samples during times of rapidly changing glucose, or alert users about possible different values at these times.

Recommended labeling precautions include these statements:

- Alternative site results may be different than the fingertip when glucose levels are changing rapidly (for example, after a meal, taking insulin, or during or after exercise).

- Do not test at an alternative site, but use samples taken from the fingertip, if you think your blood sugar is low, you are not aware of symptoms when you become hypoglycemic, or the site results do not agree with the way you feel.

Minimally Invasive and Non-Invasive Glucose Meters

Researchers are exploring new technologies for glucose testing that avoid fingersticks. One of these is based on near-infrared spectroscopy for measurement of glucose. Essentially, this amounts to measuring glucose by shining a beam of light on the skin. It is painless. There are increasing numbers of reports in the scientific literature on the challenges, strengths, and weaknesses of this and other new approaches to testing glucose without fingersticks.

FDA has approved one "minimally invasive" meter and one "non-invasive" glucose meter. Neither of these should replace standard glucose testing. They are used to obtain additional glucose values between fingerstick tests. Both devices require daily calibration using standard fingerstick glucose measurements and both remain the subject of continuing studies to find how they are best used as tools for diabetes management.

MiniMed Continuous Glucose Monitoring System: The Mini-Med system consists of a small plastic catheter (very small tube) inserted just under the skin. The catheter collects small amounts of liquid that is passed through a "biosensor" to measure the amount of glucose present.

MiniMed is intended for occasional use and to discover trends in glucose levels during the day. It does not give you readings for individual tests and therefore you can't use it for typical day-to-day monitoring. The device collects measurements over a 72-hour period and then must be downloaded by the patient or healthcare provider. Understanding trends over time might help patients know the best time to do their standard fingerstick tests. You need a prescription to buy MiniMed.

Cygnus GlucoWatch Biographer: GlucoWatch is worn on the arm like a wristwatch. It pulls tiny amounts of fluid from the skin and measures the glucose in the fluid without puncturing the skin. The device requires three hours to warm up after it is put on. After this, it can provide up to three glucose measurements per hour for 12 hours. Unlike the MiniMed device, the GlucoWatch displays results that can be read by the wearer, although like the MiniMed device, these readings are not meant to be used as replacements for fingerstick-based tests. The results are meant to show trends and patterns in glucose levels rather than report any one result alone. It is useful for detecting and evaluating episodes of hyperglycemia and hypoglycemia. However, you must confirm its results with a standard glucose meter before you take corrective action. You need a prescription to buy GlucoWatch.

Chapter 21

Insulin

Characteristics

The three characteristics of insulin are:

- **Onset:** The length of time before insulin reaches the blood-stream and begins lowering blood glucose.

- **Peak time:** The time during which insulin is at its maximum strength in terms of lowering blood glucose levels.

- **Duration:** How long the insulin continues to lower blood glucose.

Kinds

Here is a brief look at the kinds of insulins available. Remember, each person has his or her unique response to insulin, so the times mentioned here are approximate.

Rapid-acting insulins, such as insulin lispro (Humalog by Eli Lilly), insulin aspart (NovoLog by Novo Nordisk), and insulin glulisine (Apidra) begin to work about 15 minutes or less after they are injected, peak in about an hour, and continue to work for two to four hours. (Be sure to check the package inserts on rapid-acting insulins for product-specific directions, because they vary slightly.) In fact, you should never delay eating after using insulin lispro, insulin aspart, or insulin glulisine.

Also, because these insulins leave the bloodstream quickly, there is less chance of hypoglycemia (low blood glucose) several hours after the meal. Insulin lispro, insulin aspart, and insulin glulisine are only available by prescription. All are very similar in their activity, but you should not use them interchangeably unless advised to do so by your doctor.

After-meal use of rapid-acting insulins may also be of some benefit to young children, because their caloric intake is often difficult to predict before meals. After-meal use can also benefit those who have delayed stomach emptying (gastroparesis).

Regular or short-acting insulin (human) usually reaches the bloodstream within 30 minutes after injection. It peaks anywhere from two to three hours after injection and is effective for approximately three to six hours. Typically, the higher the dose of regular insulin, the greater the effect.

Intermediate-acting insulin (human) generally reaches the bloodstream about two to four hours after it is injected. It peaks four to 12 hours later, and is effective for about 12 to 18 hours. NPH is an intermediate-acting insulin, and it is often used in combination with regular insulin. (See "Insulins Commonly Used in the United States" and Table 21.1 near the end of this chapter.)

Long-acting insulins insulin glargine (trade name Lantus) and insulin detemir (trade name Levemir) have continuous, "peakless" action that mimics natural basal (background) insulin secretion. Although it provides a long-lasting effect, insulin glargine's onset is between two and four hours. Insulin glargine has been clinically proven to reduce low blood glucose, especially during the night.

Insulin glargine is clear in appearance. However, insulin glargine must not be mixed with any other type of insulin and should not be administered intravenously. Insulin detemir is a new, long-acting insulin that lasts up to 24 hours. It is a clear, ready-to-inject solution that can lower blood glucose with a decreased risk of hypoglycemia.

Many people use both rapid- or short-acting insulins and insulin glargine or insulin detemir in an effort to mimic the body's natural insulin secretion. Because insulin glargine has no peak, injections of rapid-acting or short-acting regular insulin must be given before all meals to provide bolus coverage for food intake. Both types of insulin are clear in appearance. If you are on this type of dual insulin therapy, it is very important that you choose the correct insulin from the correct vial. (One distinguishing factor is that insulin glargine vials are taller and narrower than those of other insulins.) Insulin glargine can be injected any time during the day, as long as it is taken around the same time each day.

Premixed insulins may be convenient for those who mix NPH and regular into one syringe. Often, the insulin is premixed in a prefilled insulin pen, a portable and accurate means of administering insulin, replacing the traditional vial and syringe.

The most typical mixture is 70 percent NPH and 30 percent regular. A mixture of 75 percent insulin lispro protamine and 25 percent insulin lispro, known on the market as the Humalog Mix 75/25, combines intermediate-acting insulin and rapid-acting mealtime insulin. Humalog 50/50 and Humulin 50/50 are additional mixtures that are available. Likewise, a mixture of 70 percent insulin aspart protamine and 30 percent insulin aspart (NovoLog Mix 70/30) is available.

Premixed insulin can be helpful for people who have trouble drawing up insulin out of two different bottles and reading the correct dosages. It's useful for those who have poor eyesight or dexterity and is convenient for people whose diabetes has been stabilized on this combination. Insulin pens are also useful for those with dexterity problems or poor eyesight.

Sources

Today, recombinant DNA human insulins are the most widely used insulins in this country. Through genetic engineering, bacteria, or yeast they are transformed into little "factories" that produce synthetic human insulin. Years ago, the most commonly used insulins were pork, beef, and beef-pork combinations.

The source of an insulin is important because it affects how quickly the insulin will be absorbed, peak, and last.

Strength

All insulins come dissolved or suspended in liquids, but the solutions have different strengths. The most commonly used strength in the United States today is U-100. That means it has 100 units of insulin per milliliter of fluid (100 units per cc). Not used in the United States, but still used in Europe and Latin America, is U-40, which has 40 units of insulin per milliliter of liquid.

If you are traveling, it's essential that you purchase the correct strength of insulin. And because different syringes are used for different insulin strengths (for example, U-40 syringes deliver U-40 insulin and U-100 syringes deliver U-100 insulin), it's essential that your syringe match your insulin.

U-500 insulin can be purchased in the United States, but it is rarely used. It is available by prescription only.

If you take U-500 insulin, you will have to use a tuberculin syringe, which is designed for very small doses. When discussing your insulin dosage with a new health care provider—for example, if you are in the hospital—be sure to specify that you use U-500 insulin.

Mixing Insulins

Often people will be instructed to take a given amount of rapid-acting and a given amount of another type of insulin. NPH insulins mix easily with regular, insulin aspart, insulin lispro, and insulin glulisine. Please note that mixtures containing insulin aspart, insulin lispro, or insulin glulisine should be injected immediately after mixing and that these insulins should be mixed with NPH only under the advice and instruction of your doctor.

Additives

All insulins have added ingredients. These prevent bacteria from growing and help maintain a neutral balance between acids and bases.

In addition, intermediate- and long-acting insulins also contain ingredients that prolong their actions.

In some rare cases, the additives can bring on an allergic reaction.

Consumer Advice

Convenience: In selecting a pharmacy for purchasing your insulin and diabetes supplies, consider one that is close to you and open during the hours you want to shop.

Service: Those who order insulin by mail should consider the effect of shipping during hot summer months in the South or freezing winter months in the North. Ask the distributor how the bottles will be kept cool and inspect the bottles carefully when they arrive.

If you choose to use a local pharmacy, look for one that makes deliveries. This can be helpful when you are ill or busy.

Professional pharmacist: Use a store where a pharmacist is available, and get to know him or her. Make sure the pharmacist will take an interest in your medical needs, be available to answer questions, and tell you what problems to watch for.

Check labels: Don't just ask for "NPH insulin"; look at the full brand name, strength, and kind. In fact, you might bring a used bottle with you to make sure you get the same exact insulin you got before. Then, before you pay, check the insulin label to make sure you have the correct insulin and the correct directions.

Expiration date: Make sure you will be using all the insulin you are buying before its expiration date.

Quantity purchases: Inquire whether buying more than one bottle of insulin at a time would be cheaper than buying it by the bottle. Of course, keep the expiration date in mind.

Keep alert: On the rare occasion that insulin lots must be recalled, check to see if the control number on any of your bottles matches that of the recalled lot.

Price: It does pay to shop around for your insulin. Prices can vary by several dollars a bottle depending on where it's sold. (Note: Don't switch brands or types of insulin without your doctor's advice.) However, it is important to get all of your prescriptions at one pharmacy to ensure that there is one central source for all your medications.

Storage and Safety

Although manufacturers recommend storing your insulin in the refrigerator, injecting cold insulin can sometimes make the injection more painful. To counter that, many providers recommend storing the bottle of insulin you are using at room temperature. Most believe that insulin kept at room temperature will last about a month.

Remember, though, if you buy more than one bottle at a time—a possible money-saver—store the extra bottles in the refrigerator. Then, take out the bottle ahead of time so it is ready for your next injection.

Don't store insulin at extreme temperatures. Never store insulin in the freezer, direct sunlight, or the glove compartment of a car.

Before you use any insulin, especially if you have had it awhile, check the expiration date. Don't use any insulin beyond its expiration date. And examine the bottle closely to make sure the insulin looks normal before you draw the insulin into the syringe. If you use regular, insulin aspart, insulin lispro, insulin glargine, insulin glulisine, or insulin detemir, make sure the insulin is clear. Check for particles or discoloration of the insulin.

If you find any of these in your insulin, do not use it, and return the unopened bottle to the pharmacy for exchange or refund.

Insulin Commonly Used in the United States (as of September 1, 2006)

The information that follows is presented in this form:

- Generic name (Brand Name), form, Manufacturer, cloudy or clear

Rapid Acting

- insulin glulisine (Apidra*), analog, Sanofi-Aventis, clear
- insulin lispro (Humalog*), analog, Eli Lilly and Company, clear
- insulin aspart (NovoLog*), analog, Novo Nordisk, Inc., clear

Regular

- regular (Humulin R), human, Eli Lilly and Company, clear
- regular (Novolin R*, ReliOn [Wal-Mart], human, Novo Nordisk, Inc., clear

Intermediate-Acting

- NPH (Humulin N*), human, Eli Lilly and Company, cloudy
- NPH (Novolin N*, ReliOn [Wal-Mart], human, Novo Nordisk, Inc., cloudy

Long-Acting

- insulin detemir (Levemir*), analog, Novo Nordisk, Inc., clear
- insulin glargine (Lantus*), analog, Sanofi-Aventis, clear

Table 21.1. Human and Analog Insulin: Time of Action

Insulin	Onset	Peak (hours)	Duration (hours)
lispro, aspart, glulisine	<15 minutes	1–2	3–4
regular	0.5–1 hour	2–3	3–6
detemir	0.8–2 hours	relatively flat	up to 24
NPH	2–4 hours	4–10	10–16
glargine	2–4 hours	peakless	20–24

Mixtures

- 50% lispro protamine, 50% insulin lispro (Humalog Mix 50/50*), analog, Eli Lilly and Company, cloudy

- 70% NPH/30% regular (Humulin 70/30*), human, Eli Lilly and Company, cloudy

- 70% NPH/30% regular (Novolin 70/30*†, ReliOn [Wal-Mart]), human, Novo Nordisk, Inc., cloudy

- 75% lispro protamine/(NPL) 25% lispro (Humalog Mix 75/25*), analog, Eli Lilly and Company, cloudy

- 70% aspart protamine/30% aspart (NovoLog Mix 70/30*†), analog, Novo Nordisk, Inc., cloudy

*available in prefilled, disposable pens or cartridges for reusable pens. Apidra is available in pens, pumps, or infusion sets.

† Note difference between Novolin 70/30 (70% NPH/30% regular) and NovoLog Mix 70/30 (70% aspart-protamine/30% aspart).

Less Commonly Used Insulins

The information that follows is presented in this form:

- Generic name (Brand Name), form, Manufacturer

- regular (*Humulin R, u-500), human, Eli Lilly and Company

- 50% NPH/50% regular (Humulin 50/50), human, Eli Lilly and Company

*Humulin R, u-500 is used in the rare patient who is extremely insulin resistant. Otherwise in the United States, insulin is standardized to U-100 (100 units per cc). U-40 insulin is used in some countries and requires syringes designed for that strength of insulin.

Other Injectable Drugs

Byetta (exenatide)

Manufacturer: Amylin Pharmaceuticals and Eli Lilly and Company

For use only by those with type 2 diabetes who take metformin, a sulfonylurea, or both. Enhances insulin secretion in the presence of high blood glucose. Available in 5- and 10-microgram pens.

When to take: twice daily within 60 minutes before the morning and evening meals.

Side effects: nausea, vomiting, and hypoglycemia. May need to reduce sulfonylurea dose.

Symlin (pramlintide acetate)

Manufacturer: Amylin Pharmaceuticals

Prescription-only injectable drug for people with diabetes (type 1 or type 2) who take mealtime insulin. It helps keep after-meal glucose levels from going too high.

When to take: Take before a meal that has at least 250 calories or 30 g or more of carbohydrates. Cannot be mixed with insulin so it must be taken as a separate shot. When starting Symlin, it is recommended to reduce mealtime insulin by half.

Side effects: hypoglycemia and nausea. To limit nausea, start with a low dose.

Chapter 22

Insulin Delivery Devices

Chapter Contents

Section 22.1—Syringes, Pumps, Injectors, and More 226

Section 22.2—Can I Reuse My Insulin Syringe? 250

Section 22.3—Safe Needle Disposal 251

Section 22.1

Syringes, Pumps, Injectors, and More

Syringes

Today's syringes are smaller and have finer points and special coatings that work to make injecting as easy and painless as possible. When insulin injections are done properly, most people discover they are relatively painless.

Check with your doctor or diabetes educator and test several brands before you buy. Your equipment should suit your needs.

Questions to Ask

- Does the syringe dose match your insulin strength? If you take U-100 insulin, use U-100 syringes. (Note: All insulin syringes in the United States take U-100 insulin.)

- Does your syringe match your insulin dosage? If you take 30 units or less of insulin, you may use the 3/10-cc syringe. The 1/2-cc syringe may be used by those taking 50 units or less, and the 1-cc syringe is designed for those needing up to 100 units of insulin. If your insulin needs have been increasing, you might want to buy syringes that give you an opportunity to increase your dose if need be. For example, if you take 29 units, consider buying a 50-unit syringe. Using a syringe that more closely matches your dose may help you more accurately draw up your insulin. If you are changing the syringe you use, check dosage lines carefully. In some syringes, one line is equal to one unit of insulin, but in others, each line is equal to two units of insulin.

  - Be familiar with the gauge of your needle and what it means. The higher the gauge number of your needle, the thinner it is.

- Can you easily draw up your dosage in a particular syringe? Does the syringe barrel have the kind of markings you can read easily— or are they too close together? Does having a plunger that's a different color make it easier for you?

- Would a shorter needle be a better choice for you or your child with diabetes? Some syringes now have shorter needles that many people find to be more comfortable. However, the depth of the injection can change the rate of absorption. Ask your doctor or diabetes educator to assess whether this would be a good alternative to your current syringe.

- Does this brand come packaged as you prefer? Cost is another factor because many stores use insulin syringes as key sale items. Shop around for a good price, but ask yourself: Is giving up a good local pharmacist to save $2 at an out-of-the-way store worth the money?

You may be interested in reusing your syringes. Most manufacturers do not recommend this, and there may be some increased risk to patients (i.e., needle dullness causing discomfort, possible infection, or tissue damage). While this practice remains controversial, many patients reuse syringes without any problems. Once again, your health care team can advise you on the practice. (Pen needles, however, should always be removed immediately after use; when left in place, they create an open passage to the insulin chamber. The open passage may allow bacteria into the chamber or fluid to leak out, which may alter the strength of the insulin.)

And please, always follow appropriate guidelines when disposing of your syringes and lancets. Some states have very specific laws governing disposal of such items, while others lack guidelines. Even if no guidelines exist in your state, you should be considerate of those who could possibly come in contact with used syringes and lancets. Used syringes and lancets can be safely placed in a puncture-proof container that can be sealed shut before it is placed in the trash. (Label the container "USED SHARPS" with a heavy magic marker.)

Miscellaneous Syringe Products

- **BD Home Sharps Container (BD):** For disposal of used insulin syringes, pen needles, and lancets. Holds 70 to 100 syringes or 300 pen needles.

227

Table 22.1. Syringes (U-100) (continued on next page)

Manufacturer/ Distributor and Name	Needle Gauge	Needle Size	Packaging
1-cc syringes			
Abbott Laboratories			
Pharmacy brands*	29G	1/2"	100 (individually sterile wrapped)
Precision Sure Dose	29G	1/2"	100 (individually sterile wrapped)
Precision Sure Dose	28G	1/2"	100 (individually sterile wrapped)
Aimsco Ultra Thin II Short	30G	5/16"	100 (individually sterile wrapped)
Aimsco Ultra Thin II	29G	1/2"	100 (10 packs of 10 individually wrapped)
Aimsco Maxi Comfort	28G	1/2"	100 (10 packs of 10 individually wrapped)
Aimsco Uni Body Ultra II	29G	1/2"	100 (10 packs of 10)
Aimsco Uni Body Ultra II	28G	1/2"	100 (10 packs of 10)
Aimsco Safety Syringe	29G	1/2"	100 (individually sterile wrapped)
Allison Medical, Inc.			
SureComfort	31G	5/16"	100 (10 packs of 10)
SureComfort	30G	1/2"	100 (10 packs of 10)
SureComfort	30G	5/16"	100 (10 packs of 10)
SureComfort	29G	1/2"	100 (10 packs of 10)
SureComfort	28G	1/2"	100 (10 packs of 10)
BD SafetyGlide Syringe	29G	1/2"	100 (individually sterile wrapped) safety-engineered
BD Safety-Lok Syringe	29G	1/2"	100 (individually sterile wrapped) safety-engineered
BD Integra Syringe	29G	1/2"	100 (individually sterile wrapped) safety-engineered
BD Ultra-Fine II Short	31G	5/16"	100 (10 packs of 10)
BD Ultra-Fine	30G	1/2"	100 (10 packs of 10)
BD Micro-Fine IV	28G	1/2"	100 (10 packs of 10)
Can-Am Care Corp.			
Monoject Ultra Comfort Short	31G	5/16"	100 (individually sterile wrapped)
Monoject Ultra Comfort Short	30G	5/16"	100 (individually sterile wrapped)
Monoject Ultra Comfort 29	29G	1/2"	100 (individually sterile wrapped)
Monoject Ultra Comfort 28	28G	1/2"	100 (individually sterile wrapped)
Various store brands†	31G	5/16"	100 (individually sterile wrapped)
Various store brands†	30G	5/16"	100 (individually sterile wrapped)
Various store brands†	29G	1/2"	100 (individually sterile wrapped)
Various store brands†	28G	1/2"	100 (individually sterile wrapped)
Medicore Lite Touch	30G	5/16"	100 (10 packs of 10)
Medicore Lite Touch	29G	1/2"	100 (10 packs of 10)
Medicore Lite Touch	28G	1/2"	100 (10 packs of 10)

Table 22.1. Syringes (U-100) (continued on next page)

Manufacturer/ Distributor and Name	Needle Gauge	Needle Size	Packaging
1-cc syringes (continued)			
UltiMed, Inc.			
UltiCare, UltiSmooth	28G	1/2"	100 (10 packs of 10)
UltiCare, UltiFine	29G	1/2"	100 (10 packs of 10)
UltiCare, UltiThin	30G	1/2"	100 (10 packs of 10)
UltiCare, UltiThin Short	30G	5/16"	100 (10 packs of 10)
UltiCare, UltiFine II Short	31G	5/16"	100 (10 packs of 10)
UltiGuard, UltiFine**	29G	1/2"	100 (10 packs of 10) with disposable container
UltiGuard, UltiThin**	30G	1/2"	100 (10 packs of 10) with disposable container
UltiGuard, UltiThin Short**	30G	5/16"	100 (10 packs of 10) with disposable container
UltiGuard, UltiFine II Short**	31G	5/16"	100 (10 packs of 10) with disposable container
1/2-cc syringes			
Abbott Laboratories			
Pharmacy brands*	30G	3/8"	100 (individually sterile wrapped)
Pharmacy brands*	29G	1/2"	100 (individually sterile wrapped)
Precision Sure Dose	30G	5/16"	100 (individually sterile wrapped)
Precision Sure Dose	29G	1/2"	100 (individually sterile wrapped)
Precision Sure Dose	28G	1/2"	100 (individually sterile wrapped)
Aimsco Ultra Thin II Short	31G	5/16"	100 (10 packs of 10 individually wrapped)
Aimsco Ultra Thin II Short	30G	5/16"	100 (individually sterile wrapped)
Aimsco Ultra Thin II	29G	1/2"	100 (10 packs of 10 individually wrapped)
Aimsco Maxi Comfort	28G	1/2"	100 (10 packs of 10 individually wrapped)
Aimsco Uni Body Ultra II	29G	1/2"	100 (10 packs of 10)
Aimsco Uni Body Ultra II	28G	1/2"	100 (10 packs of 10)
Allison Medical, Inc.			
SureComfort	31G	5/16"	100 (10 packs of 10)
SureComfort	30G	1/2"	100 (10 packs of 10)
SureComfort	30G	5/16"	100 (10 packs of 10)
SureComfort	29G	1/2"	100 (10 packs of 10)
SureComfort	28G	1/2"	100 (10 packs of 10)
BD SafetyGlide Syringe	29G	1/2"	100 (individually sterile wrapped) safety-engineered
BD Safety-Lok Syringe	29G	1/2"	100 (individually sterile wrapped) safety-engineered
BD Ultra-Fine II Short	31G	5/16"	100 (10 packs of 10)
BD Ultra-Fine	30G	1/2"	100 (10 packs of 10)

Table 22.1. (continued) Syringes (U-100) (continued on next page)

Manufacturer/ Distributor and Name	Needle Gauge	Needle Size	Packaging
1/2-cc syringes (continued)			
BD Micro-Fine IV	28G	1/2"	100 (10 packs of 10)
Can-Am Care, LLC			
Monoject Ultra Comfort Short	31G	5/16"	100 (individually sterile wrapped)
Monoject Ultra Comfort Short	30G	5/16"	100 (individually sterile wrapped)
Monoject Ultra Comfort 29	29G	1/2"	100 (individually sterile wrapped)
Monoject Ultra Comfort 28	28G	1/2"	100 (individually sterile wrapped)
Various store brands†	31G	5/16"	100 (individually sterile wrapped)
Various store brands†	30G	5/16"	100 (individually sterile wrapped)
Various store brands†	29G	1/2"	100 (individually sterile wrapped)
Various store brands†	28G	1/2"	100 (individually sterile wrapped)
Medicore Lite Touch	30G	5/16"	100 (10 packs of 10)
Medicore Lite Touch	29G	1/2"	100 (10 packs of 10)
Medicore Lite Touch	28G	1/2"	100 (10 packs of 10)
UltiMed, Inc.			
UltiCare, UltiSmooth	28G	1/2"	100 (10 packs of 10)
UltiCare, UltiFine	29G	1/2"	100 (10 packs of 10)
UltiCare, UltiThin	30G	1/2"	100 (10 packs of 10)
UltiCare, UltiThin Short***	30G	5/16"	100 (10 packs of 10)
UltiCare, UltiFine II Short***	31G	5/16"	100 (10 packs of 10)
UltiGuard, UltiFine**	29G	1/2"	100 (10 packs of 10) with disposable container
UltiGuard, UltiThin**	30G	1/2"	100 (10 packs of 10) with disposable container
UltiGuard, UltiThin Short**	30G	5/16"	100 (10 packs of 10) with disposable container
UltiGuard, UltiFine II Short**	31G	5/16"	100 (10 packs of 10) with disposable container
3/10-cc syringes			
Abbott Laboratories			
Pharmacy brands*	30G	3/8"	100 (individually sterile wrapped)
Pharmacy brands*	29G	1/2"	100 (individually sterile wrapped)
Precision Sure Dose	30G	5/16"	100 (individually sterile wrapped) 1/2-unit barrel markings
Precision Sure Dose	30G	5/16"	100 (individually sterile wrapped)
Precision Sure Dose	29G	1/2"	100 (individually sterile wrapped)
Aimsco Ultra Thin II Short	31G	5/16"	100 (10 packs of 10 individually wrapped)
Aimsco Ultra Thin II Short	30G	5/16"	100 (10 packs of 10)
Aimsco Ultra Thin II	29G	1/2"	100 (10 packs of 10)

Table 22.1. Syringes (U-100) (continued)

Manufacturer/ Distributor and Name	Needle Gauge	Needle Size	Packaging
3/10-cc syringes (continued)			
Allison Medical, Inc.			
SureComfort	31G	5/16"	100 (10 packs of 10)
SureComfort	30G	1/2"	100 (10 packs of 10)
SureComfort	30G	5/16"	100 (10 packs of 10)
SureComfort	29G	1/2"	100 (10 packs of 10)
BD SafetyGlide Syringe	29G	1/2"	100 (individually sterile wrapped) safety-engineered
BD Safety-Lok Syringe	29G	1/2"	100 (individually sterile wrapped) safety-engineered
BD Ultra-Fine II Short	31G	5/16"	100 (10 packs of 10)
BD Ultra-Fine	30G	1/2"	100 (10 packs of 10)
BD Micro-Fine IV	28G	1/2"	100 (10 packs of 10)
Can-Am Care LLC			
Monoject Ultra Comfort Short	31G	5/16"	100 (individually sterile wrapped)
Monoject Ultra Comfort Short	30G	5/16"	100 (individually sterile wrapped)
Monoject Ultra Comfort 29	29G	1/2"	100 (individually sterile wrapped)
Various store brands†	31G	5/16"	100 (individually sterile wrapped)
Various store brands†	30G	5/16"	100 (individually sterile wrapped)
Various store brands†	29G	1/2"	100 (individually sterile wrapped)
UltiMed, Inc.			
UltiCare, UltiFine	29G	1/2"	100 (10 packs of 10)
UltiCare, UltiThin	30G	1/2"	100 (10 packs of 10)
UltiCare, UltiThin Short	30G	5/16"	100 (10 packs of 10)
UltiCare, UltiFine II Short	31G	5/16"	100 (10 packs of 10)
UltiGuard, UltiFine**	29G	1/2"	100 (10 packs of 10) with disposable container
UltiGuard, UltiThin**	30G	1/2"	100 (10 packs of 10) with disposable container
UltiGuard, UltiThin Short**	30G	5/16"	100 (10 packs of 10) with disposable container
UltiGuard, UltiFine II Short**	31G	5/16"	100 (10 packs of 10) with disposable container

*Sold at Brooks Pharmacy and CVS stores.

†Sold at Albertson's, Wal-Mart (ReliOn), Medicine Shoppe, Kroger, Leader, Longs, Kmart (Value Plus), Meijer, Sunmark, Brite Life, Good Neighbor, Family Pharmacy, Shop Rite, Preferred Plus, Winn Dixie.

**Sold under CareOne Rx brand at Stop & Shop, Giant, and Tops.

***Sold under Schnuck's brand.

- **BD Safe-Clip (BD):** Needle clipping and storage device. Clips and stores up to 1,500 needles. Portable.

- **BD Sharps Disposal by Mail (BD):** For disposal of insulin syringes, pen needles, and lancets by mail. Holds 70 to 100 syringes or 300 pen needles.

- **UltiGuard Syringes and Disposable Container Unit (UltiMed, Inc.):** UltiGuard syringe line combines 100 syringes with a syringe dispenser and disposal unit. UltiGuard syringe sizes include 1-cc, 1/2-cc, and 1/3-cc syringes in 29G, 30G, and 31G.

Pumps

The insulin pump is not an artificial pancreas (because you still have to monitor your blood glucose level), but pumps can help some people achieve better control, and many people prefer this continuous system of insulin delivery over injections.

Insulin pumps are computerized devices, about the size of a callbeeper, that you can wear on your belt or in your pocket. They deliver insulin in two ways: in a steady, measured, and continuous dose (the "basal" insulin) and as a surge ("bolus") dose, at your direction, around mealtime. Doses are delivered through a flexible plastic tube called a catheter. With the aid of a small needle, the catheter is inserted through the skin into the fatty tissue and is taped in place. In the newer products, the needle is removed and only a soft catheter remains in place.

If you use rapid-acting insulins, you can direct your pump to release a bolus dose close to mealtime to blunt the rise in blood glucose after a meal. If you use regular insulin, you would usually take the bolus dose about 30 minutes before you eat.

Because the pump also releases incredibly small doses of insulin continuously, this delivery system most closely mimics the body's normal release of insulin. Also, pumps deliver very precise insulin doses for different times of day, which in many instances are necessary to correct for situations like the dawn phenomenon, the rise of blood glucose that occurs in the hours before and after waking.

Many people have chosen the insulin pump because it enables them to enjoy a more flexible lifestyle. To use a pump, however, you must be willing to check your blood glucose frequently and learn how to make adjustments in insulin, food, and physical activity in response to those test results. (These things should be done with insulin injections as well!)

You'll want to check with your insurance carrier before you buy a pump and all the supplies. Although most carriers do cover these items, some do not. (Please note: Medicare now covers pumps and supplies for people with diabetes (both type 1 and type 2) who meet its eligibility requirements, including those regarding fasting C-peptide levels.)

If you are interested in using a pump, talk to your health care team to see if one might be appropriate for you. Your health care team can provide the forms and letters needed to start the process. Pump company representatives can also help with the process. You and your team can select the brand. For more information on the basic features of each pump see below.

Animas IR 1250

- **Manufacturer:** Animas Corporation
- **Size (inches):** 2.9 × 2.0 × 0.76
- **Weight:** 3.13 oz. with battery and full cartridge
- **Battery type/life:** (1) AA lithium (1.5 volt) 6–8 weeks; can use AA alkaline (shorter life)
- **Infusion set:** All commercially available sets with standard Luer connection.
- **Basal #:** Up to 12 basal rates in four personalized programs, plus a temporary basal rate; the duration of temporary rates can be adjusted from 30 minutes to 24 hours in 30-minute intervals; 10 percent increments.
- **Basal range:** 0.025–25 U/hr
- **Smallest bolus:** 0.05 units
- **Occlusion alarm:** Patented sensor and algorithm to detect occlusions promptly.
- **Over-delivery alarm:** Prevented by continuous self-tests, layers of redundancies, and other safeguards.
- **Near-empty alarm:** Yes. User set: 10, 20, 30, 40, or 50 units.
- **Warranty:** 4 years.
- **Features:** CarbSmart stores up to 500 food items from CalorieKing database on the pump. Personalize food lists. Calculator features for carbohydrates, blood glucose corrections, and insulin on board; large 992-mm display screen; reminders for time of day and blood glucose check, waterproof tested to 12 feet/24

hours; ezBolus, audio bolus, combo bolus, PrimeSmart step-by-step priming for safety; history includes boluses, TDD, alarm, prime, suspend, basal; precise basal rate adjustment in 0.025-unit increments; interchangeable color covers; 24-hour, toll-free customer service; PC download and upload with ezManager Plus. Available in Spanish.

CozMore Insulin Technology System

- **Manufacturer:** Smiths Medical MD, Inc.
- **Size (inches):** 3.2 × 1.8 × 0.9
- **Weight:** 3.3 oz. with battery and insulin
- **Battery type/life:** (1) AAA
- **Infusion set:** All standard luer-lock infusion sets.
- **Basal #:** Four programmable basal patterns. Temporary basal set in either percent or U/hr, for 30 minutes to 72 hours.
- **Basal range:** 0.05–35 U/hr
- **Smallest bolus:** 0.05 units
- **Occlusion alarm:** Yes
- **Over-delivery alarm:** Yes
- **Near-empty alarm:** Yes
- **Warranty:** 4 years.
- **Features:** All-in-one pump and blood glucose meter. Cozmonitor snaps onto the Cozmo pump and uses FreeStyle test strips. Blood glucose results are displayed on the Cozmo screen. Bolus calculation based on grams of carbohydrate eaten and personalized insulin to carb ratios. Continuously calculates insulin delivery from previous boluses to prevent overdosing. Special alerts (adjustable sound levels) for eight specific reminders can be set daily or for a one-time event. Up to 12 custom meal boluses. Waterproof. CoZmanager PC communications download programs to view all blood glucose, carbohydrate, bolus, and basal history. 24-hour toll-free help line; insurance reimbursement support; customer training plan; key pad lockout feature; screen backlight; personalized duration of insulin action.

DANA Diabecare II

- **Manufacturer:** Sooil Development

- **Size (inches):** 2.95 × 1.77 × 0.74
- **Weight:** 1.8 oz.
- **Battery type/life:** (1) 3.6-volt DC (2- to 3-month life)
- **Infusion set:** Proprietary sets, including cannula and needle, straight and angled insertion available in 27" and 43" inch tubing.
- **Basal #:** 24 basal rates plus temporary basal in 10 percent increments +/- 100 percent in 60-minute durations up to 12 hours.
- **Basal range:** 0.00–16 U/hr in 0.1-unit increments smallest bolus: 0.1 units
- **Occlusion alarm:** Yes
- **Over-delivery alarm:** Yes; internal cross checks.
- **Near-empty alarm:** Yes; audible alerts at 20 units.
- **Warranty:** 4 years.
- **Features:** Light, watertight, 300-U capacity. Icon-driven programming with PIN access. Pre-setting of meal-specific, default, or extended boluses. Bolus frequency may be limited and a "lock-out" feature can be enabled. Features selection of eight languages, 24-hour toll free technical support.

Medtronic MiniMed Paradigm 515/715

- **Manufacturer:** Medtronic Diabetes
- **Size (inches):** 3.0 × 2.0 × 0.8 (515 model); 3.6 × 2.0 × 0.8 (715 model)
- **Weight:** 3.5 oz. (515 with battery and full reservoir); 3.8 oz. (715 with battery and full reservoir)
- **Battery type/life:** 1 standard AAA battery
- **Infusion set:** 23" and 43" lengths: Quick set (6 mm or 9 mm; at-site disconnect); Sof-set (6 mm or 9 mm away-from-body disconnect); Silhouette (at site disconnect). Serters available for each set.
- **Basal #:** Three patterns; up to 48 basal rates per pattern; temporary basal rate (fixed rate or percent of basal pattern for 30 minutes to 24 hours in 30-minute increments).
- **Basal range:** 0.05–35.0 U/hr
- **Smallest bolus:** 0.1 units
- **Occlusion alarm:** Yes

235

- **Over-delivery alarm:** Yes. Integrated safety check motor with Bio-Pulse helps ensure no over-delivery.

- **Near-empty alarm:** Yes; by time or volume remaining (user-settable). Alarm repeats with 50 percent of user-defined, set-point remaining.

- **Warranty:** 4 years.

- **Features:** In-warranty upgrade program available. Model 515 reservoir size is 176 units; model 715 reservoir size is 176 or 300 units. Bolus Wizard Calculator uses blood glucose readings and food entries to estimate food and correction boluses; monitor wirelessly beams test results to pump; multiple bolus options include normal, square wave, dual wave, Easy Bolus; self-test features; downloadable memory includes approximately 90-day delivery history; web-based CareLink Therapy Management System charts A1C, blood glucose, carbohydrates, and other trends to optimize therapy; 24-hour toll-free help line; free video, educational materials, and insurance assistance.

MiniMed Paradigm 522/722

- **Manufacturer:** Medtronic Diabetes

- **Size (inches):** 3.0 × 2.0 × 0.8 (522 model); 3.6 × 2.0 × 0.8 (722 model)

- **Weight:** 3.5 oz. (522 with battery; 176 unit reservoir); 3.8 oz. (722 with battery; 300 unit reservoir)

- **Battery type/life:** (1) AAA

- **Infusion set:** 23" and 43" lengths; serters available: Quick set (6 mm or 9 mm; at-site disconnect); Sof-set (6 mm or 9 mm; away-from-body disconnect); Silhouette (13 mm or 17 mm; at-site disconnect). Sure-T (6 mm; steel needle; away-from-body disconnect; 23: length only; no serter available).

- **Basal #:** Three patterns; up to 48 basal rates per pattern; temporary basal rate (fixed rate or percent of basal pattern for 30 minutes to 24 hours in 30-minute increments).

- **Basal range:** 0.05–35.0 U/hr

- **Smallest bolus:** 0.1 units

- **Occlusion alarm:** Yes

- **Over-delivery alarm:** Yes. Integrated safety check motor with Bio-Pulse helps ensure no over-delivery.

- **Near-empty alarm:** Yes; by time or volume (user settable).
- **Warranty:** 4 years.
- **Features:** Displays readings every five minutes. Alarms alert user to low and high glucose levels. Bolus Wizard calculator suggests an appropriate bolus amount. Multiple bolus options include normal, square wave, and dual wave. The web-based CareLink Therapy Management System transforms downloadable data (up to 90 days) into charts, graphs, and tables to help optimize therapy. Works with the Paradigm REAL-Time Continuous Glucose monitoring kit (purchased separately) or as a stand-alone pump. Paradigm Pathway in-warranty upgrade program available. Low-battery warning; keypad lockout; and remote control.

OmniPod Insulin Management System

- **Manufacturer:** Insulet Corporation
- **Size (inches):** OmniPod: 1.6 × 2.4 × 0.7; Personal Diabetes Manager (PDM): 2.6 × 4.3 × 1.0
- **Weight:** 1.2 oz. OmniPod (with full reservoir); 4.0 oz. PDM (with batteries)
- **Battery type/life:** OmniPod batteries are integrated into each pod; PDM (2) AAA (up to 4 weeks life)
- **Infusion set:** Integrated infusion set with automated cannula insertion and no tubing.
- **Basal #:** Seven basal programs with up to 24 rates per program; temporary basal rates can be set in either percentage or U/hr for 30 minutes to 12 hours in 30-minute increments.
- **Basal range:** 0.05–30.0 U/hr
- **Smallest bolus:** 0.05 units
- **Occlusion alarm:** Yes
- **Over-delivery alarm:** Yes. Comprehensive safety systems monitor delivery.
- **Near-empty alarm:** Yes, with adjustable user settings.
- **Warranty:** 4 years.
- **Features:** OmniPod Insulin Management System consists of two components: OmniPod and PDM. Integrated infusion set; inserter and insulin reservoir; automated cannula insertion; no tubing. The PDM incorporates blood glucose monitoring technology;

a food database with 1000+ common food items; setup wizard; suggested bolus calculator; and memory to store 90 days of data or 5,400 records. Other features include insulin on-board calculation; adjustable reverse corrections; adjustable duration of insulin action; programmable reminders and alerts; personalized ratios/factors/targets/presets; adjustable auto off; LCD backlight; and child lock-out feature.

Insulin Pump Supplies

- **Accu-Chek Rapid-D (Disetronic/Roche Diagnostics):** Infusion set
- *Features:* 90° insertion angle, surgical stainless steel needle infusion set with 28-gauge needle. Works with all standard luer-lock pumps. 6-, 8-, and 10-mm needle lengths with 24", 31", or 43" tubing.

- **Accu-Chek Tender** (Disetronic/Roche Diagnostics): Infusion set
- *Features:* Infusion set 20° to 45° insertion set with a soft Teflon cannula. 13- and 17-mm cannula lengths. Works with all standard luer-lock pumps. Available with 24", 31", or 43" tubing.

- **Accu-Chek Tender Mini** (Disetronic/Roche Diagnostics): Infusion set
- *Features:* Infusion set 13-mm cannula version of the Tender infusion set. Works with all standard luer-lock pumps. Available with 24", 31", or 43" tubing.

- **Accu-Chek UltraFlex** (Disetronic/Roche Diagnostics): Infusion set
- *Features:* Infusion set 90° insertion angle with disconnect at site. Tapered Teflon cannula for quick insertion. Works with all standard luer-lock pumps. 8- and 10-mm cannula lengths with 24", 31", or 43" tubing.

- **Cleo 90** (Smiths Medical): Infusion set
- *Features:* Insertion needle automatically retracts into the insertion device, standard luer connection, transparent skin adhesive, Flex-Attach system for 360° site connection and rotation, straight in (90°) soft cannula in 6-mm and 9-mm lengths.

- **Quick Set with Quick-serter** (Medtronic Diabetes): Infusion set compatible with automatic insertion device
- *Features:* 90° insertion angle with 6-mm or 9-mm soft, tapered cannula. No overtaping needed; built-in adhesive; at-site disconnect. Available with 23" and 43" tubing. Can be inserted manually or via the Quick-serter insertion device.

- **Silhouette with Sil-sertable** (Medtronic Diabetes): Infusion set compatible with automatic insertion device
- *Features:* Variable insertion angle with 13 mm and 17 mm soft, tapered cannula. It flexes to conform to the body's twists and bends. No overtaping needed; built-in adhesive; at-site disconnect. Available with 23" and 43" tubing. Optional Sil-serter insertion device.

- **SimpleChoice Easy** (SpectRx, Inc.): Infusion set
- *Features:* 30° or "variable angled" infusion set for Medtronic MiniMed, Animas, and CozMore insulin pumps. Compatible with Sil-serter insertion device, 12-mm and 17-mm catheters, water-resistant tape, stable connect and release at insertion site, and small, portable packaging.

- **SimpleChoice Easy Pro** (SpectRx, Inc.): Infusion set
- *Features:* 30° or "variable angled" infusion set for use with Medtronic MiniMed Paradigm pump. Compatible with Sil-serter insertion device, 12-mm and 17-mm catheters, water-resistant tape, stable connect and release at insertion site, and small, portable packaging.

- **SimpleChoice Reservoir** (SpectRx, Inc.): Insulin cartridge
- *Features:* Disposable, single-use insulin reservoir for use with Medtronic MiniMed 504, 507, 507c, and 508 insulin pumps.

- **SimpleChoice Reservoir Pro** (SpectRx, Inc.): Insulin cartridge
- *Features:* Disposable, single-use insulin reservoir for use with Medtronic MiniMed Paradigm insulin pumps. 1.8-ml and 3-ml capacity.

- **SimpleChoice Twist** (SpectRx, Inc.): Infusion set
- *Features:* 90° insertion angle infusion set for use with Medtronic MiniMed, Animas, Roche, and CozMore insulin pumps. 360°

239

rotation at the site, compatible with Quick-serter insertion device, 5-mm and 9-mm catheters, and small, portable packaging.

- **SimpleChoice Twist Pro** (SpectRx, Inc.): Infusion set
- *Features:* 90° insertion angle infusion set for use with Medtronic MiniMed Paradigm insulin pumps. 360° rotation at the site, compatible with Quick-serter insertion device, 5-mm and 9-mm catheters, and small, portable packaging.

- **Soft-set with Sof-serter** (Medtronic Diabetes): Infusion set with automatic insertion device
- *Features:* Soft Teflon catheter remains in place after insertion. Disconnectable. Placement at optimal depth for insulin absorption.

- **Sure-T** (Medtronic Diabetes): Infusion set
- *Features:* 90° insertion angle with 6-mm fine steel needle. Low profile design. No overtaping needed; built-in adhesive. Tubing disconnects 4 inches from insertion site for easy detachment from pump.

Injection Aids and Alternatives

This category includes devices that make giving injections easier as well as syringe alternatives.

Talk with your doctor or diabetes educator about these kinds of products. Oftentimes, they will make sample products available to you before you make a purchase. You'll want to look for an item that is easy for you to use and is durable. Some items require more skill and dexterity on the part of the user than others, so try several before you buy.

Make sure that the injection aid you purchase works with your brand of syringe and needle length. Some injection aids have adapters for short needles.

Insertion aids: These devices accelerate needle insertion into the skin. Some even aid in pushing down the plunger. Most are spring-loaded and hide the needle from view.

Syringe alternatives: At present, this category includes insulin pens, infusers, and jet injectors.

Carrying around an insulin pen is like having an old-fashioned cartridge pen in your pocket—only instead of a writing point, there's a needle, and instead of an ink cartridge, there's an insulin cartridge. Disposable insulin pens are also available. These devices are convenient, accurate, and often used by people on a multidose regimen. Insulin cartridges can be prefilled with regular, NPH, insulin lispro, insulin aspart, insulin glulisine, or 70/30 or 75/25 premixed insulin. They are particularly useful for people whose coordination or vision is impaired or for people who are on the go.

If you are using a pen with NPH, 70/30, or 75/25, it is important to tip the pens back and forth at least 10 times to ensure the insulin is well mixed.

Infusers create "portals" into which you inject insulin. With an infuser, a needle or catheter is inserted into subcutaneous tissues and remains taped in place, usually on the abdomen, for 48–72 hours. The insulin is injected into it, rather than directly through the skin into the fatty tissue. Some people are prone to infections with this type of product, so be sure to discuss the necessary cleaning procedures with your health care team.

Jet injectors release a tiny jet stream of insulin, which is forced through the skin with pressure, not a puncture. These devices have no needles. However, they can sometimes cause bruising.

You will need to work with your health care team to ensure good blood glucose control while you adjust to one of these devices.

You'll want to ask manufacturers about training on the use of a jet injector, as well as how to clean it and how to troubleshoot. If jet injectors interest you, discuss their use with your health care team. Before buying, check to be sure your insurance covers jet injectors.

Injection Aids

- **Autoject, Autoject 2 (Owen Mumford, Inc.):** Spring-loaded plastic syringe holder positioned over skin. Press device against site, push button to insert needle automatically without seeing the needle penetrate the skin to deliver the dose.
- *Syringe Used:* Autoject: most 1-cc, 1/2-cc, and 3/10-cc plastic syringes; Autoject 2: Abbott Labs, Precision Sure Dose 1-cc, 1/2-cc; BD 1-cc, 1/2-cc
- *Needle Visible:* No
- *Adjustable Depth of Skin Penetration:* Yes
- *Comments:* Increases injection site alternatives.

241

- **BD Inject-Ease Automatic Injector (BD):** Spring-loaded plastic syringe holder positioned over skin. Insert syringe needle at the touch of a button. Designed for those who have anxiety about injections.
- *Syringe Used:* BD 1-cc, 1/2-cc, and 3/10-cc syringes
- *Needle Visible:* No
- *Adjustable Depth of Skin Penetration:* Yes (one adjustment)
- *Comments:* Increases injection site alternatives, 5-year guarantee.

- **Inject-Ease (Palco Labs, Inc.):** Spring-loaded plastic syringe holder designed to shield injection from view and reduce pain of injection. One-handed use helps reach alternative sites. Single-button activation inserts needle at proper angle.
- *Syringe Used:* BD 1-cc, 1/2-cc, and 3/10-cc syringes
- *Needle Visible:* No
- *Adjustable Depth of Skin Penetration:* Yes (two adjustments)
- *Comments:* Includes clear plunger cap to preload syringes.

- **Instaject (Medicool, Inc.):** Combination syringe injector and blood lancet device. Button-activated.
- *Syringe Used:* Most 1-cc, 1/2-cc, and 3/10-cc syringes
- *Needle Visible:* No
- *Adjustable Depth of Skin Penetration:* Yes
- *Comments:* Self-contained as injector. Lancet adapter only.

- **NeedleAid (Needle Aid, Ltd.):** Stabilizing guide for injection using an insulin pen or syringe. Broad base hides the needle, masks the sensation of needle entry, provides safety as needle is automatically withdrawn, and ensures injection at the proper angle and to proper depth. Insulin is injected manually. Needle is hidden from view to reduce fear and pain perception.
- *Syringe Used:* FlexPen, NovoPen 4, 3, 1.5, Junior, Novo Nordisk disposable pens; Lilly insulin pens; most 1-, 1/2-, 3/10-cc syringes
- *Needle Visible:* No
- *Adjustable Depth of Skin Penetration:* No
- *Comments:* Appropriate for needle phobia, visually impaired, beginning insulin users, and home care.

- **NovoPen 3 PenMate (Novo Nordisk, Inc.):** Attachment to conceal the needle to help reduce pain perception.
- *Syringe Used:* Fits NovoPen Junior and NovoPen 3 insulin-delivery systems
- *Needle Visible:* No

Insulin Pens

Autopen (Owen Mumford, Inc.): Automatic side injection for delivery from 1.5- or 3-ml insulin cartridge. Available in four models. The Autopen AN 3000 (1.5 ml) delivers 2–32 units in 2-unit increments. The Autopen AN 3100 (1.5 ml) administers 1–16 units in 1-unit increments. The AN 3800 (3 ml) delivers 2–42 units in 2-unit increments. The AN 3810 (3 ml) delivers 1–21 units in 1-unit increments; compatible with Eli Lilly 3-ml cartridge.

Humalog Mix 75/25 Pen (Eli Lilly and Company): Same as Humalog Pen (see below).

Humalog Pen 50/50 Pen (Eli Lilly and Company): Same as Humalog Pen (see below).

Humalog Pen (Eli Lilly and Company): Prefilled, disposable insulin delivery device that holds 3 ml (300 units) of insulin. Knob can be dialed forward or backward in single-unit increments until the number of units appears in the magnifying dose window. No refrigeration needed after first use.

Humulin 70/30 Pen (Eli Lilly and Company): Same as Humalog Pen.

Humulin N Pen (Eli Lilly and Company): Same as Humalog Pen.

Levemir FlexPen (Novo Nordisk): Prefilled disposable insulin pen that contains 3 ml (300 units) of Levemir. Dose steps are in 1-unit increments for up to 60 units. Large dialing window and audible clicks. Dose dial can be turned backward or forward for dose correction. Dose scale resets to "0" during injection. Designed for use with the NovoFine 30G or 31G disposable needles.

NovoLog FlexPen (Novo Nordisk): Prefilled disposable insulin pen that contains 3 ml (300 units) of NovoLog. Dose steps are in 1-unit increments. Large dialing window and audible clicks. Dose dial can be turned backward or forward for dose correction. Dose scale resets to zero after injection. Designed for use with the NovoFine 30G or 31G disposable needles.

NovoLog Mix 70/30 FlexPen (Novo Nordisk): Prefilled disposable insulin pen that contains 3 ml (300 units) of NovoLog Mix 70/30. Dose steps are in 1-unit increments. Has large dialing window and audible clicks. Dose dial can be turned backward or forward for dose correction. Dose scale resets to zero after injection. Designed for use with NovoFine disposable needles.

NovoPen Junior (Novo Nordisk): Insulin delivery in 1/2-unit increments. Provides precision dosing. Color-coded options provide flexibility for various types of insulin regimens. Designed for use with all Novo Nordisk PenFill 3-ml (300-unit) cartridges and NovoFine 30G or 31G disposable needles.

NovoPen 3 (Novo Nordisk): Durable insulin pen that delivers insulin in precise 1-unit increments from 2 to 70 units; large, easy-to-read dose indicator for dose setting; designed for use with all Novo Nordisk PenFill 3-ml (300-unit) insulin cartridges and NovoFine 30G or 31G disposable needles.

OptiClik (Sanofi-Aventis): Reusable insulin delivery device (insulin pen) for use with 3-ml Lantus (insulin glargine [rDNA origin] injection) cartridge (U-100) system or 3-ml Apidra (insulin glulisine [rDNA origin] injection) Cartridge U-100 system.

Pen Needles

BD Ultra-Fine Original Pen Needles (BD): BD's widest inner diameter insulin needle (29G, 12.7 mm [1/2"]) makes it easier to press the push button and expel insulin. BD-engineered point geometry and patented, micro-bonded needle lubricant for maximum comfort during injection. Recommended for people who take large doses or those with limited manual dexterity. Paper tab and inner shield are color-coded pink for easy size/gauge recognition. Can be used with all makes of diabetes pens and dosers sold in the United States.

BD Ultra-Fine III Mini Pen Needles (BD): Shortest, thinnest needle available (31G, 5 mm [3/16"]); eliminates the need to "pinch up." Can be safely used by both children and adults. BD-engineered point geometry and patented, micro-bonded needle lubricant for maximum comfort during injection. Paper tab and inner shield are color-coded purple for easy size/gauge recognition. Can be used with all makes of diabetes pens and dosers sold in the United States.

BD Ultra-Fine III Short Pen Needles (BD): BD's thinnest needle (31G, 8 mm [5/16"]). "Short" offers the best size for most adults. BD-engineered point geometry and patented, micro-bonded needle lubricant for maximum comfort during injection. Paper tab and inner shield are color-coded blue for easy size/gauge recognition. Can be used with all makes of diabetes pens and dosers sold in the United States.

NovoFine 30 Disposable (Novo Nordisk): 30G, 8-mm disposable insulin needles. Thin-wall technology and ultra-sharp points designed to help increase injection comfort. For use with the Novo Nordisk line of insulin-delivery systems.

NovoFine 31 Disposable (Novo Nordisk): 31G, 6-mm disposable insulin needles. Thin-wall technology and ultra-sharp points designed to help increase injection comfort. For use with the Novo Nordisk line of insulin-delivery systems.

Pen Needles (Can Am Care, LLC): Universal pen needles available in 50-count boxes in 29G/12-mm needles or 31G/8 mm. "Snap on" feature makes application to an insulin pen easier. Sold under various store brands.

UltiCare/Private Label Pen Needles (UltiMed, Inc.): UltiCare and private label pen needles available in mini (6 mm, 31G), short (8 mm, 31G), and original (12 mm, 29G). Compatible with all brand name insulin delivery pens. Available in 100- and 50-count boxes.

Unifine Pentips Pen Needles (Owen Mumford, Inc.): Ultra-thin lubricated pen needles compatible with all brand name reusable and disposable cartridge pens. 31G available in short (8-mm) and ultra-short (6-mm) lengths in boxes of 100. 29G available in original (12-mm) length. Available in 100-count box.

Other Delivery Systems

InnoLet (Novo Nordisk): A prefilled disposable insulin doser. Features include a large dial with easy-to-read numbers for dosage selection, dials forward and back to add and subtract units of insulin, support shoulder for consistent injection depth, and audible clicks for each unit of insulin set and delivered. Available in human insulin formulations Novolin 70/30, Novolin NPH, and Novolin R. Designed for use with NovoFine 30G or 31G disposable needles.

Innovo (Novo Nordisk): Insulin-delivery system. Insulin can be dosed in 1-unit increments, from 1 to 70 units. Large display features a memory function, which indicates when the last insulin dose was taken and the number of units of the last dose. In addition, a 6-second countdown display indicates when the entire insulin dose has been delivered and the needle may be withdrawn. Designed for use with all Novo Nordisk PenFill 3-ml insulin cartridges (including NovoLog; NovoLog Mix 70/30; and Novolin R, N, and 70/30) and NovoFine disposable needles.

Aids for People with Visual Impairments

There are several products designed to make injections easier for people who are visually impaired. Some products handle more than one task.

- **Nonvisual insulin measurement:** Helps you measure an accurate dose of insulin. Some "click" at each 1- or 2-unit increment of insulin.

- **Needle guides and vial stabilizers:** Help you insert the needle into the correct insulin vial for drawing up an injection.

- **Syringe magnifiers:** Enlarge the measure marks on a syringe barrel.

It's important to note that some of these aids fit only with specific brands of syringes, so check to be sure the product you want works with your syringe.

Syringe Magnifiers

BD Magni-Guide (BD): Syringe is slipped into curved channel of Magni-Guide. At opposite end, insulin vial is snapped into collar. Guide magnifies entire scale 1.7 times. Uses BD 1-cc, 1/2-cc, or 3/10-cc syringe. Available from BD; local pharmacies; Medicool, Inc.; Gemco Medical.

Syringe Magnifier (Apothecary Products): Clips firmly to syringe barrel. Easy calibration readings of 1/2-cc and 1-cc syringes. Uses any standard-size syringe. Available from local pharmacies.

Tru-Hand (Whittier Medical): Insulin bottle holder/syringe guide/ magnifier. Locks in syringes with direct guide into vial stopper. Magnifies entire scale. Insulin bottles can be changed without removing syringe from device. Uses BD, Terumo, and Monoject (all sizes). Available from local pharmacies.

Nonvisual Insulin Measurement

Count-a-Dose (Medicool, Inc.): Syringe-filling device. Empty syringe secured in easy-to-locate platform; slide moves syringe plunger to control insulin intake. Click wheel activates slide to ensure accurate dosage in 1-unit increments. Click heard and felt as wheel is rotated. Holds one or two bottles of insulin for mixed doses. Use with BD U-100, 1/2-cc Lo-Dose syringe. Available from Medicool, Inc., and Science Products.

Needle Guides and Vial Stabilizers

Holdease (Meditec, Inc.): Needle guide and syringe/vial holder. Unit holds syringe and insulin together in easy-to-handle unit while user fills syringe.

Inject Assist (Apothecary Products): Holds syringe and insulin bottle steady as syringe is filled. Preset dosage guide for accuracy. Holds U-100, U-80, and U-40 syringes.

Injection Safety Guard (Apothecary Products): Protects hands from accidental injection. Fits over the top of insulin vial, allowing user to place hands underneath safety guard and begin filling the syringe.

NeedleAid (NeedleAid, Ltd.): Stabilizing guide for injection using an insulin pen or syringe. The broad base indicates where the injection will be made. Ensures injection at the proper angle and to proper depth. Shields the needle for increased safety. Suitable for use with one hand. Insulin is injected manually. Needle is hidden from view to reduce needle fear and pain perception.

Vial Syringe Guides

Bioject Vial Adapter (Bioject, Inc.): Allows home-injection patients to reconstitute and/or draw up medication using any syringe with a standard luer-style tip. Does not contain sharps. Disposable in regular trash.

Vial Syringe Guide (Apothecary Products): Eliminates blunted or broken needles by safely connecting syringe to insulin bottle.

Voice Modules and Synthesizers

Accu-Chek Voicemate (Roche Diagnostics): Hand-held voice synthesizer incorporating an Accu-Chek Advantage blood glucose monitor and Accu-Chek Comfort Curve touchable test strips to integrate blood glucose monitoring and insulin identification. Talks user through blood glucose monitoring and reads bar-coded labels of Eli Lilly-brand insulin vials aloud. Also available with Spanish voice prompts. Special order through local pharmacies or durable medical equipment suppliers.

Digi-Voice Deluxe, Mini-DV (Captek/Science Products): Speech module plugs into data jack on LifeScan Basic and SureStep monitors. Talks user through self-test procedure. Repeat feature. Earphone, cassette instructions. Mini-DV is a smaller version of the Digi-Voice. Other languages available.

Jet Injectors

- **Advanta Jet** (Activa Brand Products, Inc.)
- *Size:* 6" × 1"
- *Weight:* 5.6 oz.
- *Features:* Standard model injector for the average skin type. Delivers from 1/2 to 50 units of all types and mixes of U-100 insulin; 14 comfort settings; 2-year warranty; tactile indents for visually impaired; lifetime benefit program available to all users; video included; toll-free help line; immediate service.

- **Advanta Jet ES** (Activa Brand Products, Inc.)
- *Size:* 6" × 1"
- *Weight:* 5.6 oz.
- *Features:* An extra strength Advanta Jet for those whose skin conditions require additional power from an injector; same features as Advanta Jet.

- **Gentle Jet** (Activa Brand Products, Inc.)
- *Size:* 6" × 1"
- *Weight:* 5.6 oz.

- *Features:* A lower-power model Activa Jet specifically designed for children and those with low levels of subcutaneous tissue; 2-year warranty; same features as Advanta Jet.

- **Medi-Jector Vision** (Antares Pharma, Inc.)
- *Size:* 6" × 1/2"
- *Weight:* 4.6 oz.
- *Features:* Compact, needle-free injector with needle-free syringes reusable for up to 21 injections. Delivers single or mixed doses from two to 50 units of all types of U-100 insulin; includes manual, video, carrying case, disposable adapters, and needle-free syringes. 30-day trial period; 2-year warranty.

- **Vitajet 3** (Bioject, Inc.)
- *Size:* 6" × 1"
- *Weight:* 5.6 oz.
- *Features:* Personal insulin system lets you draw up and inject needle-free. Adjustable pressure for comfort level. Crystal Check nozzle lets patients see insulin dose prior to injection and to verify complete delivery. Delivers from two to 50 units of insulin per injection. Carrying pouch; disposable nozzles, vial adapter, and training video; 2-year warranty; 30-day money-back guarantee.

Section 22.2

Can I Reuse My Insulin Syringe?

"Can I Reuse My Insulin Syringe?" © Michigan Diabetes
Research and Training Center (www.med.umich.edu/mdrtc).
Reprinted with permission.

For years, people with diabetes were told to use their insulin syringes only once and then discard them to reduce the risk of getting an infection. However, research indicates that the risk of getting an infection from reusing a syringe is really very small. In fact, many people safely give their shots through clothing. According to a recent statement from the American Diabetes Association, "for many patients it appears both safe and practical for the syringe to be reused if the patient so desires."

The advantages to reusing a syringe generally outweigh the disadvantages. The main disadvantage to reusing a syringe is the very slight risk of getting an infection. Even this slight risk can be reduced by following the guidelines for syringe reuse listed below. Another disadvantage is that the needle may become dull after several uses. Also, the lines that show the unit markings may wear off after a while, making it hard to draw up the right dose.

The most obvious advantage in reusing syringes is to save money. If a syringe that costs 20 cents each is used once a day, the total cost for a year is $73. If you take two injections a day and use a new syringe for each injection the cost is $146 a year, and if you take three injections a day and use a new syringe every time the cost is $219 a year. However, if you make each syringe last one week, you pay only about $10 a year. This means that, depending on how many injections of insulin you take, you could save from $63 to $209 a year by making each syringe last one week. Another reason for reusing plastic syringes is for the environment waste. Plastic syringes do not biodegrade, and since no one else should ever use your syringe, they can not be recycled either. Every syringe that is thrown away becomes garbage. So every time a syringe is reused there is a little less pollution in the world and a little more money in your pocket.

Guidelines for Reuse of Syringes:

If you decide to reuse your syringes, we suggest that you follow these American Diabetes Association (ADA) guidelines:

- Store the syringe to be reused (dry) at room temperature.

- Recap the needle to store it.

- If the needle touches anything except your skin at the injection site and the top of the insulin bottle, throw it away.

- Do not clean the needle with alcohol. (This wipes off the coating that makes it less painful to stick yourself.)

- Do not reuse a needle that is bent or dull.

- Never use anyone else's syringe and never let anyone else use yours.

Section 22.3

Safe Needle Disposal

From "Protect Yourself, Protect Others: Safe Options
for Home Needle Disposal," U.S. Environmental Protection
Agency (www.epa.gov), June 2006.

Why are used needles dangerous?

Used needles and lancets are dangerous because they can injure people, spread germs, and spread diseases such as HIV/AIDS, hepatitis, tetanus, and syphilis.

All needles should be treated as if they carry a disease. That means that if someone gets stuck with a needle, they have to get expensive medical tests and worry about whether they have caught a harmful or deadly disease. Be sure you get rid of your used needles the safe way to avoid exposing other people to harm.

Don't

- Throw loose needles in the garbage
- Flush used needles down the toilet
- Put needles in recycling containers

Do

- Use one of the recommended disposal methods in this chapter

Remember, not all of the options listed in this brochure are available in all areas. Check carefully to see what options are available near you—it could save a life!

Recommended Needle Disposal Options for Self-Injectors

Community Services National Services

Drop-off collection sites: Some communities offer collection sites that accept used needles—often for free. These collection sites may be at local hospitals, doctors' offices, health clinics, pharmacies, health departments, community organizations, police and fire departments, and medical waste facilities. Don't just leave your needles at one of these places—make sure the site accepts them, and be sure to put needles in the right place.

"Household hazardous waste" centers: Many communities have a disposal site already set up that accepts "household hazardous waste" items like used oil, batteries, and paint. In some places, these centers also accept used needles. If your area has a hazardous household waste center, be sure it accepts used needles before you go, and put needles in the right place when you drop them off.

Residential "special waste" pickup service: Some communities offer a "special waste" pickup service that collects your full container of used needles from your house. Some services require you to call for a pickup, while others collect used needles on a regular schedule.

How Can I Find More Information?

- Call your trash or public health department, listed in the city or county government (blue) pages in your phone book, to find out about programs available in your area.

252

- Check the Centers for Disease Control and Prevention (CDC) website at http://www.cdc.gov/needledisposal for a list of needle disposal rules in your state, along with needle disposal programs near you.

- Ask your health care provider or local pharmacist if they can dispose of your used needles, or if they know of safe disposal programs near you.

- Contact the Coalition for Safe Community Needle Disposal at (800) 643-1643 or visit the website at http://www.safeneed ledisposal.org to find out about safe disposal programs near you.

- Visit the Earth 911 website at http://www.earth911.org. You can go to the "Household Hazardous Waste" section of the site and search for a needle disposal program near you by entering your ZIP code.

- To learn more about rules regarding medical waste disposal, consult EPA's Medical Waste website at http://www.epa.gov/ epaoswer/other/medical.

National Services

Mail-back service: You can buy this service, which comes with a needle container and mail-back packaging. You fill the needle container with your used needles and mail it back in the package that is provided by the company. You have to pay for this service, and the price usually depends on the size of the container you pick.

For a list of mail-back service companies, contact the Coalition for Safe Community Needle Disposal at 800-643-1643 or visit the website at http://www.safeneedledisposal.org. When contacting a mail-back service company, be sure to ask them if the service is approved by the U.S. Postal Service.

Home needle destruction devices: Several manufacturers offer products for sale that allow you to destroy needles at home by burning, melting, or cutting off the needle—making it save to throw in the garbage. Prices vary depending on the product.

Before buying any medical device for home use, be sure it's been approved by the U.S. Food and Drug Administration (FDA).

For information pertaining to needle destruction devices, please see FDA's website at: http://www.fda.gov/diabetes/lancing.html#5.

Traveling with Needles

Don't forget, safe needle disposal is important no matter where you are—at home, at work, or on the road. Never place used needles in the trash in hotel rooms, on airplanes, or in public restrooms, where they could injure the cleaning staff or other people.

Sharps and Air Travel

Before you fly, check the Transportation Security Administration (TSA) website (http://www.tsa.gov) for up-to-date rules on what to do with your needles when you travel. To make your trip through airport security easier, make sure your medicines are labeled with the type of medicine and the manufacturer's name or a drug store label, and bring a letter from your doctor. Be prepared—ask about options for safe needle disposal when you make travel reservations, board an airplane, or check into a hotel or cruise ship. If you aren't sure that needle containers will be available where you're going, be sure to buy a needle container that you can take with you to hold your used needles until you can throw them away the right way.

Chapter 23

Oral Medications for Type 2 Diabetes

Chapter Contents

Section 23.1—Classes of Diabetes Medications 256

Section 23.2—Metformin May Offer Important
 Advantages 262

Section 23.3—Diabetes and Incretin-Based Therapy 264

Section 23.4—Stronger Heart Warning on Some Diabetes
 Drugs 267

Section 23.1

Classes of Diabetes Medications

With type 1 diabetes, the root of the problem is clear: the pancreas no longer makes any insulin.

Type 2 diabetes is not as easy to understand. If you're a typical person with type 2, your blood glucose levels are high because you have:

- a pancreas that doesn't make enough insulin to control your blood glucose;

- a liver that releases glucose inappropriately;

- muscle cells that don't easily take in glucose.

Here's how things worked before you developed type 2 diabetes:

You ate. Your blood glucose level started to go up. When your pancreas sensed the glucose, it sent out insulin. When your muscle and fat cells sensed the insulin, they let in glucose.

Your liver helped control your blood glucose levels, too. It tracked insulin levels in your blood. Under normal conditions, when there was insulin in your blood, glucose levels were high, too. Your liver would say, "Oh, good, the body just ate. No need for me to send out glucose."

But when you didn't eat for hours (like when you were sleeping), your liver sensed the lack of insulin in your blood. It then released glucose to keep your level from dropping too low.

But today you have type 2 diabetes. If your diabetes is typical, it began like this:

You'd eat. Your blood glucose levels would go up. Your pancreas would put out the right amount of insulin. But your muscle cells couldn't sense the insulin. So they didn't take in much glucose.

Your liver may have failed to sense the insulin, too. It would think, "Hmm, no insulin means the body hasn't eaten recently. I'd better put out glucose."

Your pancreas would sense that there was still a lot of glucose in your blood, so it would produce extra insulin. This may have gone on for years. When your system could no longer keep up with the extra demand, your blood glucose levels went up and stayed up. And you were told you had diabetes.

So type 2 diabetes involves several problems, and there are a number of potential solutions. One may be insulin injections. These can overcome insulin resistance. There are also five classes of diabetes pills. Each class acts in a different way to control blood glucose levels.

Many people benefit from taking two or more diabetes drugs, each of which addresses a different problem. Such combination therapy is so common that some drug companies now market combination pills.

No matter which diabetes pill you use, you'll still also need insulin—whether natural or injected—in your body to move glucose into your cells.

Oral Agents for Type 2

Alpha-Glucosidase Inhibitors

- *Generic Name:* Acarbose
- *Available as a Generic:* No
- *Brand Names:* Precose
- *Comments/Cautions:* Take with the first bite of each meal. Advantages: Acarbose and miglitol don't cause weight gain. Side Effects: Include gas, bloating, and diarrhea. To minimize side effects, ask your doctor about starting with a low dose and building up slowly. Who shouldn't take: Because these medications work directly in the intestines, people with inflammatory bowel disease, other intestinal diseases, or obstructions should not take them. Hypoglycemia: Acarbose and miglitol don't cause hypoglycemia (low blood glucose) when used alone. When used in combination with certain other diabetes medications, hypoglycemia can occur. In these cases, treat hypoglycemia with pure glucose, such as glucose tablets or gels. Acarbose and miglitol slow the breakdown of many other carbohydrates, so those carbs won't work as fast to treat a low blood glucose.

- *Generic Name:* Miglitol
- *Available as a Generic:* No
- *Brand Name:* Glyset

257

Biguanides

- *Generic Name:* Metformin
- Available as a Generic : Yes
- *Brand Name:* Glucophage
- *Comments/Cautions:* Advantages: Metformin doesn't promote weight gain and may improve cholesterol levels. Common Side Effects: When starting metformin are nausea, diarrhea, or loss of appetite, but these should subside within a few weeks. To minimize these side effects, take with meals. Lactic Acidosis: Is a rare but serious side effect of using metformin. This can occur in people whose kidneys don't function well or who have severe respiratory disease. Metformin may not be right for you if you have kidney problems, severe respiratory problems, if you are 80 or older, if you are taking medication for heart failure, if you have a history of liver disease, if you drink alcohol excessively, or if you are hospitalized. If you are scheduled for any medical testing or surgical procedures where you will have to fast or have an iodinated dye injected into your veins, you must inform the doctor in charge that you take metformin.

- *Generic Name:* Metformin (long-acting)
- *Available as a Generic:* Yes
- *Brand Name:* Glucophage XR

- *Generic:* Metformin (liquid)
- *Available as a Generic:* No
- *Brand Name:* Riomet

Meglitinides

These drugs could cause low blood glucose, but the risk is lower than with sulfonylureas.

- *Generic Name:* Nateglinide
- *Available as a Generic:* No
- *Brand Name:* Starlix
- *Comments/Cautions:* Take right before meals. Don't take either drug if you are skipping a meal.

- *Generic Name:* Repaglinide
- *Available as a Generic:* No
- *Brand Name:* Prandin

Sulfonylureas

These drugs can cause low blood glucose.

- *Generic Name:* Acetohexamide
- *Available as a Generic:* Yes
- *Brand Name:* Generic only

- *Generic Name:* Chlorpropamide
- *Available as a Generic:* Yes
- *Brand Name:* Diabinese
- *Comments/Cautions:* Longest-acting drug in this class, so it has a higher potential to cause low blood glucose. Not recommended for elderly patients and those with kidney disease. May cause low blood sodium levels, jaundice, and possibly skin rashes.

- *Generic Name:* Glimepiride
- *Available as a Generic:* Yes
- *Brand Name:* Amaryl
- *Comments/Cautions:* Probably safe in people with kidney disease, but a patient with kidney disease or who is elderly should be started on a lower-than-usual dose.

- *Generic Name:* Glipizide
- *Available as a Generic:* Yes
- *Brand Name:* Glucotrol
- *Comments/Cautions:* Appears to be more effective when taken a half hour before meals.

- *Generic Name:* Glipizide (long-acting)
- *Available as a Generic:* Yes
- *Brand Name:* Glucotrol XL
- *Comments/Cautions:* Can be taken with a meal.

- *Generic Name:* Glyburide
- *Available as a Generic:* Yes
- *Brand Name:* DiaBeta, Micronase
- *Comments/Cautions:* Intermediate-acting, but effects may last entire day.

- *Generic Name:* Glyburide (micronized)
- *Available as a Generic:* Yes
- *Brand Name:* Glynase PresTab

- *Comments/Cautions:* More readily absorbed than regular glyburide, so the strengths of the tablets are different.

- *Generic Name:* Tolazamide
- *Available as a Generic:* Yes
- *Brand Name:* Generic only
- *Comments/Cautions:* Patients with kidney disease may need smaller doses.

- *Generic Name:* Tolbutamide
- *Available as a Generic:* Yes
- *Brand Name:* Generic only
- *Comments/Cautions:* Short-acting sulfonylurea. Less potential for low blood glucose. May be good choice for elderly patients or those with liver or kidney disease. Not a good choice if you often forget to take pills.

Thiazolidinediones (TZDs)

- *Generic Name:* Pioglitazone
- *Available as a Generic:* No
- *Brand Name:* Actos
- *Comments/Cautions:* Often used in combination with other medications but may be used alone. Typically takes four to six weeks to see an effect on your blood glucose. May cause weight gain. Liver Tests: Another drug in this class (troglitazone, Rezulin) was taken off the market due to reports of serious liver damage. Your doctor may check your liver function prior to starting these medications and periodically throughout your treatment. Symptoms of liver damage include nausea, vomiting, abdominal pain, fatigue, loss of appetite, and dark urine. Call your doctor immediately if you experience any of these symptoms. Who Shouldn't Take: These medications may cause fluid retention or swelling. Therefore, they are not recommended for people with heart failure. Women: These medications may cause women who are not ovulating and haven't gone through menopause to begin ovulating again, enabling them to conceive. Also, oral contraceptives may be less effective when taking these medications. Women should discuss this issue with their doctors.

- *Generic Name:* Rosiglitazone
- *Available as a Generic:* No
- *Brand Name:* Avandia

Combination Pills

- *Generic Name:* Metformin + glyburide
- *Available as a Generic:* Yes
- *Brand Name:* Glucovance
- *Comments / Cautions:* See cautions for each drug in the combination, above.

- *Generic Name:* Metformin + rosiglitazone
- *Available as a Generic:* No
- *Brand Name:* Avandamet
- *Comments / Cautions:* See cautions for each drug in the combination, above.

- *Generic Name:* Metformin + glipizide
- *Available as a Generic:* No
- *Grand Name:* Metaglip
- *Comments / Cautions:* See cautions for each drug in the combination, above.

- *Generic Name:* Metformin + pioglitazone
- *Available as a Generic:* No
- *Brand Name:* Actoplus Met
- *Comments / Cautions:* See cautions for each drug in the combination, above.

- *Generic Name:* Rosiglitazone + glimepiride
- *Available as a Generic:* No
- *Brand Name:* Avandaryl
- *Comments / Cautions:* See cautions for each drug in the combination, above.

Section 23.2

Metformin May Offer Important Advantages

"While Most Diabetes Drugs Provide Similar Glucose Control, Some
Offer Important Advantages, New Review Shows," Press Release, Agency
for Healthcare Research and Quality, Rockville, MD, July 16, 2007.

Most oral medications prescribed for type 2 diabetes are similarly
effective for reducing blood glucose, but the drug metformin is less
likely to cause weight gain and may be more likely than other treatments to decrease so-called bad cholesterol, according to a report
funded by the Department of Health and Human Services' (HHS)
Agency for Healthcare Research and Quality (AHRQ). A version of the
analysis was posted in the online version of *Annals of Internal Medicine* on July 16, 2007.

The federally funded analysis is based on scientific evidence found
in 216 published studies. The report summarizes the effectiveness,
risks, and estimated costs for 10 drugs: acarbose (sold as Precose),
glimepiride (Amaryl), glipizide (Glucotrol), glyburide (Micronase,
DiaBeta, Glynase PresTab), metformin (Glucophage, Riomet, Fortamet),
miglitol (Glyset), nateglinide (Starlix), pioglitazone (Actos), repaglinide
(Prandin), and rosiglitazone (Avandia).

Type 2 diabetes is an increasingly common chronic disease that
occurs in people who have difficulty converting glucose (a sugar) into
energy. Blood glucose levels are high either because their cells are
resistant to insulin (a hormone that helps convert glucose into energy)
or because their pancreas does not produce enough insulin. Diabetes
can cause severe problems with the heart, eyes, kidneys, and nerves.
Obesity increases the risks of developing type 2 diabetes. From 1980
through 2005, the number of Americans diagnosed with diabetes
soared from 5.6 million to 15.8 million.

"As more people are diagnosed with type 2 diabetes and with the
growing array of treatment choices, this is a landmark review," said
AHRQ Director Carolyn M. Clancy, M.D. "This summary of scientific
evidence is not only an important tool for clinicians and patients seeking the most appropriate therapy, but it also points out in what areas we need more research to confront this disease."

As new classes of oral diabetes medications have become available, patients and clinicians have faced a growing list of treatment options. Earlier scientific reviews have highlighted some differences between medications, but AHRQ's new analysis is the first to summarize evidence on the effectiveness and adverse events for all approved oral medications commonly used in the United States for type 2 diabetes.

Diabetes patients typically are monitored with tests that check the percentage of hemoglobin A1C (HbA1c) in their blood. Checking for HbA1c is a more reliable indicator of chronic high blood sugar than checking blood glucose itself. According to the AHRQ review, most diabetes drugs offer about a one point absolute reduction in HbA1c. In those cases, for example, a diabetes patient's HbA1c might drop from eight to seven (with five being normal in patients who don't have diabetes). Nateglinide, acarbose, and miglitol lower HbA1c by about half that much. Combining diabetes medications, evidence shows, often works better at reducing HbA1c.

AHRQ's analysis of published studies, completed by the Agency's Johns Hopkins University Evidence-based Practice Center in Baltimore, also concluded:

- Metformin and acarbose do not increase weight among diabetes patients. Other diabetes drugs (glimepiride, glipizide, glyburide, pioglitazone, repaglinide, and rosiglitazone) have been shown to increase weight by an average of two pounds to 11 pounds.

- Blood levels of low-density lipoprotein, which is known as "bad cholesterol" because it may amplify risks of heart attack and stroke, consistently decrease (by about 10 milligrams per deciliter) in patients taking metformin and increase (by similar amounts) in patients taking rosiglitazone and pioglitazone.

- Pioglitazone and rosiglitazone cause a small but significant increase in high-density lipoprotein, often called "good cholesterol" because it promotes the breakdown and removal of cholesterol from the body.

- Glimepiride, glipizide, glyburide, and repaglinide are associated with hypoglycemia (when blood glucose levels go too low) more than other diabetes drugs.

- Metformin and acarbose are generally more likely than other diabetes medications to cause gastrointestinal problems such as diarrhea. Patients who used metformin alone were more likely to experience problems than those using the drug at a lower dose in combination with glimepiride, glipizide, glyburide, pioglitazone, or rosiglitazone.

• Patients who take pioglitazone and rosiglitazone have a greater risk of congestive heart failure compared with those who take metformin, glimepiride, glipizide, or glyburide. While one recent analysis raised the possibility that rosiglitazone may also increase heart attack risks, authors of the AHRQ analysis concluded that current evidence is not sufficient to make a meaningful assessment.

• More, longer studies are needed to understand the impact of oral diabetes drugs on patients' quality of life and whether longterm use causes adverse side effects or reduces important complications of diabetes such as heart disease and kidney disease. Additional research is needed to study interactions between the drugs and to compare therapeutic combinations of the drugs, according to the report.

Section 23.3

Incretin-Based Therapy

What is diabetes and what are the risks?

Diabetes is a disease characterized by levels of glucose (sugar) in the bloodstream that are higher than normal. Glucose is produced by the body from the foods that you eat. Insulin, which is produced by the pancreas (an organ located in your abdomen), takes the glucose from the bloodstream and carries it into your cells where it is used for energy.

Diabetes occurs when the pancreas does not produce insulin (called type 1, or insulin-dependent, diabetes) or when the body becomes resistant to the effects of insulin (called type 2, or non-insulin-dependent, diabetes). In either case, the result is that glucose does not enter the cells and builds up in the bloodstream.

How is diabetes treated?

Keeping blood sugar levels as close to normal is key to the prevention of a number of serious complications from diabetes including heart disease, stroke, kidney disease, blindness, and nerve damage.

Treatment for diabetes depends on the type of diabetes you have and how well you respond to treatments. To keep blood glucose levels as close to normal the most common treatment options are:

- lifestyle changes (diet and exercise);
- oral (by mouth) medications;
- insulin therapy.

Recently, attention has turned to a new line of therapy using substances called incretins for patients with type 2 diabetes. GLP-1 is an important incretin hormone that helps normalize blood sugar levels.

How do incretins affect blood sugar levels?

After you eat, your intestines release incretins such as GLP-1 into the bloodstream. GLP-1 affects blood sugar by:

- increasing insulin produced by your pancreas.
- decreasing glucagon release (Glucagon is a hormone that controls the release of glucose, or sugar, from the liver after meals.).
- promoting a feeling of fullness after a meal, which means that you eat less.
- slowing the emptying of the stomach's contents into the intestines, which lowers blood sugar levels after a meal.

What is incretin-based therapy?

There are two types of incretin-based drugs that improve the effects of GLP-1 in controlling blood sugar—incretin mimetics and DPP-IV inhibitors.

Incretin mimetics: An incretin mimetic, such as exenatide, copies (or mimics) the action of GLP-1 that is produced by your body. The difference between the two is that exenatide last about 10 hours, whereas GLP-1 only lasts about two minutes. Exenatide has been shown to improve diabetes control and to produce weight loss in most patients (average of six to ten pounds).

Exenatide is used alone or in combination with other antidiabetic drugs, such metformin and sulfonylureas. It may also be used with insulin. Exenatide is given by injection twice a day, usually before breakfast and dinner. The main side effect is nausea. There's also a possible risk of low blood sugar, especially when exenatide is used in combination with a sulfonylurea or insulin.

DPP-IV inhibitors: GLP-1 is rapidly inactivated in the blood by an enzyme called DPP-IV. DPP-IV inhibitors work by stopping the breakdown of GLP-1. This makes GLP-1 last longer and, in turn, increases the levels of GLP-1 in your blood. DPP-IV inhibitors (for example, sitagliptin and vildagliptin) may be used alone or in combination with other antidiabetic drugs. These drugs are fairly well tolerated by most patients, have minimal side effects and are usually not associated with weight changes during therapy.

When is incretin-based therapy used?

Both exenatide and DPP-IV inhibitors may be used in people with poorly controlled diabetes. They are used alone or in combination with other antidiabetic medications. Both lower blood sugar levels; in addition, exenatide may be associated with some weight loss.

What should you do with this information?

If you have type 2 diabetes and want to know if incretin-based therapy might benefit you, talk with your doctor. An endocrinologist, an expert in hormones, can help diagnose, treat, and manage your diabetes.

No matter what the treatment plan, managing your diabetes requires that you maintain a healthy lifestyle that includes a balanced meal plan and regular exercise. Follow your doctor's recommendations for treatment and regularly monitor your blood sugar to avoid high or low blood sugar.

Section 23.4

Stronger Heart Warning on Some Diabetes Drugs

"Stronger Heart Warning on Diabetes Drugs," Consumer Update, U.S. Food and Drug Administration (www.fda.gov), August 15, 2007.

The U.S. Food and Drug Administration (FDA) announced today that manufacturers of certain drugs approved to treat type 2 (non-insulin-dependent) diabetes have agreed to add the agency's strongest warning—"boxed"—on the risk of heart failure. This cardiovascular condition occurs when the heart does not adequately pump blood.

Which drugs will receive the warning?

The upgraded warning emphasizes that the following medications in the class of antidiabetic drugs (thiazolidinediones) may cause or worsen heart failure in certain patients:

- Avandia (rosiglitazone)
- Actos (pioglitazone)
- Avandaryl (rosiglitazone and glimepiride)
- Avandamet (rosiglitazone and metformin)
- Duetact (pioglitazone and glimepiride)

These drugs are used together with diet and exercise to improve blood sugar control in adults with type 2 diabetes.

What does the warning mean?

- Addresses FDA's concerns that despite the warnings and information already listed in the drug labels, these drugs are still being prescribed to patients without careful monitoring for signs of heart failure.

- Advises health care professionals to watch patients carefully for signs and symptoms of heart failure, including excessive, rapid

267

weight gain, shortness of breath, and swelling (edema), after starting drug therapy.

- Advises patients with these symptoms to seek immediate medical attention. Patients with questions about starting or continuing use of these drugs should contact their health care professional to discuss their individual treatment options.

- States that these drugs should not be used by people with serious or severe heart failure who have marked limits on their activity, are comfortable only at rest, or are confined to bed or a chair.

Concerns about Heart Failure vs. Heart Attacks

The boxed warning action above is a separate issue from FDA's ongoing review of Avandia and the possible increased risk of heart attacks (ischemic risks). But the two issues are often confused.

The agency's Endocrine and Metabolic Advisory Committee and Drug Safety and Risk Management Advisory Committee recommended on July 30, 2007, that Avandia continue to be marketed, and further recommended that information be added to the labeling for risk of heart attacks (ischemic risks). FDA also will provide updates on this issue as information becomes available.

Chapter 24

Flu Shots and Other Vaccinations Recommended for People with Diabetes

Influenza Vaccine

For people with diabetes, the flu can be more than aches and pains. It can mean longer illness, hospitalization, and even death because diabetes can make the immune system more vulnerable to severe cases of the flu. In fact, people with diabetes are almost three times more likely to die with influenza ("the flu") or pneumonia.

Flu vaccines are available at little or no cost—in fact, they're covered by Medicare, Part B—at doctors' offices, clinics, pharmacies, and grocery stores before flu season starts in the fall. But talk to your doctor first. Some people shouldn't get vaccinated.

Take Control

Consider the odds:

- During flu epidemics, deaths among people with diabetes increase 5–15%.

- People with diabetes are six times more likely to be hospitalized with flu complications.

This chapter includes "If You Have Diabetes, a Flu Shot Could Save Your Life" and an excerpt from Chapter 11 of "Take Charge of Your Diabetes," Centers for Disease Control and Prevention (www.cdc.gov/diabetes), 1998 and January 31, 2005.

- Each year, 10–30,000 deaths among people with diabetes are associated with influenza and pneumonia.

When you live with diabetes, you watch your diet, exercise, and see your doctor regularly. Now you can add an annual flu vaccine to your routine. It's one more way to stay in control of your diabetes.

Can a flu shot give me the flu?

No. Flu vaccines do not contain a live virus, so they cannot infect you. Some people coincidentally catch a cold a week or two following immunization. This is not a result of their flu vaccine—the flu is not a cold.

If you do develop the flu despite vaccination, the vaccine will still help prevent lower respiratory tract involvement or other secondary complications, reducing the risk of hospitalization and death.

Do I need a flu shot every year?

Yes. Flu viruses vary from year to year, so it's important to get a shot every year to be sure you're protected.

Does my family need flu shots too?

Yes. The flu is highly contagious, so immunizing your family not only keeps them healthy, it decreases your chances of catching the flu from your loved ones.

Pneumococcal Vaccine

Pneumococcal disease is a major source of illness and death. It can cause serious infections of the lungs (pneumonia), the blood (bacteremia), and the covering of the brain (meningitis). Pneumococcal polysaccharide vaccine (often called PPV) can help prevent this disease.

PPV can be given at the same time as the flu vaccine—or at any time of the year. Most people only have to take PPV once in their life. Ask your health care provider whether you might need a second vaccination. This vaccine is fully covered under Medicare Part B.

Tetanus/Diphtheria (Td) Toxoid

Tetanus (or lockjaw) and diphtheria are serious diseases. Tetanus is caused by a germ that enters the body through a cut or wound.

Diphtheria spreads when germs pass from one person to the nose or throat of others.

You can help prevent tetanus and diphtheria with a combined shot called Td toxoid. Most people get Td toxoid as part of their routine childhood vaccinations, but all adults need a Td booster shot every 10 years. Other vaccines may be given at the same time as Td toxoid.

Other Vaccines

You may need vaccines to protect you against other illnesses. Ask your health care provider if you need any of these:

- Measles/mumps/rubella vaccine

- Hepatitis A and B vaccines

- Varicella (chicken pox) vaccine

- Polio vaccine

- Vaccines for travel to other countries

How to Get More Information

Call the immunization program in your state health department to find out where you can get vaccinations in your area. Keep your vaccination records up-to-date so you and your health care provider will know what vaccines you may need.

For more information on vaccination, call the CDC National Immunization Hotline at 800-232-2522 (English) or 800-232-0233 (Spanish). These are toll-free calls.

Chapter 25

Complementary and Alternative Medical Therapies for Diabetes

The National Center for Complementary and Alternative Medicine, part of the National Institutes of Health, defines complementary and alternative medicine as a "group of diverse medical and health care systems, practices, and products that are not presently considered to be part of conventional medicine." Complementary medicine is used with conventional therapy, whereas alternative medicine is used instead of conventional medicine.

Some people with diabetes use complementary or alternative therapies to treat diabetes. Although some of these therapies may be effective, others can be ineffective or even harmful. Patients who use complementary and alternative medicine need to let their health care providers know what they are doing.

Some complementary and alternative medicine therapies are discussed below. For more information, talk with your health care provider.

Does acupuncture help with diabetes?

Acupuncture is a procedure in which a practitioner inserts needles into designated points on the skin. Some scientists believe that acupuncture triggers the release of the body's natural painkillers. Acupuncture

This chapter includes: "Complementary and Alternative Medical Therapies for Diabetes," National Diabetes Information Clearinghouse, National Institute of Diabetes and Digestive and Kidney Diseases, May 2004; and "Treating Type 2 Diabetes with Dietary Supplements," National Center for Complementary and Alternative Medicines, June 2005.

has been shown to offer relief from chronic pain. Acupuncture is sometimes used by people with neuropathy, the painful nerve damage of diabetes.

Can biofeedback be used by people with diabetes?

Biofeedback is a technique that helps a person become more aware of and learn to deal with the body's response to pain. This alternative therapy emphasizes relaxation and stress-reduction techniques. Guided imagery is a relaxation technique that some professionals who use biofeedback do. With guided imagery, a person thinks of peaceful mental images, such as ocean waves. A person may also include the images of controlling or curing a chronic disease, such as diabetes. People using this technique believe their condition can be eased with these positive images.

Does ginseng help lower blood glucose?

Several types of plants are referred to as ginseng but most studies of ginseng and diabetes have used American ginseng. Those studies have shown some glucose-lowering effects in fasting and post-prandial (after meal) blood glucose levels as well as in A1C levels (average blood glucose levels over a three-month period). However, larger and more long-term studies are needed before general recommendations for use of ginseng can be made. Researchers also have determined that the amount of glucose-lowering compound in ginseng plants varies widely.

Does vanadium help control blood glucose?

Vanadium is a compound found in tiny amounts in plants and animals. Early studies showed that vanadium normalized blood glucose levels in animals with type 1 and type 2 diabetes. A recent study found that when people with diabetes were given vanadium, they developed a modest increase in insulin sensitivity and were able to decrease their insulin requirements. Currently researchers want to understand how vanadium works in the body, discover potential side effects, and establish safe dosages.

Treating Type 2 Diabetes with Dietary Supplements

- There is limited scientific evidence on the effectiveness of dietary supplements as complementary and alternative medicine (CAM) for type 2 diabetes. The evidence that is available is not sufficiently strong to prove that any of the six supplements discussed in this section have benefits for type 2 diabetes or its complications. A possible exception may be the use of omega-3 fatty acids (essential nutrients that the body cannot make on its own but can obtain from foods such as fish and flaxseed, or from dietary supplements) to lower triglyceride levels.

- It is very important not to replace conventional medical therapy for diabetes with an unproven CAM therapy.

- To ensure a safe and coordinated course of care, people should inform their health care providers about any CAM therapy that they are currently using or considering.

- The six dietary supplements reviewed in this section appear to be generally safe at low-to-moderate doses. However, each can interact with various prescription medications, affecting the action of the medications. People with type 2 diabetes need to know about these risks and discuss them with their health care provider. Prescribed medicines may need to be adjusted if a person is also using a CAM therapy.

How is diabetes managed in conventional medicine?

In conventional medicine's approach, people with diabetes learn to keep their blood glucose in as healthy a range as possible. They do this by following a healthy food plan, being physically active, controlling their weight, and testing their blood glucose regularly. Some people also need to take medicine, such as insulin injections or prescription diabetes pills. When lifestyle changes and medical treatment are combined to rigorously maintain and control blood sugar in the normal range, this approach to managing type 2 diabetes minimizes the serious complications of the disease. This enables patients to lead productive, full lives.

It is important to note that conventional medicine is medicine as practiced by holders of M.D. (medical doctor) or D.O. (doctor of osteopathy) degrees and by their allied health professionals, such as nurses, physical therapists, and dietitians. Complementary and alternative medicine (CAM) is a group of diverse medical and health care systems, practices, and products that are not presently considered to be part of conventional medicine. Complementary medicine is used along with conventional medicine, and alternative medicine is used instead of conventional medicine. Some practitioners of conventional medicine are also practitioners of CAM.

What CAM therapies are discussed in this section?

There are many different CAM therapies used for diabetes and its complications, and it is beyond the scope of this chapter to discuss them all. Scientific information on any CAM therapy for diabetes can be sought in the PubMed database on the internet and from the National Center for Complementary and Alternative Medicine (NCCAM) Clearinghouse. Overall, there have been few rigorous studies published on the use of CAM approaches for type 2 diabetes. Most of the literature has looked at herbal or other dietary supplements, which reflects the tradition in certain whole medical systems of using plant products with claimed effects on blood sugar. This section focuses on six of the dietary supplements that people try for diabetes: alpha-lipoic acid (ALA), chromium, coenzyme Q10, garlic, magnesium, and omega-3 fatty acids.

What should people do if they have diabetes and are considering using any CAM therapy?

- People with diabetes need to be under the care of a physician or other health care provider who will help them learn to manage their diabetes and will monitor their efforts to control it. Dietitians and diabetes educators help people learn and use the skills needed for managing diabetes on a daily basis. In addition, many patients need to be under the care of one or more specialists, such as an endocrinologist, an ophthalmologist, or a podiatrist.

- It is important to not replace scientifically proven treatments for diabetes with CAM treatments that are unproven. The consequences of not following one's prescribed medical regimen for diabetes can be very serious, even life-threatening.

- People with diabetes should tell their health care provider about any dietary supplements or medications (prescription or over-the-counter) that they are using or considering. Prescribed medicines for diabetes and all other major health conditions may need to be adjusted if a person is also using a CAM therapy. Pharmacists can be another helpful source of information about dietary supplements.

- If they decide to use supplements, they should know that what they see on the label may not accurately reflect what is in the bottle. Some herbal supplements, for example, have been found to be contaminated; some tests of dietary supplements have found that the contents did not match the labeled dose on the bottle.

276

- Women who are pregnant or nursing, or people who are thinking of using supplements to treat a child, should use extra caution and be sure to consult their health care provider.

- If people with diabetes decide to use a supplement and notice any unusual effects, they should stop and contact their health care provider.

What is known about the safety and effectiveness of these six dietary supplements as CAM treatments for diabetes?

Below is a brief overview of each dietary supplement and what is known from research about its effectiveness and safety in use for diabetes.

Alpha-Lipoic Acid

Alpha-lipoic acid (ALA, also known as lipoic acid or thioctic acid) is a chemical that is similar to a vitamin. It is an antioxidant—a substance that prevents cell damage caused by substances called free radicals in a process called oxidative stress. High levels of blood glucose are one cause of oxidative stress. ALA is found in some foods, such as liver, spinach, broccoli, and potatoes. ALA can also be made in the laboratory. ALA supplements are marketed as tablets or capsules. It is theorized that ALA may be beneficial because of its antioxidant activity.

Summary of the research findings: The evidence on ALA for type 2 diabetes and obesity is limited. There are a number of small studies in animals and in people that have shown hints of beneficial effects. In a few of these studies, some possible benefit from ALA was seen in glucose uptake in muscle; sensitivity of the body to insulin; diabetic neuropathy; or weight loss. More research is needed to document whether there is any benefit of ALA in diabetes and to better understand how ALA works.

Side effects and possible risks: While ALA appears to be safe for the general adult population, people with diabetes need to know that ALA might lower blood sugar too much, and thus they would need to monitor their blood sugar level especially carefully. ALA may also lower blood levels of minerals, such as iron; interact with some medicines, such as antacids; and decrease the effectiveness of some anti-cancer drugs. Other possible side effects of ALA include headache, skin rash, and stomach upset.

Chromium

Chromium is a metal and an essential trace mineral. Chromium is found in some foods, such as meats, animal fats, fish, brown sugar, coffee, tea, some spices, whole-wheat and rye breads, and brewer's yeast. It is marketed in supplement form (capsules and tablets) as chromium picolinate, chromium chloride, and chromium nicotinate.

Summary of the research findings: There are scientific controversies about the use or need for chromium supplementation by persons with diabetes. First, it is difficult to determine, including through tests, whether a person has a chromium deficiency. Second, it is not known whether it is beneficial to take chromium supplementation in diabetes, and there is a lack of rigorous basic science studies to explain or support any evidence of benefit. In sum, there is not enough evidence to show that taking chromium supplements is beneficial for diabetes.

Side effects and other risks: At low doses, short-term use of chromium appears to be safe in the general adult population. However, chromium can add to insulin in its effects on blood sugar; this might cause the blood sugar to go too low. Possible side effects at low doses include weight gain, headache, insomnia, skin irritation, sleep problems, and mood changes. High doses can cause serious side effects. The foremost concern for persons with diabetes who use chromium is the development of kidney problems. Other possible effects include vomiting, diarrhea, bleeding into the gastrointestinal tract, and worsening of any behavioral or psychiatric problems.

Coenzyme Q10

Coenzyme Q10, often referred to as CoQ10 (sometimes written as CoQ10; other names include ubiquinone and ubiquinol) is a vitamin-like substance. CoQ10 helps cells make energy and acts as an antioxidant. Meats and seafood contain small amounts of CoQ10. Supplements are marketed as tablets and capsules.

Summary of the research findings: There have been few studies on CoQ10 and type 2 diabetes so far. The evidence is not sufficient to evaluate CoQ10's effectiveness as a CAM therapy in diabetes. CoQ10 has not been shown to affect blood glucose control. In theory, it might have use against heart disease in people with diabetes, but well-designed studies looking at heart disease outcomes are needed to answer this question.

Side effects and other risks: CoQ10 appears to be safe for most of the adult population. However, it may interact with and affect the action of some medicines, including warfarin (a blood thinner) and medicines used for high blood pressure or cancer chemotherapy. Other possible side effects of CoQ10 include nausea, vomiting, diarrhea, loss of appetite, and heartburn.

Garlic

Garlic (*Allium sativum*) is an herb used to flavor food. Garlic can also be processed and made into dietary supplements. In some cultures, garlic is used for medicinal purposes. The chemical in garlic of most interest for health purposes is allicin, which gives garlic its strong taste and odor. One of the claims for garlic is that the rates of certain diseases are lower in countries where lots of garlic is consumed. However, it has not been proven that garlic (and not some other factor such as lifestyle) is the reason.

Summary of the research findings: Few rigorous studies have been conducted on garlic, allicin, or both, for type 2 diabetes. In the studies that have been done, findings have been mixed. There are some intriguing basic science studies that suggest that garlic has some biological activities that are relevant to the treatment of diabetes. However, the evidence so far does not support that there is any benefit from garlic for type 2 diabetes.

Side effects and other risks: Garlic is safe for most adults. However, garlic appears to interact with various types of drugs. For example, when combined with certain medicines used to treat HIV/AIDS (non-nucleoside reverse transcriptase inhibitors and saquinavir), garlic may decrease their effectiveness. Garlic may also interact with and affect the action of birth control pills, cyclosporine, medications that are broken down by the liver, and blood thinners (including warfarin). Other possible side effects of garlic include an odor on the breath or skin, an allergic reaction, stomach disorders, diarrhea, and skin rash.

Magnesium

Magnesium is a mineral. Foods high in magnesium include green leafy vegetables, nuts, seeds, and some whole grains. Various supplemental forms of magnesium are marketed as tablets, capsules, or liquids.

Magnesium has many important functions in the body, including in the heart, nerves, muscles, bones, handling glucose, and making proteins. Low levels of magnesium are commonly seen in people with diabetes. Scientists have studied the relationship between magnesium and diabetes for a long time, but it is not yet fully understood.

Summary of the research findings: There have been a handful of studies on magnesium and type 2 diabetes, many of them very small in size and/or short in length and primarily looking at blood glucose control. The results have been mixed, with most finding that magnesium did not affect blood glucose control. Some studies have suggested that low magnesium levels may make glucose control worse in type 2 diabetes (interrupting insulin secretion in the pancreas and increasing insulin resistance) and contribute to diabetes complications. There is evidence that magnesium supplementation may be helpful for insulin resistance. Additional controlled studies are needed to establish firmly whether magnesium supplements have any role or benefit as a CAM therapy for type 2 diabetes.

Side effects and other risks: Magnesium supplements appear to be safe for most adults at low doses. High doses can be unsafe and cause such problems as nausea, diarrhea, loss of appetite, muscle weakness, difficulty breathing, extremely low blood pressure, irregular heart rate, and confusion. Magnesium can interact with and affect the action of certain drugs, including some antibiotics, drugs to prevent osteoporosis, certain high blood pressure medicines (calcium channel blockers), muscle relaxants, and diuretics ("water pills").

Omega-3 Fatty Acids

Omega-3 fatty acids (omega-3s, for short) are a group of polyunsaturated fatty acids that come from food sources, such as fish, fish oil, some vegetable oils (primarily canola and soybean), walnuts, wheat germ, and certain dietary supplements. As supplements, omega-3s are marketed as capsules or oils, often as fish oil.

Omega-3s are important in a number of bodily functions, including moving calcium and other substances in and out of cells, the relaxation and contraction of muscles, blood clotting, digestion, fertility, cell division, and growth. Omega-3s have been the subject of much media attention in recent years, because of studies finding they may be useful for such purposes as decreasing the rate of heart disease, reducing inflammation, and lowering triglyceride levels. Some countries and organizations have issued formal recommendations on the intake of omega-3s, through meals, oils, and possibly supplementation. Omega-3s have been of interest for diabetes primarily because having diabetes increases a person's risk for heart disease and stroke.

Summary of the research findings: Randomized clinical trials have found that omega-3 supplementation reduces the incidence of cardiovascular disease and events (such as heart attack and stroke) and slows the progression of atherosclerosis (hardening of the arteries). However, these studies were not done in populations that were at higher risk, such as those with type 2 diabetes.

With regard to studies on omega-3 supplementation for type 2 diabetes, there is somewhat more literature available than for most other CAM therapies for this condition. A 2001 analysis was published by the Cochrane Collaboration, of 18 randomized placebo-controlled trials on fish oil supplementation in type 2 diabetes. The authors found that fish oil lowered triglycerides and raised LDL cholesterol but had no significant effect on fasting blood glucose, HbA1c, total cholesterol, or HDL cholesterol. (The authors did not identify and include studies with cardiovascular outcomes, but noted that this is an area for further research.) Another analysis was published in 2004 by the Agency for Healthcare Research and Quality, of 18 studies on omega-3 fatty acids for a number of measurable outcomes in type 2 diabetes. This study confirmed virtually all the Cochrane authors' findings, except for finding no significant effect on LDL cholesterol.

Additional studies are needed to determine whether omega-3 supplements are safe and beneficial for heart problems in people with type 2 diabetes. Studies that look specifically at heart disease outcomes in this population are needed.

Side effects and possible risks: Omega-3s appear to be safe for most adults at low-to-moderate doses. There have been some safety questions raised about fish oil supplements, because certain species of fish can be contaminated with substances from the environment, like mercury, pesticides, or PCBs. Fish oil is on the list of food substances that the U.S. Food and Drug Administration considers to be "generally recognized as safe." How well a product is prepared is another factor for consumers to consider. Women who are pregnant or breastfeeding should not take fish oil supplements. Fish oil in high doses can possibly interact with, and affect the action of, certain medications, including blood-thinning drugs and drugs for high blood pressure. Potential side effects of fish oil include a fishy aftertaste, belching, stomach disturbances, and nausea.

What research is being done on CAM therapies for diabetes?

Recent NCCAM-supported research projects are studying the effects of:

- chromium on high blood glucose levels;
- yoga on glucose control in people at risk for diabetes;
- ginkgo biloba extract on diabetes medicines.

Also, researchers in the Diabetes Unit of NCCAM's Division of Intramural Research are studying many aspects of diabetes, including what happens when the body does not properly react to insulin. Recent clinical trials, for example, have been studying whether vitamin C supplements are beneficial in diabetes, the safety of glucosamine with respect to insulin resistance, and whether dark chocolate lowers blood pressure and improves insulin sensitivity. Diabetes Unit staff note that a category of functional foods containing polyphenols (also available as extracts) may be of benefit for further study in diabetes, including green tea (*Epigallocatechin gallate*), dark chocolate (epicatechin), and red wine (resveratrol).

Part Four

Diabetes Complications
and Co-Occurring Conditions

Chapter 26

Hypoglycemia

Hypoglycemia, also called low blood sugar, occurs when your blood glucose (blood sugar) level drops too low to provide enough energy for your body's activities. In adults or children older than 10 years, hypoglycemia is uncommon except as a side effect of diabetes treatment, but it can result from other medications or diseases, hormone or enzyme deficiencies, or tumors.

Glucose, a form of sugar, is an important fuel for your body. Carbohydrates are the main dietary sources of glucose. Rice, potatoes, bread, tortillas, cereal, milk, fruit, and sweets are all carbohydrate-rich foods.

After a meal, glucose molecules are absorbed into your bloodstream and carried to the cells, where they are used for energy. Insulin, a hormone produced by your pancreas, helps glucose enter cells. If you take in more glucose than your body needs at the time, your body stores the extra glucose in your liver and muscles in a form called glycogen. Your body can use the stored glucose whenever it is needed for energy between meals. Extra glucose can also be converted to fat and stored in fat cells.

When blood glucose begins to fall, glucagon, another hormone produced by the pancreas, signals the liver to break down glycogen and release glucose, causing blood glucose levels to rise toward a normal

"Hypoglycemia," National Diabetes Information Clearinghouse, National Institute of Diabetes and Digestive and Kidney Diseases, NIH Pub. No. 03-3926, March 2003.

level. If you have diabetes, this glucagon response to hypoglycemia may be impaired, making it harder for your glucose levels to return to the normal range.

Symptoms

Symptoms of hypoglycemia include the following:

- Hunger
- Nervousness and shakiness
- Perspiration
- Dizziness or light-headedness
- Sleepiness
- Confusion
- Difficulty speaking
- Feeling anxious or weak

Hypoglycemia can also happen while you are sleeping. You might cry out or have nightmares, find that your pajamas or sheets are damp from perspiration, or feel tired, irritable, or confused when you wake up.

Hypoglycemia: A Side Effect of Diabetes Medications

Hypoglycemia can occur in people with diabetes who take certain medications to keep their blood glucose levels in control. Usually hypoglycemia is mild and can easily be treated by eating or drinking something with carbohydrate. But left untreated, hypoglycemia can lead to loss of consciousness. Although hypoglycemia can happen suddenly, it can usually be treated quickly, bringing your blood glucose level back to normal.

Causes of Hypoglycemia

In people taking certain blood-glucose lowering medications, blood glucose can fall too low for a number of reasons:

- Meals or snacks that are too small, delayed, or skipped
- Excessive doses of insulin or some diabetes medications, including sulfonylureas and meglitinides (Alpha-glucosidase

inhibitors, biguanides, and thiazolidinediones alone should not cause hypoglycemia but can when used with other diabetes medicines.)

- Increased activity or exercise
- Excessive drinking of alcohol

Prevention

Your diabetes treatment plan is designed to match your medication dosage and schedule to your usual meals and activities. If you take insulin but then skip a meal, the insulin will still lower your blood glucose, but it will not find the food it is designed to break down. This mismatch might result in hypoglycemia.

To help prevent hypoglycemia, you should keep in mind several things:

- Your diabetes medications. Some medications can cause hypoglycemia. Ask your health care provider if yours can. Also, always take medications and insulin in the recommended doses and at the recommended times.

- Your meal plan. Meet with a registered dietitian and agree on a meal plan that fits your preferences and lifestyle. Do your best to follow this meal plan most of the time. Eat regular meals, have enough food at each meal, and try not to skip meals or snacks.

- Your daily activity. Talk to your health care team about whether you should have a snack or adjust your medication before sports or exercise. If you know that you will be more active than usual or will be doing something that is not part of your normal routine—shoveling snow, for example—consider having a snack first.

- Alcoholic beverages. Drinking, especially on an empty stomach, can cause hypoglycemia, even a day or two later. If you drink an alcoholic beverage, always have a snack or meal at the same time.

- Your diabetes management plan. Intensive diabetes management—keeping your blood glucose as close to the normal range as possible to prevent long-term complications—can increase the risk of hypoglycemia. If your goal is tight control, talk to your health care team about ways to prevent hypoglycemia and how best to treat it if it does occur.

Treatment

If you think your blood glucose is too low, use a blood glucose meter to check your level. If it is 70 mg/dL or below, have one of these "quick fix" foods right away to raise your blood glucose:

- 2 or 3 glucose tablets
- ½ cup (4 ounces) of any fruit juice
- ½ cup (4 ounces) of a regular (not diet) soft drink
- 1 cup (8 ounces) of milk
- 5 or 6 pieces of hard candy
- 1 or 2 teaspoons of sugar or honey

After 15 minutes, check your blood glucose again to make sure that it is no longer too low. If it is still too low, have another serving. Repeat these steps until your blood glucose is at least 70. Then, if it will be an hour or more before your next meal, have a snack.

If you take insulin or a diabetes medication that can cause hypoglycemia, always carry one of the quick-fix foods with you. Wearing a medical identification bracelet or necklace is also a good idea.

Exercise can also cause hypoglycemia. Check your blood glucose before you exercise.

Severe hypoglycemia can cause you to lose consciousness. In these extreme cases when you lose consciousness and cannot eat, glucagon can be injected to quickly raise your blood glucose level. Ask your health care provider if having a glucagon kit at home and at work is appropriate for you. This is particularly important if you have type 1 diabetes. Your family, friends, and co-workers will need to be taught how to give you a glucagon injection in an emergency.

Prevention of hypoglycemia while you are driving a vehicle is especially important. Checking blood glucose frequently and snacking as needed to keep your blood glucose above 70 mg/dL will help prevent accidents.

Hypoglycemia and Diabetes: Doing Your Part

Signs and symptoms of hypoglycemia can vary from person to person. Get to know your own signs and describe them to your friends and family so they will be able to help you. If your child has diabetes, tell school staff about hypoglycemia and how to treat it.

If you experience hypoglycemia several times a week, call your health care provider. You may need a change in your treatment plan:

less medication or a different medication, a new schedule for your insulin shots or medication, a different meal plan, or a new exercise plan.

Hypoglycemia in People Who Do Not Have Diabetes

Two types of hypoglycemia can occur in people who do not have diabetes: reactive (postprandial, or after meals) and fasting (postabsorptive). Reactive hypoglycemia is not usually related to any underlying disease; fasting hypoglycemia often is.

Symptoms

Symptoms of both types resemble the symptoms that people with diabetes and hypoglycemia experience: hunger, nervousness, perspiration, shakiness, dizziness, light-headedness, sleepiness, confusion, difficulty speaking, and feeling anxious or weak.

If you are diagnosed with hypoglycemia, your doctor will try to find the cause by using laboratory tests to measure blood glucose, insulin, and other chemicals that play a part in the body's use of energy.

Reactive Hypoglycemia

In reactive hypoglycemia, symptoms appear within four hours after you eat a meal. To diagnose reactive hypoglycemia, your doctor may ask you about signs and symptoms; test your blood glucose while you are having symptoms*; or check to see whether your symptoms ease after your blood glucose returns to 70 or above (after eating or drinking). *The doctor will take a blood sample from your arm and send it to a laboratory for analysis. A personal blood glucose monitor cannot be used to diagnose reactive hypoglycemia.

A blood glucose level of less than 70 mg/dL at the time of symptoms and relief after eating will confirm the diagnosis.

The oral glucose tolerance test is no longer used to diagnose hypoglycemia; experts now know that the test can actually trigger hypoglycemic symptoms.

Causes and treatment: The causes of most cases of reactive hypoglycemia are still open to debate. Some researchers suggest that certain people may be more sensitive to the body's normal release of the hormone epinephrine, which causes many of the symptoms of hypoglycemia. Others believe that deficiencies in glucagon secretion might lead to hypoglycemia.

A few causes of reactive hypoglycemia are certain, but they are uncommon. Gastric (stomach) surgery, for instance, can cause hypoglycemia because of the rapid passage of food into the small intestine. Also, rare enzyme deficiencies diagnosed early in life, such as hereditary fructose intolerance, may cause reactive hypoglycemia.

To relieve reactive hypoglycemia, some health professionals recommend taking the following steps:

- Eat small meals and snacks about every three hours
- Exercise regularly
- Eat a variety of foods, including meat, poultry, fish, or nonmeat sources of protein; starchy foods such as whole-grain bread, rice, and potatoes; fruits; vegetables; and dairy products
- Choose high-fiber foods
- Avoid or limit foods high in sugar, especially on an empty stomach

Your doctor can refer you to a registered dietitian for personalized meal planning advice. Although some health professionals recommend a diet high in protein and low in carbohydrates, studies have not proven the effectiveness of this kind of diet for reactive hypoglycemia.

Fasting Hypoglycemia

Fasting hypoglycemia is diagnosed from a blood sample that shows a blood glucose level of less than 50 mg/dL after an overnight fast, between meals, or after exercise.

Causes and treatment: Causes include certain medications, alcohol, critical illnesses, hormonal deficiencies, some kinds of tumors, and certain conditions occurring in infancy and childhood.

Medications, including some used to treat diabetes, are the most common cause of hypoglycemia. Other medications that can cause hypoglycemia include:

- salicylates, including aspirin, when taken in large doses;
- sulfa medicines, which are used to treat infections;
- pentamidine, which treats a very serious kind of pneumonia;
- quinine, which is used to treat malaria.

If using any of these medications causes your blood glucose to drop, your doctor may advise you to stop using the drug or change the dosage.

Drinking, especially binge drinking, can cause hypoglycemia because your body's breakdown of alcohol interferes with your liver's efforts to raise blood glucose. Hypoglycemia caused by excessive drinking can be very serious and even fatal.

Some illnesses that affect the liver, heart, or kidneys can cause hypoglycemia. Sepsis (overwhelming infection) and starvation are other causes of hypoglycemia. In these cases, treatment targets the underlying cause.

Hormonal deficiencies may cause hypoglycemia in very young children, but usually not in adults. Shortages of cortisol, growth hormone, glucagon, or epinephrine can lead to fasting hypoglycemia. Laboratory tests for hormone levels will determine a diagnosis and treatment. Hormone replacement therapy may be advised.

Insulinomas, insulin-producing tumors, can cause hypoglycemia by raising your insulin levels too high in relation to your blood glucose level. These tumors are very rare and do not normally spread to other parts of the body. Laboratory tests can pinpoint the exact cause. Treatment involves both short-term steps to correct the hypoglycemia and medical or surgical measures to remove the tumor.

Conditions Occurring in Infancy and Childhood

Children rarely develop hypoglycemia. If they do, causes may include:

- Brief intolerance to fasting, often in conjunction with an illness that disturbs regular eating patterns. Children usually outgrow this tendency by age 10.

- Hyperinsulinism, which is the excessive production of insulin. This condition can result in transient neonatal hypoglycemia, which is common in infants of mothers with diabetes. Persistent hyperinsulinism in infants or children is a complex disorder that requires prompt evaluation and treatment by a specialist.

- Enzyme deficiencies that affect carbohydrate metabolism. These deficiencies can interfere with the body's ability to process natural sugars, such as fructose and galactose, glycogen, or other metabolites.

- Hormonal deficiencies such as lack of pituitary or adrenal hormones.

Points to Remember

Diabetes-Related Hypoglycemia

- If you think your blood glucose is low, check it and treat the problem right away.

- To treat hypoglycemia, have a serving of a quick-fix food, wait 15 minutes, and check your blood glucose. Repeat the treatment until your blood glucose is above 70.

- Keep quick-fix foods in the car, at work—anywhere you spend time.

- Be careful when you are driving. Check your blood glucose frequently and snack as needed to keep your level above 70 mg/dL.

Hypoglycemia Unrelated to Diabetes

- In reactive hypoglycemia, symptoms occur within four hours of eating. People with this condition are usually advised to follow a healthy eating plan recommended by a registered dietitian.

- Fasting hypoglycemia can be caused by certain medications, critical illnesses, hereditary enzyme or hormonal deficiencies, and some kinds of tumors. Treatment targets the underlying problem.

Chapter 27

Diabetes and Obesity

Obesity and Diabetes: The Link

The prevalence of obesity is rising to epidemic proportions worldwide. In some countries, an astonishing half of the population is overweight. Being overweight or obese seriously increases an individual's risk of developing other health problems such as type 2 diabetes, coronary heart disease, and some forms of cancer.

In both men and women, the more overweight an individual is, the greater the risk of developing type 2 diabetes. The means by which excessive body fat causes type 2 diabetes is not clearly defined, but it appears that excess fat increases insulin resistance, raising blood glucose levels, and the likelihood of developing diabetes. People with a greater amount of abdominal fat have a higher risk of developing the condition.

Diabetes is the most preventable consequence of the obesity epidemic. Figures from the International Obesity Task Force (IOTF) suggest that up to 1.7 billion of the world's population are already at a heightened risk of weight-related non-communicable diseases such as type 2 diabetes and cardiovascular disease. In fact, the risk in type 2 diabetes appears to be mainly related to the increasing prevalence of overweight and obese individuals worldwide. One in three Americans born today is predicted to develop diabetes as a consequence of obesity.

Prevention

Although obesity can affect anyone, the main risk factors are high-fat, high-energy dense diets, and physical inactivity. Growing trends in many countries portray an 'obesogenic' society where the consumption of high-fat, high energy dense food is preferred to healthy fresh fruit and vegetables, and where the level of physical activity has dramatically been reduced or substituted by the constant usage of motor vehicles.

The importance of eating a low-fat, low-energy dense diet, and participating in physical activity should be greatly promoted in order to reduce the risks of becoming overweight or obese. If these habits are introduced in children, there is a greater chance that they will continue into adulthood.

Public health programs should stress the importance of a healthy environment, promoting improved diet and activity throughout communities. National programs should be especially aimed at improving education and awareness of obesity and its consequences in schools and in youth recreational centers.

Treatment Options

Weight management is the best strategy to prevent the development of type 2 diabetes. Research has shown that even a small amount of weight loss can decrease or slow down the risk of developing type 2 diabetes. Group therapy is advised to improve the psychological approach to weight loss, and to maintain an appropriate weight. Drugs to assist weight loss play a role in individuals for whom lifestyle changes alone may be insufficient to produce the required weight loss.

Facts

- The prevalence of obesity is rising to epidemic proportions at an alarming rate in both developed and developing countries worldwide.

- Overweight and obesity affect over half the world's population and diabetes rates are climbing to 20% of all adults in many Middle Eastern, Asian, and Latin American countries.

- Two thirds of adult men and women in the US with type 2 diabetes have a BMI of 27 or greater.

- It is estimated that at least half of all diabetes cases would be eliminated if weight gain in adults could be prevented.

- Non-communicable diseases such as diabetes now account for more deaths each year worldwide than AIDS.

- The twin epidemics of obesity and diabetes already represent the biggest public health challenge of the 21st century.

- Lifestyle interventions, including diet and moderate physical activity, can reduce the risk of developing type 2 diabetes by as much as 40–60%.

Chapter 28

Diabetes, Heart Disease, and Stroke

Having diabetes or pre-diabetes puts you at increased risk for heart disease and stroke. You can lower your risk by keeping your blood glucose (also called blood sugar), blood pressure, and blood cholesterol close to the recommended target numbers—the levels suggested by diabetes experts for good health. Reaching your targets also can help prevent narrowing or blockage of the blood vessels in your legs, a condition called peripheral arterial disease. You can reach your targets by choosing foods wisely, being physically active, and taking medications if needed.

If you have already had a heart attack or a stroke, taking care of yourself can help prevent future health problems.

What is the connection between diabetes, heart disease, and stroke?

If you have diabetes, you are at least twice as likely as someone who does not have diabetes to have heart disease or a stroke. People with diabetes also tend to develop heart disease or have strokes at an earlier age than other people. If you are middle-aged and have type 2 diabetes, some studies suggest that your chance of having a heart attack is as high as someone without diabetes who has already had one heart attack. Women who have not gone through menopause usually have less risk of heart disease than men of the same age. But women of all ages with

Excerpted from "Diabetes, Heart Disease, and Stroke," National Diabetes Information Clearinghouse, National Institute of Diabetes and Digestive and Kidney Diseases, NIH Pub. No. 06-5094, December 2005.

diabetes have an increased risk of heart disease because diabetes cancels out the protective effects of being a woman in her child-bearing years.

People with diabetes who have already had one heart attack run an even greater risk of having a second one. In addition, heart attacks in people with diabetes are more serious and more likely to result in death. High blood glucose levels over time can lead to increased deposits of fatty materials on the insides of the blood vessel walls. These deposits may affect blood flow, increasing the chance of clogging and hardening of blood vessels (atherosclerosis).

What are the risk factors for heart disease and stroke in people with diabetes?

Diabetes itself is a risk factor for heart disease and stroke. Also, many people with diabetes have other conditions that increase their chance of developing heart disease and stroke. These conditions are called risk factors. One risk factor for heart disease and stroke is having a family history of heart disease. If one or more members of your family had a heart attack at an early age (before age 55 for men or 65 for women), you may be at increased risk.

You can't change whether heart disease runs in your family, but you can take steps to control the other risk factors for heart disease listed here:

- Having central obesity. Central obesity means carrying extra weight around the waist, as opposed to the hips. A waist measurement of more than 40 inches for men and more than 35 inches for women means you have central obesity. Your risk of heart disease is higher because abdominal fat can increase the production of LDL (bad) cholesterol, the type of blood fat that can be deposited on the inside of blood vessel walls.

- Having abnormal blood fat (cholesterol) levels.

  - LDL cholesterol can build up inside your blood vessels, leading to narrowing and hardening of your arteries—the blood vessels that carry blood from the heart to the rest of the body. Arteries can then become blocked. Therefore, high levels of LDL cholesterol raise your risk of getting heart disease.

  - Triglycerides are another type of blood fat that can raise your risk of heart disease when the levels are high.

  - HDL (good) cholesterol removes deposits from inside your blood vessels and takes them to the liver for removal. Low levels of HDL cholesterol increase your risk for heart disease.

- Having high blood pressure. If you have high blood pressure, also called hypertension, your heart must work harder to pump blood. High blood pressure can strain the heart, damage blood vessels, and increase your risk of heart attack, stroke, eye problems, and kidney problems.

- Smoking. Smoking doubles your risk of getting heart disease. Stopping smoking is especially important for people with diabetes because both smoking and diabetes narrow blood vessels. Smoking also increases the risk of other long-term complications, such as eye problems. In addition, smoking can damage the blood vessels in your legs and increase the risk of amputation.

What is metabolic syndrome and how is it linked to heart disease?

Metabolic syndrome is a grouping of traits and medical conditions that puts people at risk for both heart disease and type 2 diabetes. It is defined by the National Cholesterol Education Program as having any three of the five traits and medical conditions listed in Table 28.1.

What can I do to prevent or delay heart disease and stroke?

Even if you are at high risk for heart disease and stroke, you can help keep your heart and blood vessels healthy. You can do so by taking the following steps:

Make sure that your diet is "heart-healthy": Meet with a registered dietitian to plan a diet that meets these goals:

- Include at least 14 grams of fiber daily for every 1,000 calories consumed. Foods high in fiber may help lower blood cholesterol. Oat bran, oatmeal, whole-grain breads and cereals, dried beans and peas (such as kidney beans, pinto beans, and black-eyed peas), fruits, and vegetables are all good sources of fiber. Increase the amount of fiber in your diet gradually to avoid digestive problems.

- Cut down on saturated fat. It raises your blood cholesterol level. Saturated fat is found in meats, poultry skin, butter, dairy products with fat, shortening, lard, and tropical oils such as palm and coconut oil. Your dietitian can figure out how many grams of saturated fat should be your daily maximum amount.

- Keep the cholesterol in your diet to less than 300 milligrams a day. Cholesterol is found in meat, dairy products, and eggs.

- Keep the amount of trans fat in your diet to a minimum. It's a type of fat in foods that raises blood cholesterol. Limit your intake of crackers, cookies, snack foods, commercially prepared baked goods, cake mixes, microwave popcorn, fried foods, salad dressings, and other foods made with partially hydrogenated oil. In addition, some kinds of vegetable shortening and margarines have trans fat. Check for trans fat in the Nutrition Facts section on the food package.

Make physical activity part of your routine: Aim for at least 30 minutes of exercise most days of the week. Think of ways to increase physical activity, such as taking the stairs instead of the elevator. If you haven't been physically active recently, see your doctor for a checkup before you start an exercise program.

Reach and maintain a healthy body weight: If you are overweight, try to be physically active for at least 30 minutes a day, most

Table 28.1. Metabolic Syndrome

Traits and Medical Conditions	Definition
Elevated waist circumference	Waist measurement of 40 inches or more in men and 35 inches or more in women
Elevated levels of triglycerides	150 mg/dL or higher or taking medication for elevated triglyceride levels
Low levels of HDL (good) cholesterol	Below 40 mg/dL in men and below 50 mg/dL in women, or taking medication for low HDL cholesterol levels
Elevated blood pressure levels	130 mm Hg or higher for systolic blood pressure or 85 mm Hg or higher for diastolic blood pressure, or taking medication for elevated blood pressure levels
Elevated fasting blood glucose levels	100 mg/dL or higher or taking medication for elevated blood glucose levels

Source: Grundy SM, et al. Diagnosis and Management of the Metabolic Syndrome: An American Heart Association/National Heart, Lung, and Blood Institute Scientific Statement. *Circulation.* 2005;112:2735–2752.

days of the week. Consult a registered dietitian for help in planning meals and lowering the fat and calorie content of your diet to reach and maintain a healthy weight. Aim for a loss of no more than one to two pounds a week.

If you smoke, quit: Your doctor can help you find ways to quit smoking.

Ask your doctor whether you should take aspirin: Studies have shown that taking a low dose of aspirin every day can help reduce the risk of heart disease and stroke. However, aspirin is not safe for everyone. Your doctor can tell you whether taking aspirin is right for you and exactly how much to take.

Get prompt treatment for transient ischemic attacks (TIAs): Early treatment for TIAs, sometimes called mini-strokes, may help prevent or delay a future stroke. Signs of a TIA are sudden weakness, loss of balance, numbness, confusion, blindness in one or both eyes, double vision, difficulty speaking, or a severe headache.

How will I know whether my diabetes treatment is working?

You can keep track of the ABCs of diabetes to make sure your treatment is working. Talk with your health care provider about the best targets for you.

"A" stands for A1C (a test that measures blood glucose control). Have an A1C test at least twice a year. It shows your average blood glucose level over the past three months. Talk with your doctor about whether you should check your blood glucose at home and how to do it.

- A1C target: Below 7 percent
- Blood glucose targets: Before meals—90 to 130 mg/dL; one to two hours after the start of a meal—less than 180 mg/dL

"B" is for blood pressure. Have it checked at every office visit.

- Blood pressure target: Below 130/80 mm Hg

"C" is for cholesterol. Have it checked at least once a year.

- Blood fat (cholesterol) targets: LDL (bad) cholesterol—under 100 mg/dL; triglycerides—under 150 mg/dL; HDL (good) cholesterol—for men above 40 mg/dL and for women above 50 mg/dL

Control of the ABCs of diabetes can reduce your risk for heart disease and stroke. If your blood glucose, blood pressure, and cholesterol levels aren't on target, ask your doctor what changes in diet, activity, and medications can help you reach these goals.

What types of heart and blood vessel disease occur in people with diabetes?

Two major types of heart and blood vessel disease, also called cardiovascular disease, are common in people with diabetes: coronary artery disease (CAD) and cerebral vascular disease. People with diabetes are also at risk for heart failure. Narrowing or blockage of the blood vessels in the legs, a condition called peripheral arterial disease, can also occur in people with diabetes.

Coronary artery disease: Coronary artery disease, also called ischemic heart disease, is caused by a hardening or thickening of the walls of the blood vessels that go to your heart. Your blood supplies oxygen and other materials your heart needs for normal functioning. If the blood vessels to your heart become narrowed or blocked by fatty deposits, the blood supply is reduced or cut off, resulting in a heart attack.

Cerebral vascular disease: Cerebral vascular disease affects blood flow to the brain, leading to strokes and TIAs. It is caused by narrowing, blocking, or hardening of the blood vessels that go to the brain or by high blood pressure.

Stroke: A stroke results when the blood supply to the brain is suddenly cut off, which can occur when a blood vessel in the brain or neck is blocked or bursts. Brain cells are then deprived of oxygen and die. A stroke can result in problems with speech or vision or can cause weakness or paralysis. Most strokes are caused by fatty deposits or blood clots—jelly-like clumps of blood cells—that narrow or block one of the blood vessels in the brain or neck. A blood clot may stay where it formed or can travel within the body. People with diabetes are at increased risk for strokes caused by blood clots.

A stroke may also be caused by a bleeding blood vessel in the brain. Called an aneurysm, a break in a blood vessel can occur as a result of high blood pressure or a weak spot in a blood vessel wall.

TIAs: TIAs are caused by a temporary blockage of a blood vessel to the brain. This blockage leads to a brief, sudden change in brain function, such as temporary numbness or weakness on one side of the body. Sudden changes in brain function also can lead to loss of balance, confusion, blindness in one or both eyes, double vision, difficulty speaking, or a severe headache. However, most symptoms disappear quickly and permanent damage is unlikely. If symptoms do not resolve in a few minutes, rather than a TIA, the event could be a stroke. The occurrence of a TIA means that a person is at risk for a stroke sometime in the future.

Heart failure: Heart failure is a chronic condition in which the heart cannot pump blood properly—it does not mean that the heart suddenly stops working. Heart failure develops over a period of years, and symptoms can get worse over time. People with diabetes have at least twice the risk of heart failure as other people. One type of heart failure is congestive heart failure, in which fluid builds up inside body tissues. If the buildup is in the lungs, breathing becomes difficult.

Blockage of the blood vessels and high blood glucose levels also can damage heart muscle and cause irregular heart beats. People with damage to heart muscle, a condition called cardiomyopathy, may have no symptoms in the early stages, but later they may experience weakness, shortness of breath, a severe cough, fatigue, and swelling of the legs and feet. Diabetes can also interfere with pain signals normally carried by the nerves, explaining why a person with diabetes may not experience the typical warning signs of a heart attack.

Peripheral arterial disease: Another condition related to heart disease and common in people with diabetes is peripheral arterial disease (PAD). With this condition, the blood vessels in the legs are narrowed or blocked by fatty deposits, decreasing blood flow to the legs and feet. PAD increases the chances of a heart attack or stroke occurring. Poor circulation in the legs and feet also raises the risk of amputation. Sometimes people with PAD develop pain in the calf or other parts of the leg when walking, which is relieved by resting for a few minutes.

How will I know whether I have heart disease?

One sign of heart disease is angina, the pain that occurs when a blood vessel to the heart is narrowed and the blood supply is reduced. You may feel pain or discomfort in your chest, shoulders, arms, jaw, or back, especially when you exercise. The pain may go away when you rest or take angina medicine. Angina does not cause permanent

303

damage to the heart muscle, but if you have angina, your chance of having a heart attack increases.

A heart attack occurs when a blood vessel to the heart becomes blocked. With blockage, not enough blood can reach that part of the heart muscle and permanent damage results. During a heart attack, you may have the following:

- Chest pain or discomfort

- Pain or discomfort in your arms, back, jaw, neck, or stomach

- Shortness of breath

- Sweating

- Nausea

- Light-headedness

Symptoms may come and go. However, in some people, particularly those with diabetes, symptoms may be mild or absent due to a condition in which the heart rate stays at the same level during exercise, inactivity, stress, or sleep. Also, nerve damage caused by diabetes may result in lack of pain during a heart attack.

Women may not have chest pain but may be more likely to have shortness of breath, nausea, or back and jaw pain. If you have symptoms of a heart attack, call 911 right away. Treatment is most effective if given within an hour of a heart attack. Early treatment can prevent permanent damage to the heart.

Your doctor should check your risk for heart disease and stroke at least once a year by checking your cholesterol and blood pressure levels and asking whether you smoke or have a family history of premature heart disease. The doctor can also check your urine for protein, another risk factor for heart disease. If you are at high risk or have symptoms of heart disease, you may need to undergo further testing.

What are the treatment options for heart disease?

Treatment for heart disease includes meal planning to ensure a heart-healthy diet and physical activity. In addition, you may need medications to treat heart damage or to lower your blood glucose, blood pressure, and cholesterol. If you are not already taking a low dose of aspirin every day, your doctor may suggest it. You also may need surgery or some other medical procedure.

How will I know whether I have had a stroke?

The following signs may mean that you have had a stroke:

- Sudden weakness or numbness of your face, arm, or leg on one side of your body

- Sudden confusion, trouble talking, or trouble understanding

- Sudden dizziness, loss of balance, or trouble walking

- Sudden trouble seeing out of one or both eyes or sudden double vision

- Sudden severe headache

If you have any of these symptoms, call 911 right away. You can help prevent permanent damage by getting to a hospital within an hour of a stroke. If your doctor thinks you have had a stroke, you may have tests such as a neurological examination to check your nervous system, special scans, blood tests, ultrasound examinations, or x rays. You also may be given medication that dissolves blood clots.

What are the treatment options for stroke?

At the first sign of a stroke, you should get medical care right away. If blood vessels to your brain are blocked by blood clots, the doctor can give you a "clot-busting" drug. The drug must be given soon after a stroke to be effective. Subsequent treatment for stroke includes medications and physical therapy, as well as surgery to repair the damage. Meal planning and physical activity may be part of your ongoing care. In addition, you may need medications to lower your blood glucose, blood pressure, and cholesterol and to prevent blood clots.

Chapter 29

Diabetic Vascular Disease

What Is Peripheral Vascular Disease?

An estimated 10 million Americans, most over age 50, suffer from peripheral vascular disease (PVD), or narrowing of peripheral (i.e., outside of the heart and brain) blood vessels or arteries (the latter is a subtype of PVD known as peripheral artery disease, or PAD). This narrowing reduces blood flow, depriving tissue and organs of oxygen and potentially causing tissue death. Symptoms of PVD most often occur in the legs and feet, resulting in pain, numbness, and other problems.

Over time, high blood sugars can cause blood vessel narrowing, and so can high cholesterol levels. High cholesterol can leave fatty deposits in the blood vessels (arteriosclerosis); sometimes these fatty deposits harden or combine with calcium deposits (creating plaques) and "hardening of the arteries" (arteriosclerosis) is the result.

Other potential causes include blood clots, inflammation of the arteries (vasculitis), infection, and traumatic injury to blood vessels.

Symptoms

The primary symptom of PVD is pain in the buttocks, calves, and/ or thighs (and less commonly, in the arms), particularly when standing, walking, or exercising. Other symptoms may include:

- Cold feet and legs;
- Numbness in feet and legs;
- Bluish or reddish skin coloring on the legs or feet;
- Leg wounds gets to your legs that won't heal properly;
- Calf and leg cramps when walking (i.e., intermittent claudication);
- A weak or absent pulse in the arms or legs.

Treatment and Prevention

In some cases, angioplasty (either with or without stenting) may be recommended to open blocked arteries. Angioplasty is a surgical procedure involving inserting a balloon-tipped catheter into an artery and expanding the balloon at the point of the arterial blockage to try and reopen it. A stent, a tube-shaped device designed to prevent reblockage of the artery, may be placed at the time of the angioplasty.

Another surgical option for PVD is an arterial bypass, in which a section of healthy artery (harvested from elsewhere in the patient's body) is grafted on to the diseased artery to bypass the blockage and shuttle blood around it. In some cases, a surgery may use a piece of synthetically produced artery for the bypass.

Pentoxifylline (Trental) and cilostazol (Pletal) are two medications that have been approved for the treatment of intermittent claudication by the U.S. Food and Drug Administration. Other drugs used to treat PVD by improving blood flow include antiplatelet drugs (e.g., aspirin), anticoagulants (e.g., warfarin), and thrombolytics. Thrombolytic drugs, also known as "clot busters," are only administered in a hospital setting.

To prevent PVD, patients with diabetes should focus on the basics for good diabetes control and heart health—controlling blood glucose and cholesterol levels, quitting smoking, maintaining good nutrition and exercise habits, and keeping blood pressure in a safe range.

Chapter 30

Foot Ulcers

What is a diabetic foot ulcer?

A diabetic foot ulcer is an open sore or wound that most commonly occurs on the bottom of the foot in approximately 15 percent of patients with diabetes. Of those who develop a foot ulcer, six percent will be hospitalized due to infection or other ulcer-related complication.

Diabetes is the leading cause of nontraumatic lower extremity amputations in the United States, and approximately 14 to 24 percent of patients with diabetes who develop a foot ulcer have an amputation. Research, however, has shown that the development of a foot ulcer is preventable.

Who can get a diabetic foot ulcer?

Anyone who has diabetes can develop a foot ulcer. Native Americans, African Americans, Hispanics, and older men are more likely to develop ulcers. People who use insulin are at a higher risk of developing a foot ulcer, as are patients with diabetes-related kidney, eye, and heart disease. Being overweight and using alcohol and tobacco also play a role in the development of foot ulcers.

"Your Podiatric Physician Talks About Diabetic Wound Care." Reprinted with permission from the American Podiatric Medical Association, www.apma.org. © 2007 APMA. All rights reserved.

309

How do diabetic foot ulcers form?

Ulcers form due to a combination of factors, such as lack of feeling in the foot, poor circulation, foot deformities, irritation (such as friction or pressure), and trauma, as well as duration of diabetes. Patients who have diabetes for many years can develop neuropathy, a reduced or complete lack of feeling in the feet due to nerve damage caused by elevated blood glucose levels over time. The nerve damage often can occur without pain and one may not even be aware of the problem. Your podiatric physician can test feet for neuropathy with a simple and painless tool called a monofilament.

Vascular disease can complicate a foot ulcer, reducing the body's ability to heal and increasing the risk for an infection. Elevations in blood glucose can reduce the body's ability to fight off a potential infection and also retard healing.

What is the value of treating a diabetic foot ulcer?

Once an ulcer is noticed, seek podiatric medical care immediately. Foot ulcers in patients with diabetes should be treated for several reasons such as reducing the risk of infection and amputation, improving function and quality of life, and reducing health care costs.

How should a diabetic foot ulcer be treated?

The primary goal in the treatment of foot ulcers is to obtain healing as soon as possible. The faster the healing, the less chance for an infection.

There are several key factors in the appropriate treatment of a diabetic foot ulcer:

- Prevention of infection
- Taking the pressure off the area, called "off-loading"
- Removing dead skin and tissue, called "debridement"
- Applying medication or dressings to the ulcer
- Managing blood glucose and other health problems

Not all ulcers are infected; however if your podiatric physician diagnoses an infection, a treatment program of antibiotics, wound care, and possibly hospitalization will be necessary.

There are several important factors to keep an ulcer from becoming infected:

- Keep blood glucose levels under tight control.
- Keep the ulcer clean and bandaged.
- Cleanse the wound daily, using a wound dressing or bandage.
- Do not walk barefoot.

For optimum healing, ulcers, especially those on the bottom of the foot, must be "off-loaded." Patients may be asked to wear special footgear, or a brace, specialized castings, or use a wheelchair or crutches. These devices will reduce the pressure and irritation to the ulcer area and help to speed the healing process.

The science of wound care has advanced significantly over the past ten years. The old thought of "let the air get at it" is now known to be harmful to healing. We know that wounds and ulcers heal faster, with a lower risk of infection, if they are kept covered and moist. The use of full strength Betadine, peroxide, whirlpools and soaking are not recommended, as this could lead to further complications.

Appropriate wound management includes the use of dressings and topically applied medications. These range from normal saline to advanced products, such as growth factors, ulcer dressings, and skin substitutes that have been shown to be highly effective in healing foot ulcers.

For a wound to heal there must be adequate circulation to the ulcerated area. Your podiatrist can determine circulation levels with noninvasive tests.

Controlling blood glucose: Tightly controlling blood glucose is of the utmost importance during the treatment of a diabetic foot ulcer. Working closely with a medical doctor or endocrinologist to accomplish this will enhance healing and reduce the risk of complications.

Surgical options: A majority of noninfected foot ulcers are treated without surgery; however, when this fails, surgical management may be appropriate. Examples of surgical care to remove pressure on the affected area include shaving or excision of bone(s) and the correction of various deformities, such as hammertoes, bunions, or bony "bumps."

Healing factors: Healing time depends on a variety of factors, such as wound size and location, pressure on the wound from walking or standing, swelling, circulation, blood glucose levels, wound care, and what is being applied to the wound. Healing may occur within weeks or require several months.

311

How can a foot ulcer be prevented?

The best way to treat a diabetic foot ulcer is to prevent its development in the first place. Recommended guidelines include seeing a podiatrist on a regular basis. He or she can determine if you are at high risk for developing a foot ulcer and implement strategies for prevention.

You are at high risk if you:

- have neuropathy,
- have poor circulation,
- have a foot deformity (for example, bunion, hammer toe),
- wear inappropriate shoes,
- have uncontrolled blood sugar.

Reducing additional risk factors, such as smoking, drinking alcohol, high cholesterol, and elevated blood glucose are important in the prevention and treatment of a diabetic foot ulcer. Wearing the appropriate shoes and socks will go a long way in reducing risks. Your podiatric physician can provide guidance in selecting the proper shoes.

Learning how to check your feet is crucial in noticing a potential problem as early as possible. Inspect your feet every day—especially between the toes and the sole—for cuts, bruises, cracks, blisters, redness, ulcers, and any sign of abnormality. Each time you visit a health care provider, remove your shoes and socks so your feet can be examined. Any problems that are discovered should be reported to your podiatrist as soon as possible, no matter how "simple" it may seem to you.

The key to successful wound healing is regular podiatric medical care to ensure the following "gold standard" of care:

- Lowering blood sugar
- Appropriate debridement of wounds
- Treating any infection
- Reducing friction and pressure
- Restoring adequate blood flow

The old saying, "an ounce of prevention is worth a pound of cure" was never as true as it is when preventing a diabetic foot ulcer.

Diabetes Tips from the American Podiatric Medical Association (PMA)

If You Have Diabetes Already...Do

- Wash feet daily. Using mild soap and lukewarm water, wash your feet in the mornings or before bed each evening. Dry carefully with a soft towel, especially between the toes, and dust your feet with talcum powder to wick away moisture. If the skin is dry, use a good moisturizing cream daily, but avoid getting it between the toes.

- Inspect feet and toes daily. Check your feet every day for cuts, bruises, sores, or changes to the toenails, such as thickening or discoloration. If age or other factors hamper self-inspection, ask someone to help you, or use a mirror.

- Lose weight. People with diabetes are commonly overweight, which nearly doubles the risk of complications.

- Wear thick, soft socks. Socks made of an acrylic blend are well suited, but avoid mended socks or those with seams, which could rub to cause blisters or other skin injuries.

- Stop smoking. Tobacco can contribute to circulatory problems, which can be especially troublesome in patients with diabetes.

- Cut toenails straight across. Never cut into the corners, or taper, which could trigger an ingrown toenail. Use an emery board to gently file away sharp corners or snags. If your nails are hard to trim, ask your podiatrist for assistance.

- Exercise. As a means to keep weight down and improve circulation, walking is one of the best all-around exercises for the diabetic patient. Walking is also an excellent conditioner for your feet. Be sure to wear appropriate athletic shoes when exercising. Ask your podiatric physician what's best for you.

- See your podiatric physician. Regular checkups by your podiatric physician—at least annually—are the best way to ensure that your feet remain healthy.

- Be properly measured and fitted every time you buy new shoes. Shoes are of supreme importance to diabetes sufferers because poorly fitted shoes are involved in as many as half of the problems that lead to amputations. Because foot size and shape may change over time, everyone should have their feet measured by an experienced shoe fitter whenever they buy a new pair of shoes.

New shoes should be comfortable at the time they're purchased and should not require a "break-in" period, though it's a good idea to wear them for short periods of time at first. Shoes should have leather or canvas uppers, fit both the length and width of the foot, leave room for toes to wiggle freely, and be cushioned and sturdy.

- Don't go barefoot. Not even in your own home. Barefoot walking outside is particularly dangerous because of the possibility of cuts, falls, and infection. When at home, wear slippers. Never go barefoot.

- Don't wear high heels, sandals, and shoes with pointed toes. These types of footwear can put undue pressure on parts of the foot and contribute to bone and joint disorders, as well as diabetic ulcers. In addition, open-toed shoes and sandals with straps between the first two toes should also be avoided.

- Don't drink in excess. Alcohol can contribute to neuropathy (nerve damage) which is one of the consequences of diabetes. Drinking can speed up the damage associated with the disease, deaden more nerves, and increase the possibility of overlooking a seemingly minor cut or injury.

- Don't wear anything that is too tight around the legs. Panty hose, panty girdles, thigh-highs, or knee-highs can constrict circulation to your legs and feet, as can men's dress socks if the elastic is too tight.

- Never try to remove calluses, corns, or warts by yourself. Commercial, over-the-counter preparations that remove warts or corns should be avoided because they can burn the skin and cause irreplaceable damage to the foot of a diabetic sufferer. Never try to cut calluses with a razor blade or any other instrument because the risk of cutting yourself is too high, and such wounds can often lead to more serious ulcers and lacerations. See your podiatric physician for assistance in these cases.

Chapter 31

Hypertension and Diabetes

Often diabetes and high blood pressure (hypertension) go hand-in-hand. It is thought that more than 70% of people with diabetes have high blood pressure as well. High blood pressure, like diabetes, is a lifelong disease. It can be treated but not cured. If you have both diabetes and high blood pressure, it will be especially important to work closely with your doctor and other health care professionals to manage both.

Blood pressure is the amount of force your blood exerts against the walls of your blood vessels. Blood pressure is usually measured as two numbers, such as 120/80 (normal blood pressure). The first and larger number (systolic pressure) is the blood pressure during a contraction (beat) of the heart. The second and smaller number (diastolic pressure) is the blood pressure when the heart is at rest (between beats). Your blood pressure can change many times during the day depending on physical activity, emotional state, and other reasons. Therefore a number of blood pressure readings are needed before a diagnosis of high blood pressure (hypertension) can be made. Blood pressure readings above 140/90 on two or more occasions mean you have high blood pressure regardless of age. For the person with diabetes who is found to have high blood pressure too, most diabetes specialists believe that the target of treatment of that high blood pressure should be 130/80.

"Diabetes and High Blood Pressure: A Challenging Combination," © Michigan Diabetes Research and Training Center (www.med.umich.edu/mdrtc). Reprinted with permission.

Sometimes blood pressure that is too high will cause dizziness, headaches, or nosebleeds. Most often, however, high blood pressure causes no outward signs of trouble. Because of this, high blood pressure is often referred to as a "silent" disease. It can be missed in people who do not have their blood pressure checked regularly. Because usually there are no symptoms, people who have high blood pressure sometimes stop taking their medicine because they feel okay. This is a serious mistake. High blood pressure that is not treated can lead to a heart attack, stroke, or kidney failure.

If you have diabetes and high blood pressure, it is very important to take care of them both. High blood pressure can cause the complications of diabetes to be worse. High blood pressure can speed up the process of hardening of the arteries and kidney disease. This leads to an increased risk of heart attack, stroke, and kidney failure. High blood pressure further weakens damaged blood vessels in the eyes, and can make blood flow problems in the feet and legs worse. Taking good care of your diabetes and high blood pressure can decrease, delay, and sometimes prevent these problems.

The care of high blood pressure is somewhat like the care of diabetes. In fact, sometimes the same treatment works for both of them. Weight loss and regular exercise will often help control both diabetes and high blood pressure. Cutting down on salt may help lower blood pressure. People with high blood pressure also need to faithfully take any medicine or medicines prescribed. By working with your health care team and following your treatment plan, you can meet the challenge of caring for diabetes and high blood pressure.

Chapter 32

Diabetes and Kidney Disease

Chapter Contents

Section 32.1—How Can Diabetes Damage the
Kidneys? 318
Section 32.2—Proteinuria 322
Section 32.3—Amyloidosis 324
Section 32.4—Nephrotic Syndrome 327
Section 32.5—Glomerular Diseases 329

Section 32.1

How Can Diabetes Damage the Kidneys?

Excerpted from "Kidney Disease of Diabetes," National Kidney and Urologic Diseases Information Clearinghouse, National Institute of Diabetes and Digestive and Kidney Diseases, NIH Pub. No. 07-3925, October 2006.

Each year in the United States, more than 100,000 people are diagnosed with kidney failure, a serious condition in which the kidneys fail to rid the body of wastes. Kidney failure is the final stage of kidney disease, also known as nephropathy.

Diabetes is the most common cause of kidney failure, accounting for nearly 45 percent of new cases. Even when diabetes is controlled, the disease can lead to nephropathy and kidney failure. Most people with diabetes do not develop nephropathy that is severe enough to cause kidney failure. About 18 million people in the United States have diabetes, and more than 150,000 people are living with kidney failure as a result of diabetes.

People with kidney failure undergo either dialysis, which substitutes for some of the filtering functions of the kidneys, or transplantation to receive a healthy donor kidney. Most U.S. citizens who develop kidney failure are eligible for federally funded care. In 2003, care for patients with kidney failure cost the nation more than $27 billion.

African Americans, American Indians, and Hispanics/Latinos develop diabetes, nephropathy, and kidney failure at rates higher than Caucasians. Scientists have not been able to explain these higher rates. Nor can they explain fully the interplay of factors leading to diabetic nephropathy—factors including heredity, diet, and other medical conditions, such as high blood pressure. They have found that high blood pressure and high levels of blood glucose increase the risk that a person with diabetes will progress to kidney failure.

The Course of Kidney Disease

Diabetic kidney disease takes many years to develop. In some people, the filtering function of the kidneys is actually higher than normal in the first few years of their diabetes. This process has been called hyperfiltration.

Over several years, people who are developing kidney disease will have small amounts of the blood protein albumin begin to leak into their urine. At its first stage, this condition has been called microalbuminuria. The kidney's filtration function usually remains normal during this period.

As the disease progresses, more albumin leaks into the urine. This stage may be called overt diabetic nephropathy or macroalbuminuria. As the amount of albumin in the urine increases, filtering function usually begins to drop. The body retains various wastes as filtration falls. Creatinine is one such waste, and a blood test for creatinine can be used to estimate the decline in kidney filtration. As kidney damage develops, blood pressure often rises as well.

Overall, kidney damage rarely occurs in the first 10 years of diabetes, and usually 15 to 25 years will pass before kidney failure occurs. For people who live with diabetes for more than 25 years without any signs of kidney failure, the risk of ever developing it decreases.

Effects of High Blood Pressure

High blood pressure, or hypertension, is a major factor in the development of kidney problems in people with diabetes. Both a family history of hypertension and the presence of hypertension appear to increase chances of developing kidney disease. Hypertension also accelerates the progress of kidney disease when it already exists.

In the past, hypertension was defined as blood pressure exceeding 140 millimeters of mercury-systolic and 90 millimeters of mercury-diastolic. Professionals shorten the name of this limit to 140/90 or "140 over 90." The terms systolic and diastolic refer to pressure in the arteries during contraction of the heart (systolic) and between heartbeats (diastolic).

The American Diabetes Association and the National Heart, Lung, and Blood Institute recommend that people with diabetes keep their blood pressure below 130/80.

Hypertension can be seen not only as a cause of kidney disease, but also as a result of damage created by the disease. As kidney disease proceeds, physical changes in the kidneys lead to increased blood pressure. Therefore, a dangerous spiral, involving rising blood pressure and factors that raise blood pressure, occurs. Early detection and treatment of even mild hypertension are essential for people with diabetes.

Preventing and Slowing Kidney Disease

Blood Pressure Medicines

Scientists have made great progress in developing methods that slow the onset and progression of kidney disease in people with diabetes. Drugs used to lower blood pressure (antihypertensive drugs) can slow the progression of kidney disease significantly. Two types of drugs, angiotensin-converting enzyme (ACE) inhibitors and angiotensin receptor blockers (ARBs), have proven effective in slowing the progression of kidney disease. Many people require two or more drugs to control their blood pressure. In addition to an ACE inhibitor or an ARB, a diuretic is very useful. Beta blockers, calcium channel blockers, and other blood pressure drugs may also be needed.

An example of an effective ACE inhibitor is captopril, which doctors commonly prescribe for treating kidney disease of diabetes. The benefits of captopril extend beyond its ability to lower blood pressure: it may directly protect the kidney's glomeruli. ACE inhibitors have lowered proteinuria and slowed deterioration even in diabetic patients who did not have high blood pressure.

An example of an effective ARB is losartan, which has also been shown to protect kidney function and lower the risk of cardiovascular events.

Any medicine that helps patients achieve a blood pressure target of 130/80 or lower provides benefits. Patients with even mild hypertension or persistent microalbuminuria should consult a physician about the use of antihypertensive medicines.

Moderate-Protein Diets

In people with diabetes, excessive consumption of protein may be harmful. Experts recommend that people with kidney disease of diabetes consume the recommended dietary allowance for protein, but avoid high-protein diets. For people with greatly reduced kidney function, a diet containing reduced amounts of protein may help delay the onset of kidney failure. Anyone following a reduced-protein diet should work with a dietitian to ensure adequate nutrition.

Intensive Management of Blood Glucose

Antihypertensive drugs and low-protein diets can slow kidney disease when significant nephropathy is present. A third treatment, known as intensive management of blood glucose or glycemic control, has shown great promise for people with type 1 and type 2 diabetes, especially for those in early stages of nephropathy.

Intensive management is a treatment regimen that aims to keep blood glucose levels close to normal. The regimen includes testing blood glucose frequently, administering insulin frequently throughout the day on the basis of food intake and physical activity, following a diet and activity plan, and consulting a health care team frequently. Some people use an insulin pump to supply insulin throughout the day.

A number of studies have pointed to the beneficial effects of intensive management. In the Diabetes Control and Complications Trial (DCCT) supported by the National Institute of Diabetes and Digestive and Kidney Diseases (NIDDK), researchers found a 50 percent decrease in both development and progression of early diabetic kidney disease in participants who followed an intensive regimen for controlling blood glucose levels. The intensively managed patients had average blood glucose levels of 150 milligrams per deciliter—about 80 milligrams per deciliter lower than the levels observed in the conventionally managed patients. The United Kingdom Prospective Diabetes Study, conducted from 1976 to 1997, showed conclusively that, in people with improved blood glucose control, the risk of early kidney disease was reduced by a third. Additional studies conducted over the past decades have clearly established that any program resulting in sustained lowering of blood glucose levels will be beneficial to patients in the early stages of diabetic nephropathy.

Section 32.2

Proteinuria

Excerpted from "Proteinuria," National Kidney and Urologic Diseases Information Clearinghouse, National Institute of Diabetes and Digestive and Kidney Diseases, NIH Pub. No. 06-4732, September 2006.

Proteinuria describes a condition in which urine contains an abnormal amount of protein. Proteins are the building blocks for all body parts, including muscles, bones, hair, and nails. Proteins in your blood also perform a number of important functions. They protect you from infection, help your blood clot, and keep the right amount of fluid circulating throughout your body.

As blood passes through healthy kidneys, they filter the waste products out and leave in the things the body needs, like proteins. Most proteins are too big to pass through the kidneys' filters into the urine unless the kidneys are damaged. The main protein that is most likely to appear in urine is albumin. Proteins from the blood can escape into the urine when the filters of the kidney, called glomeruli, are damaged. Sometimes the term albuminuria is used when a urine test detects albumin specifically. Albumin's function in the body includes retention of fluid in the blood. It acts like a sponge, soaking up fluid from body tissues.

Inflammation in the glomeruli is called glomerulonephritis, or simply nephritis. Many diseases can cause this inflammation, which leads to proteinuria. Additional processes that can damage the glomeruli and cause proteinuria include diabetes, hypertension, and other forms of kidney diseases.

Research shows that the level and type of proteinuria (whether the urinary proteins are albumin only or include other proteins) strongly determine the extent of damage and whether you are at risk for developing progressive kidney failure.

Proteinuria is also associated with cardiovascular disease. Damaged blood vessels may lead to heart failure or stroke as well as kidney failure. If your doctor finds that you have proteinuria, do what you can to protect your health and prevent any of these diseases from developing.

Several health organizations recommend that some people be regularly checked for proteinuria so that kidney disease can be detected and treated before it progresses. A 1996 study sponsored by the National Institutes of Health determined that proteinuria is the best predictor of progressive kidney failure in people with type 2 diabetes. The American Diabetes Association recommends regular urine testing for proteinuria for people with type 1 or type 2 diabetes. The National Kidney Foundation recommends that routine checkups include testing for excess protein in the urine, especially for people in high-risk groups.

What are the signs of proteinuria and kidney failure?

Large amounts of protein in your urine may cause it to look foamy in the toilet. Also, because the protein has left your body, your blood can no longer soak up enough fluid and you may notice swelling in your hands, feet, abdomen, or face. These are signs of very large protein loss. More commonly, you may have proteinuria without noticing any signs or symptoms. Testing is the only way to find out how much protein you have in your urine.

What are the tests for proteinuria?

To test for proteinuria, you will need to give a urine sample. A strip of chemically treated paper will change color when dipped in urine that has too much protein. Laboratory tests that measure exact amounts of protein or albumin in the urine are recommended for people at risk for kidney disease, especially those with diabetes. The protein-to-creatinine or albumin-to-creatinine ratio can be measured on a sample of urine to detect smaller amounts of protein, which can indicate kidney disease. If the laboratory test shows high levels of protein, another test should be done one to two weeks later. If the second test also shows high levels of protein, you have persistent proteinuria and should have additional tests to evaluate your kidney function.

Your doctor will also test a sample of your blood for creatinine and urea nitrogen. These are waste products that healthy kidneys remove from the blood. High levels of creatinine and urea nitrogen in your blood indicate that kidney function is impaired.

How is proteinuria treated?

If you have diabetes, hypertension, or both, the first goal of treatment will be to control your blood glucose and blood pressure. If you have diabetes, you should test your blood glucose often, follow a healthy eating plan, take your medicines, and get plenty of exercise. If you have diabetes and high blood pressure, your doctor may prescribe a medicine from a class of drugs called ACE (angiotensin-converting enzyme) inhibitors or a similar class called ARBs (angiotensin receptor blockers). These drugs have been found to protect kidney function even more than other drugs that provide the same level of blood pressure control. The American Diabetes Association recommends that people with diabetes keep their blood pressure below 130/80.

To maintain this target, you may need to take a combination of two or more blood pressure medicines. Your doctor may also prescribe a diuretic in addition to your ACE inhibitor or ARB. Diuretics are also called "water pills" because they help you urinate and get rid of excess fluid in your body.

In addition to blood glucose and blood pressure control, the National Kidney Foundation recommends restricting dietary salt and protein. Your doctor may refer you to a dietitian to help you develop and follow a healthy eating plan.

Section 32.3

Amyloidosis

Excerpted from "Amyloidosis and Kidney Disease," National Kidney and Urologic Diseases Information Clearinghouse, National Institute of Diabetes and Digestive and Kidney Diseases, NIH Pub. No. 06-4694, May 2006.

Proteins are important building blocks for all body parts, including muscles, bones, hair, and nails. Proteins circulate throughout the body in the blood and are normally harmless. Occasionally, cells produce abnormal proteins that can settle in body tissue, forming deposits and causing disease. When these deposits of abnormal proteins were first discovered, they were called amyloid, and the disease process amyloidosis.

In recent years, researchers have discovered that different kinds of proteins can form amyloid deposits and have identified several types of amyloidosis. Two of these types are closely related to kidney disease. In primary amyloidosis, abnormal protein production occurs as a first step and can lead to kidney disease. Dialysis-related amyloidosis (DRA), on the other hand, is a result of kidney disease.

Primary Amyloidosis

Primary amyloidosis occurs when the body's antibody-producing cells do not function properly and produce abnormal protein fibers made of antibody fragments. Some people with primary amyloidosis have a condition called multiple myeloma. The antibody fragments come together to form amyloid deposits in different organs, including the kidneys, where they cause serious damage. Injured kidneys can't function effectively and may be unable to remove urea and other wastes from the blood. Elevated levels of these protein fibers can also damage the heart, lungs, brain, and digestive system.

One common sign of kidney amyloidosis is the presence of abnormally high levels of protein in the urine, a condition known as proteinuria. Healthy kidneys prevent protein from entering the urine, so the presence of protein may be a sign that the kidneys aren't working properly. A physician who finds large amounts of protein in the urine may also perform a biopsy—take a small sample of tissue for examination with a microscope—to confirm amyloidosis.

Current treatments are aimed at slowing the progression of amyloid build-up. Combination drug therapy with melphalan, a cancer drug, and prednisone, an anti-inflammatory steroid drug, may improve organ function and survival rates by interrupting the growth of the abnormal cells that produce amyloid protein. These are the same drugs used in chemotherapy to treat certain cancers, such as multiple myeloma, and they may have serious side effects, such as nausea and vomiting, hair loss, and fatigue.

Some clinics have reported promising results treating amyloidosis by transplanting the patient's own blood stem cells to replace diseased or damaged bone marrow. The therapy also requires high doses of melphalan, so side effects can be serious. Patients with heart problems may not be considered for this treatment.

Dialysis-Related Amyloidosis

Normal kidneys filter and remove excess small proteins from the blood, thus keeping blood levels normal. When the kidneys don't work properly, as in patients receiving dialysis, one type of small protein called beta-2-microglobulin builds up in the blood. When this occurs, beta-2-microglobulin molecules may join together, like the links of a chain, forming a few very large molecules from many smaller ones. These large molecules can form deposits and eventually damage the surrounding tissues and cause great discomfort. This condition is called dialysis-related amyloidosis (DRA).

DRA is relatively common in patients, especially older adults, who have been on hemodialysis for more than five years. Hemodialysis membranes that have been used for many years don't effectively remove the large, complex beta-2-microglobulin proteins from the bloodstream. Newer hemodialysis membranes, as well as peritoneal dialysis, remove beta-2-microglobulin more effectively, but not enough to keep blood levels normal. As a result, blood levels remain elevated, and deposits form in bone, joints, and tendons (the tissue that connects the muscle to the bone). DRA may result in pain, stiffness, and fluid in the joints. Patients with DRA may also develop hollow cavities, or cysts, in some of their bones; these may lead to unexpected bone fractures. Amyloid deposits may cause tears in ligaments and tendons. Most patients with these problems can be helped by surgical intervention.

Half of the people with DRA also develop a condition called carpal tunnel syndrome, which results from the unusual buildup of protein in the wrists. Patients with this condition may experience numbness or tingling, sometimes associated with muscle weakness, in their fingers and hands. This is a treatable condition.

Unfortunately, no cure for DRA has been found, although a successful kidney transplant may stop the disease from progressing. However, DRA has caught the attention of dialysis engineers, who are attempting to develop new dialysis membranes that can remove larger amounts of beta-2-microglobulin from the blood.

Section 32.4

Nephrotic Syndrome

Excerpted from "Nephrotic Syndrome in Adults," National Kidney and Urologic Diseases Information Clearinghouse, National Institute of Diabetes and Digestive and Kidney Diseases, NIH Pub. No. 07-4624, February 2007.

What is nephrotic syndrome?

Nephrotic syndrome is a condition marked by very high levels of protein in the urine, a condition called proteinuria; low levels of protein in the blood; swelling, especially around the eyes, feet, and hands; and high cholesterol.

What causes nephrotic syndrome?

Nephrotic syndrome results from damage to the kidneys' glomeruli—tiny blood vessels that filter wastes and excess water from the blood and send them to the bladder as urine.

When the glomeruli are working properly, they keep protein in the blood from leaking into the urine. Healthy kidneys allow less than 1 gram of protein to escape through the urine in a day. In nephrotic syndrome, the damaged glomeruli allow three grams or more of protein to leak into the urine during a 24-hour period.

As a result of this protein loss, the blood is deficient. Normal amounts of blood protein are needed to help regulate fluid throughout the body. Protein acts like a sponge to soak up fluid into the bloodstream. When blood is low in protein, fluid accumulates in the body's tissues rather than circulating. The fluid causes swelling and puffiness.

Nephrotic syndrome can occur with many diseases. In adults, the most common causes are diabetic nephropathy and membranous nephropathy. In older adults, the most common cause is amyloidosis. Prevention of nephrotic syndrome relies on controlling these diseases. Frequently, however, the cause of nephrotic syndrome is unknown.

How is nephrotic syndrome diagnosed?

Your doctor will need blood and urine samples to evaluate your condition.

A high level of protein in a spot urine sample may indicate nephrotic syndrome. The doctor may order a 24-hour collection of urine in order to get a more precise measurement.

Blood tests may show low levels of protein. If kidney damage is advanced, waste products such as creatinine and urea nitrogen may build up in the blood.

Once nephrotic syndrome is established, the doctor may recommend a kidney biopsy—a procedure in which tiny pieces of the kidney are removed for examination with a microscope. The biopsy may reveal the underlying disease so that the doctor can determine a course of treatment. If a person has had diabetes for some time, and the patient history and laboratory tests are consistent with diabetic nephropathy, a biopsy is rarely necessary.

How is nephrotic syndrome treated?

In addition to addressing the underlying cause, treatment of nephrotic syndrome focuses on reducing high cholesterol, blood pressure, and protein in urine through diet, medications, or both. Two groups of blood pressure medications—angiotensin-converting enzyme (ACE) inhibitors and angiotensin receptor blockers (ARBs)—also protect the kidneys by reducing proteinuria.

Some people may benefit from limiting protein in their diet to reduce the buildup of wastes in the blood.

Nephrotic syndrome may go away once the underlying cause, if known, has been treated. Depending on the disease, as many as half of the patients may develop chronic kidney disease that progresses to end-stage renal disease. In these cases, the kidneys gradually lose their ability to filter wastes and excess water from the blood. If kidney failure occurs, the person will need dialysis or a kidney transplant.

Section 32.5

Glomerular Diseases

Excerpted from "Glomerular Diseases," National Kidney and Urologic Diseases Information Clearinghouse, National Institute of Diabetes and Digestive and Kidney Diseases, NIH Pub. No. 06-4358, April 2006.

Many diseases affect kidney function by attacking the glomeruli, the tiny units within the kidney where blood is cleaned. Glomerular diseases include many conditions with a variety of genetic and environmental causes, but they fall into two major categories:

- **Glomerulonephritis:** describes the inflammation of the membrane tissue in the kidney that serves as a filter, separating wastes and extra fluid from the blood.

- **Glomerulosclerosis:** describes the scarring or hardening of the tiny blood vessels within the kidney.

Although glomerulonephritis and glomerulosclerosis have different causes, they can both lead to kidney failure.

What are the kidneys and what do they do?

The two kidneys are bean-shaped organs located near the middle of the back, just below the rib cage to the left and right of the spine. Each about the size of a fist, these organs act as sophisticated filters for the body. They process about 200 quarts of blood a day to sift out about two quarts of waste products and extra water that eventually leave the body as urine.

Blood enters the kidneys through arteries that branch inside the kidneys into tiny clusters of looping blood vessels. Each cluster is called a glomerulus, which comes from the Greek word meaning filter. The plural form of the word is glomeruli. There are approximately one million glomeruli, or filters, in each kidney. The glomerulus is attached to the opening of a small fluid-collecting tube called a tubule. Blood is filtered in the glomerulus, and extra water and wastes pass into the tubule and become urine. Eventually, the urine drains from the kidneys into the bladder through larger tubes called ureters.

Each glomerulus-and-tubule unit is called a nephron. Each kidney is composed of about one million nephrons. In healthy nephrons, the glomerular membrane that separates the blood vessel from the tubule allows waste products and extra water to pass into the tubule while keeping blood cells and protein in the bloodstream.

How do glomerular diseases interfere with kidney function?

Glomerular diseases damage the glomeruli, letting protein and sometimes red blood cells leak into the urine. Sometimes a glomerular disease also interferes with the clearance of waste products by the kidney, so they begin to build up in the blood. Furthermore, loss of blood proteins like albumin in the urine can result in a fall in their level in the bloodstream. In normal blood, albumin acts like a sponge, drawing extra fluid from the body into the bloodstream, where it remains until the kidneys remove it. But when albumin leaks into the urine, the blood loses its capacity to absorb extra fluid from the body. Fluid can accumulate outside the circulatory system in the face, hands, feet, or ankles and cause swelling.

What are the symptoms of glomerular disease?

The signs and symptoms of glomerular disease include the following:

- **Proteinuria:** large amounts of protein in the urine
- **Hematuria:** blood in the urine
- **Reduced glomerular filtration rate:** inefficient filtering of wastes from the blood
- **Hypoproteinemia:** low blood protein
- **Edema:** swelling in parts of the body

One or more of these symptoms can be the first sign of kidney disease. But how would you know, for example, whether you have proteinuria? Before seeing a doctor, you may not. But some of these symptoms have signs, or visible manifestations:

- Proteinuria may cause foamy urine.

- Blood may cause the urine to be pink or cola-colored.

- Edema may be obvious in hands and ankles, especially at the end of the day, or around the eyes when awakening in the morning, for example.

How is glomerular disease diagnosed?

Patients with glomerular disease have significant amounts of protein in the urine, which may be referred to as "nephrotic range" if levels are very high. Red blood cells in the urine are a frequent finding as well, particularly in some forms of glomerular disease. Urinalysis provides information about kidney damage by indicating levels of protein and red blood cells in the urine. Blood tests measure the levels of waste products such as creatinine and urea nitrogen to determine whether the filtering capacity of the kidneys is impaired. If these lab tests indicate kidney damage, the doctor may recommend ultrasound or an x-ray to see whether the shape or size of the kidneys is abnormal. These tests are called renal imaging. But since glomerular disease causes problems at the cellular level, the doctor will probably also recommend a kidney biopsy—a procedure in which a needle is used to extract small pieces of tissue for examination with different types of microscopes, each of which shows a different aspect of the tissue. A biopsy may be helpful in confirming glomerular disease and identifying the cause.

What causes glomerular disease?

A number of different diseases can result in glomerular disease. It may be the direct result of an infection or a drug toxic to the kidneys, or it may result from a disease that affects the entire body, like diabetes or lupus. Many different kinds of diseases can cause swelling or scarring of the nephron or glomerulus. Sometimes glomerular disease is idiopathic, meaning that it occurs without an apparent associated disease. Diabetic nephropathy is a form of glomerular disease that can be placed in two categories: systemic diseases, since diabetes itself is a systemic disease, and sclerotic diseases, because the specific damage done to the kidneys is associated with scarring.

What are renal failure and end-stage renal disease?

Renal failure is any acute or chronic loss of kidney function and is the term used when some kidney function remains. Total kidney failure, sometimes called end-stage renal disease (ESRD), indicates permanent loss of kidney function. Depending on the form of glomerular disease, renal function may be lost in a matter of days or weeks or may deteriorate slowly and gradually over the course of decades.

Chapter 33

Anemia and Diabetes

What is anemia?

Anemia is a below-normal level of hemoglobin or hematocrit (normal lab values: hemoglobin greater than 12 g/dL for women, greater than 14 g/dL for men; hematocrit greater than 36% for women, greater than 42% for men). Hemoglobin is the protein in red blood cells that carries oxygen to all parts of the body. Anemia can be temporary, a consequence of other health conditions or it can be a chronic problem. People with mild anemia may not have any symptoms or may have only mild symptoms. People with severe anemia may have problems carrying out routine activities and can feel tired or experience shortness of breath with activity.[1]

How common is anemia in people with diabetes?

There are over 17 million people in the United States who have diabetes. About 5–10% have type 1 diabetes and 90–95% have type 2 diabetes.[1] Diabetic kidney disease is a common cause of kidney failure. Approximately one-third of people who have type 1 diabetes for at least 15 years develop kidney disease.[2] Many people with kidney disease develop anemia.

What causes anemia in people with diabetes?

Kidney disease is a common complication of diabetes. Damaged kidneys may not produce enough erythropoietin (EPO), a hormone that regulates red blood cell production. Less EPO in turn means fewer red blood cells and their protein hemoglobin to deliver oxygen to your body's organs. If there are not enough red blood cells, your body does not get the right amount of oxygen, which causes symptoms of anemia. Other causes of anemia are low levels of iron or low levels of certain vitamins that your body needs to produce hemoglobin and make healthy red blood cells.[1]

What are the effects of untreated anemia in diabetes?

Studies show that having anemia along with diabetes may increase the likelihood of developing diabetic eye disease, developing heart disease or having a stroke.[3,4] People who have both diabetes and anemia are more likely to die early than those who have diabetes but not anemia.[1] High death rates are even more common in anemic people with diabetes who also have heart failure and/or kidney disease.[5] While appropriate management of anemia may be life saving in some circumstances, treatment has not yet been conclusively proven to guarantee a longer lifespan.

How do I know if I am anemic?

The best way to determine if you have anemia is to discuss your blood counts and changes in hemoglobin and hematocrit with your doctor. Symptoms usually develop when anemia is moderate to severe, and can include fatigue, weakness, pale skin, chest pain, dizziness, irritability, numbness or coldness in your hands and feet, trouble breathing, a fast heartbeat, and headache. It is important to see your doctor on a regular basis in order to be tested for possible anemia.

What treatments are available to help me?

Treatment will vary by the cause of the anemia. Iron or vitamin supplements may be recommended. Anemia that is associated with kidney disease often requires treatment with drugs that stimulate red blood cell production. Noteworthy though are recent studies which suggest that it is best not to try to correct the anemia to normal levels.[6] Close communication with your doctor will help him or her provide the treatment that is best for you based on what is causing the anemia.

Glossary

Diabetes: Disease which causes your body to either not make enough insulin (type 1) or not use insulin the right way (type 2).

Diabetic eye disease: Damage to small blood vessels of the retina.

Erythropoietin: Hormone that regulates red blood cell production.

Hematocrit: Percentage of red blood cells in a blood sample.

Hemoglobin: Protein carried by red blood cells that transports and delivers oxygen throughout your body.

References

1. National Anemia Action Council. *Anemia: A Hidden Epidemic*. Los Angeles, CA: HealthVizion Communications, Inc.; 2002.

2. NIDDK: Diabetes Control and Complications Trial. Available at: http://diabetes.niddk.nih.gov/dm/pubs/control/#kidney.

3. Friedman EA, et al. *Am J Kidney Dis*. 1995;26:202–208.

4. Qiao Q, et al. *J Clin Epidemiol*. 1997;50:153–158.

5. Collins A, et al. *Adv Stud Med*. 2003;3(3C);S14–S17.

6. Singh A, et al. *New Eng J Med* 2006 355:2085–2098.

Chapter 34

Sexual and Urologic Problems of Diabetes

Troublesome bladder symptoms and changes in sexual function are common health problems as people age. Having diabetes can mean early onset and increased severity of these problems. Sexual and urologic complications of diabetes are related to the nerve damage diabetes can cause. Men may have difficulty with erections or ejaculation. Women may have problems with sexual response and vaginal lubrication. Urinary tract infections and bladder problems occur more often in people with diabetes. By keeping your diabetes under control, you can lower your risk of sexual and urologic problems.

Diabetes and Sexual Problems

When you want to lift your arm or take a step, your brain sends nerve signals to the appropriate muscles. Internal organs like the heart and bladder are also controlled by nerve signals, but you do not have the same kind of conscious control over them as you do over your arms and legs. The nerves that control your internal organs are called autonomic nerves, and they signal your body to digest food and circulate blood without your having to think about it. Your body's response to sexual stimuli is also involuntary, governed by autonomic nerve signals that increase blood flow to the genitals and cause smooth muscle tissue to relax. Damage to these autonomic nerves is what can hinder normal function.

Excerpted from "Sexual and Urologic Problems of Diabetes," National Diabetes Information Clearinghouse, National Institute of Diabetes and Digestive and Kidney Diseases, NIH Pub. No. 04-5135, June 2004.

Sexual Problems in Men with Diabetes

Erectile Dysfunction

Estimates of the prevalence of erectile dysfunction in men with diabetes range from 20 to 85 percent. Erectile dysfunction is a consistent inability to have an erection firm enough for sexual intercourse. The condition includes the total inability to have an erection, the inability to sustain an erection, or the occasional inability to have or sustain an erection. A recent study of a clinic population revealed that 5 percent of the men with erectile dysfunction also had undiagnosed diabetes.

Men who have diabetes are three times more likely to have erectile dysfunction as men who do not have diabetes. Among men with erectile dysfunction, those with diabetes are likely to have experienced the problem as much as 10 to 15 years earlier than men without diabetes.

In addition to diabetes, other major causes of erectile dysfunction include high blood pressure, kidney disease, alcoholism, and blood vessel disease. Erectile dysfunction may also occur because of the side effects of medications, psychological factors, smoking, and hormonal deficiencies.

If you experience erectile dysfunction, talking to your doctor about it is the first step in getting help. Your doctor may ask you about your medical history, the type and frequency of your sexual problems, your medications, your smoking and drinking habits, and other health conditions. A physical exam and laboratory tests may help pinpoint causes. Your blood glucose control and hormone levels will be checked. The doctor may also ask you whether you are depressed or have recently experienced upsetting changes in your life. In addition, you may be asked to do a test at home that checks for erections that occur while you sleep.

Treatments for erectile dysfunction caused by nerve damage, also called neuropathy, vary widely and range from oral pills, a vacuum pump, pellets placed in the urethra, and shots directly into the penis, to surgery. All these methods have strengths and drawbacks. Psychotherapy to reduce anxiety or address other issues may be necessary. Surgery to implant a device to aid in erection or to repair arteries is another option.

Retrograde Ejaculation

Retrograde ejaculation is a condition in which part or all of a man's semen goes into the bladder instead of out the penis during ejaculation. Retrograde ejaculation occurs when internal muscles, called sphincters, do not function normally. A sphincter automatically opens or closes a passage in the body. The semen mixes with urine in the bladder and leaves the body during urination, without harming the bladder. A man experiencing retrograde ejaculation may notice that little semen is discharged during ejaculation or may become aware of the condition if fertility problems arise. His urine may appear cloudy; analysis of a urine sample after ejaculation will reveal the presence of semen.

Poor blood glucose control and the resulting nerve damage are associated with retrograde ejaculation. Other causes include prostate surgery or some blood pressure medicines.

Retrograde ejaculation caused by diabetes or surgery may be improved with a medication that improves the muscle tone of the bladder neck. A urologist experienced in infertility treatments may assist with techniques to promote fertility, such as collecting sperm from the urine and then using the sperm for artificial insemination.

Sexual Problems in Women with Diabetes

Decreased Vaginal Lubrication

Nerve damage to cells that line the vagina can result in dryness, which in turn may lead to discomfort during sexual intercourse. Discomfort is likely to decrease sexual response or desire.

Decreased or Absent Sexual Response

Diabetes or other diseases, blood pressure medications, certain prescription and over-the-counter drugs, alcohol abuse, smoking, and psychological factors such as anxiety or depression can all cause sexual problems in women. Gynecologic infections or conditions relating to pregnancy or menopause can also contribute to decreased or absent sexual response.

As many as 35 percent of women with diabetes may experience decreased or absent sexual response. Decreased desire for sex, inability to become or remain aroused, lack of sensation, or inability to reach orgasm can result.

Symptoms include the following:

- decreased or total lack of interest in sexual relations
- decreased or no sensation in the genital area
- constant or occasional inability to reach orgasm
- dryness in the vaginal area, leading to pain or discomfort during sexual relations

339

If you experience sexual problems or notice a change in your sexual response, talking to your doctor about it is the first step in getting help. Your doctor will ask you about your medical history, any gynecologic conditions or infections, the type and frequency of your sexual problems, your medications, your smoking and drinking habits, and other health conditions. A physical exam and laboratory tests may also help pinpoint causes. Your blood glucose control will be discussed. The doctor may ask whether you might be pregnant or have reached menopause and whether you are depressed or have recently experienced upsetting changes in your life.

Prescription or over-the-counter vaginal lubricant creams may be useful for women experiencing dryness.

Techniques to treat decreased sexual response include changes in position and stimulation during sexual relations. Psychological counseling, as well as Kegel exercises to strengthen the muscles that hold urine in the bladder, may be helpful. Studies of drug treatments are under way.

Diabetes and Urologic Problems

Bladder dysfunction can have a profound effect on quality of life. Diabetes can damage the nerves that control bladder function. Men and women with diabetes commonly have bladder symptoms that may include a feeling of urinary urgency, frequency, getting up at night to urinate often, or leakage of urine (incontinence). These symptoms have been called overactive bladder. Less common but more severe bladder symptoms include difficulty urinating and complete failure to empty (retention). These symptoms are called a neurogenic bladder. Some evidence indicates that this problem occurs in both men and women with diabetes at earlier ages than in those without diabetes.

Neurogenic Bladder

In neurogenic bladder, damage to the nerves that go to your bladder can cause it to release urine when you do not intend to urinate, resulting in leakage. Or damage to nerves may prevent your bladder from releasing urine properly and it may be forced back into the kidneys, causing kidney damage or urinary tract infections.

Neurogenic bladder can be caused by diabetes or other diseases, accidents that damage the nerves, or infections. Symptoms of neurogenic bladder include urinary tract infections, loss of the urge to urinate when the bladder is full, leakage of urine, and the inability to empty the bladder.

Your doctor will check both your nervous system (your brain and the nerves of the bladder) and the bladder itself. Tests may include x-rays and an evaluation of bladder function (urodynamics).

Treatment for neurogenic bladder depends on the specific problem and its cause. If the main problem is retention of urine in the bladder, treatment may involve medication to promote better bladder emptying and behavior changes to promote more efficient urination, called timed urination. Occasionally, people may need to periodically insert a thin tube called a catheter through the urethra into the bladder to drain the urine. Learning how to tell when the bladder is full and how to massage the lower abdomen to fully empty the bladder can help as well. If urinary leakage is the main problem, medications or surgery can help.

Urinary Tract Infections

Infections can occur in any part of the urinary tract. They are caused when bacteria, usually from the digestive system, reach the urinary tract. If bacteria are growing in the urethra, the infection is called urethritis. The bacteria may travel up the urinary tract and cause a bladder infection, called cystitis. An untreated infection may go farther into the body and cause pyelonephritis, a kidney infection. Some people have chronic or recurrent urinary tract infections.

Symptoms of urinary tract infections may include the following:

- a frequent urge to urinate
- pain or burning in the bladder or urethra during urination
- cloudy or reddish urine
- fatigue or shakiness
- in women, pressure above the pubic bone
- in men, a feeling of fullness in the rectum

If the infection is in your kidneys, you may be nauseous, feel pain in your back or side, and have a fever. Since frequent urination can be a sign of high blood glucose, you and your doctor should also evaluate recent blood glucose monitoring results.

Your doctor will ask for a urine sample, which will be analyzed for bacteria and pus. If you have frequent urinary tract infections, your doctor may order further tests. An ultrasound exam provides images

341

from the echo patterns of soundwaves bounced back from internal organs. An intravenous pyelogram (IVP) uses a special dye to enhance x-ray images of your urinary tract. Another test, called cystoscopy, allows the doctor to view the inside of the bladder.

Early diagnosis and treatment are important to prevent more serious infections. To clear up a urinary tract infection, the doctor will probably prescribe an antibiotic based on the bacteria in your urine. Current recommendations are for a full seven-day course of antibiotic treatment in people with diabetes, instead of the shorter course used for other people. Kidney infections are more serious and may require several weeks of antibiotic treatment. Drinking plenty of fluids will help prevent another infection.

Questions and Answers about Sexual and Urologic Problems

Will I experience sexual and urologic problems sooner or later?

Risk factors are conditions that increase your chances of getting a particular disease. The more risk factors you have, the greater your chances of developing that disease or condition. Diabetic neuropathy, including related sexual and urologic problems, appears to be more common in people who have poor blood glucose control, have high levels of blood cholesterol, have high blood pressure, are overweight, are over the age of 40, and who smoke.

What can I do to prevent diabetes-related sexual and urologic problems?

You can lower your risk of sexual and urologic problems by keeping your blood glucose, blood pressure, and cholesterol close to the target numbers your doctor recommends. Being physically active and maintaining a healthy weight can also help prevent the long-term complications of diabetes. Smoking is a particular problem, and quitting will improve your health in many ways. For example, if you quit smoking, you can lower your risk not only for nerve damage but also for heart attack, stroke, and kidney disease.

Chapter 35

Polycystic Ovary Syndrome

What is PCOS?

Polycystic ovary syndrome (PCOS) is a condition in which a woman's ovaries and, in some cases the adrenal glands, produce more androgens (a type of hormone) than normal. High levels of these hormones interfere with the development and release of eggs as part of ovulation. As a result, fluid-filled sacs or cysts can develop on the ovaries.

Because women with PCOS do not release eggs during ovulation, PCOS is the most common cause of female infertility.

How does PCOS affect fertility?

A woman's ovaries have follicles, which are tiny, fluid-filled sacs that hold the eggs. When an egg is mature, the follicle breaks open to release the egg so it can travel to the uterus for fertilization.

In women with PCOS, immature follicles bunch together to form large cysts or lumps. The eggs mature within the bunched follicles, but the follicles don't break open to release them.

As a result, women with PCOS often have menstrual irregularities, such as amenorrhea (they don't get menstrual periods) or oligomenorrhea (they only have periods now and then). Because the eggs

"Polycystic Ovary Syndrome (PCOS)," National Institute of Child Health and Human Development (www.nichd.nih.gov), May 25, 2007.

are not released, most women with PCOS have trouble getting pregnant.

What are the symptoms of PCOS?

In addition to infertility, women with PCOS may also have the following:

- pelvic pain
- hirsutism, or excess hair growth on the face, chest, stomach, thumbs, or toes
- male-pattern baldness or thinning hair
- acne, oily skin, or dandruff
- patches of thickened and dark brown or black skin

Also, women who are obese are more likely to have PCOS.

Although it is hard for women with PCOS to get pregnant, some do get pregnant, naturally or using assistive reproductive technology. Women with PCOS are at higher risk for miscarriage if they do become pregnant.

Women with PCOS are also at higher risk for associated conditions, such as diabetes; metabolic syndrome—sometimes called a precursor to diabetes, this syndrome indicates that the body has trouble regulating its insulin; and cardiovascular disease—including heart disease and high blood pressure.

What is the treatment for PCOS?

There is no cure for PCOS, but many of the symptoms can often be managed. It is important to have PCOS diagnosed and treated early to help prevent associated problems.

There are medications that can help control the symptoms, such as birth control pills to regulate menstruation, reduce androgen levels, and clear acne. Other medications can reduce cosmetic problems, such as hair growth, and control blood pressure and cholesterol.

Lifestyle changes such as regular exercise can aid weight loss and help reduce blood sugar levels and regulate insulin levels more effectively. Weight loss can help lessen many of the health conditions associated with PCOS and can make symptoms be less severe or even disappear.

Surgical treatment may also be an option, but it is not recommended as the first course of treatment.

How Is PCOS diagnosed?

Your health care provider will take a medical history and do a pelvic exam to feel for cysts on your ovaries. He or she may also do a vaginal ultrasound and recommend blood tests to measure hormone levels.

Other tests may include measuring levels of insulin, glucose, cholesterol, and triglycerides.

Chapter 36

Diabetic Neuropathies

Diabetic neuropathies are a family of nerve disorders caused by diabetes. People with diabetes can, over time, have damage to nerves throughout the body. Neuropathies lead to numbness and sometimes pain and weakness in the hands, arms, feet, and legs. Problems may also occur in every organ system, including the digestive tract, heart, and sex organs. People with diabetes can develop nerve problems at any time, but the longer a person has diabetes, the greater the risk.

An estimated 50 percent of those with diabetes have some form of neuropathy, but not all with neuropathy have symptoms. The highest rates of neuropathy are among people who have had the disease for at least 25 years.

Diabetic neuropathy also appears to be more common in people who have had problems controlling their blood glucose levels, in those with high levels of blood fat and blood pressure, in overweight people, and in people over the age of 40. The most common type is peripheral neuropathy, also called distal symmetric neuropathy, which affects the arms and legs.

Causes

The causes are probably different for different varieties of diabetic neuropathy. Researchers are studying the effect of glucose on nerves

"Diabetic Neuropathies: The Nerve Damage of Diabetes," National Institute of Diabetes and Digestive and Kidney Diseases, NIH Pub. No. 02-3185, May 2002. Editor's notes added by David A. Cooke, MD, February 2008.

to find out exactly how prolonged exposure to high glucose causes neuropathy. Nerve damage is likely due to a combination of factors:

- Metabolic factors, such as high blood glucose, long duration of diabetes, possibly low levels of insulin, and abnormal blood fat levels

- Neurovascular factors, leading to damage to the blood vessels that carry oxygen and nutrients to the nerves

- Autoimmune factors that cause inflammation in nerves

- Mechanical injury to nerves, such as carpal tunnel syndrome

- Inherited traits that increase susceptibility to nerve disease

- Lifestyle factors such as smoking or alcohol use

Symptoms

Symptoms depend on the type of neuropathy and which nerves are affected. Some people have no symptoms at all. For others, numbness, tingling, or pain in the feet is often the first sign. A person can experience both pain and numbness. Often, symptoms are minor at first, and since most nerve damage occurs over several years, mild cases may go unnoticed for a long time. Symptoms may involve the sensory or motor nervous system, as well as the involuntary (autonomic) nervous system. In some people, mainly those with focal neuropathy, the onset of pain may be sudden and severe.

Symptoms may include the following:

- Numbness, tingling, or pain in the toes, feet, legs, hands, arms, and fingers

- Wasting of the muscles of the feet or hands

- Indigestion, nausea, or vomiting

- Diarrhea or constipation

- Dizziness or faintness due to a drop in postural blood pressure

- Problems with urination

- Erectile dysfunction (impotence) or vaginal dryness

- Weakness

In addition, weight loss and depression are not due to neuropathy but nevertheless often accompany it.

Types of Diabetic Neuropathy

Diabetic neuropathies can be classified as peripheral, autonomic, proximal, and focal. Each affects different parts of the body in different ways.

- Peripheral neuropathy causes either pain or loss of feeling in the toes, feet, legs, hands, and arms.

- Autonomic neuropathy causes changes in digestion, bowel and bladder function, sexual response, and perspiration. It can also affect the nerves that serve the heart and control blood pressure. Autonomic neuropathy can also cause hypoglycemia (low blood sugar) unawareness, a condition in which people no longer experience the warning signs of hypoglycemia.

- Proximal neuropathy causes pain in the thighs, hips, or buttocks and leads to weakness in the legs.

- Focal neuropathy results in the sudden weakness of one nerve, or a group of nerves, causing muscle weakness or pain. Any nerve in the body may be affected.

Neuropathy Affects Nerves throughout the Body

- **Peripheral neuropathy:** Toes, feet, legs, hands, and arms
- **Autonomic neuropathy:** Heart and blood vessels, digestive system, urinary tract, sex organs, sweat glands, and eyes
- **Proximal neuropathy:** Thighs, hips, and buttocks
- **Focal neuropathy:** Eyes, facial muscles, ears, pelvis and lower back, thighs, and abdomen

Peripheral Neuropathy

This type of neuropathy damages nerves in the arms and legs. The feet and legs are likely to be affected before the hands and arms. Many people with diabetes have signs of neuropathy upon examination but have no symptoms at all. Symptoms of peripheral neuropathy may include the following:

- Numbness or insensitivity to pain or temperature
- A tingling, burning, or prickling sensation
- Sharp pains or cramps

- Extreme sensitivity to touch, even a light touch
- Loss of balance and coordination

These symptoms are often worse at night.

Peripheral neuropathy may also cause muscle weakness and loss of reflexes, especially at the ankle, leading to changes in gait (walking). Foot deformities, such as hammertoes and the collapse of the midfoot, may occur. Blisters and sores may appear on numb areas of the foot because pressure or injury goes unnoticed. If foot injuries are not treated promptly, the infection may spread to the bone, and the foot may then have to be amputated. Some experts estimate that half of all such amputations are preventable if minor problems are caught and treated in time.

Autonomic Neuropathy

Autonomic neuropathy affects the nerves that control the heart, regulate blood pressure, and control blood glucose levels. It also affects other internal organs, causing problems with digestion, respiratory function, urination, sexual response, and vision. In addition, the system that restores blood glucose levels to normal after a hypoglycemic episode may be affected, resulting in loss of the warning signs of hypoglycemia such as sweating and palpitations.

Unawareness of hypoglycemia: Normally, symptoms such as shakiness occur as blood glucose levels drop below 70 mg/dL. In people with autonomic neuropathy, symptoms may not occur, making hypoglycemia difficult to recognize. In people with autonomic neuropathy, symptoms may not occur making hypoglycemia difficult to recognize. However, other problems can also cause hypoglycemia unawareness so this does not always indicate nerve damage.

Heart and circulatory system: The heart and circulatory system are part of the cardiovascular system, which controls blood circulation. Damage to nerves in the cardiovascular system interferes with the body's ability to adjust blood pressure and heart rate. As a result, blood pressure may drop sharply after sitting or standing, causing a person to feel light-headed—or even to faint. Damage to the nerves that control heart rate can mean that it stays high, instead of rising and falling in response to normal body functions and exercise.

Digestive system: Nerve damage to the digestive system most commonly causes constipation. Damage can also cause the stomach to empty

Peripheral Nerves

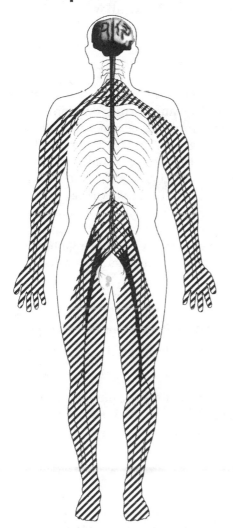

Figure 36.1. *Peripheral neuropathy affects the nerves in your arms, hands, legs, and feet.*

Autonomic Nerves

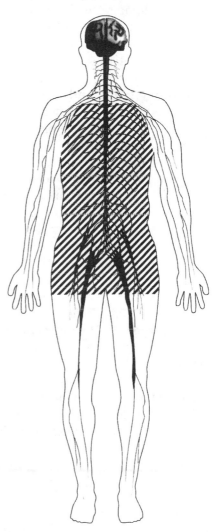

Figure 36.2. *Autonomic neuropathy affects the nerves in your lungs, heart, stomach, intestines, bladder, and sex organs.*

too slowly, a condition called gastroparesis. Severe gastroparesis can lead to persistent nausea and vomiting, bloating, and loss of appetite. Gastroparesis can make blood glucose levels fluctuate widely as well, due to abnormal food digestion.

Nerve damage to the esophagus may make swallowing difficult, while nerve damage to the bowels can cause constipation alternating with frequent, uncontrolled diarrhea, especially at night. Problems with the digestive system may lead to weight loss.

Urinary tract and sex organs: Autonomic neuropathy most often affects the organs that control urination and sexual function. Nerve damage can prevent the bladder from emptying completely, allowing bacteria to grow in the bladder and kidneys and causing urinary tract infections. When the nerves of the bladder are damaged, urinary incontinence may result because a person may not be able to sense when the bladder is full or control the muscles that release urine.

Neuropathy can also gradually decrease sexual response in men and women, although the sex drive is unchanged. A man may be unable to have erections or may reach sexual climax without ejaculating normally. A woman may have difficulty with lubrication, arousal, or orgasm.

Sweat glands: Autonomic neuropathy can affect the nerves that control sweating. When nerve damage prevents the sweat glands from working properly, the body cannot regulate its temperature properly. Nerve damage can also cause profuse sweating at night or while eating.

Eyes: Finally, autonomic neuropathy can affect the pupils of the eyes, making them less responsive to changes in light. As a result, a person may not be able to see well when the light is turned on in a dark room or may have trouble driving at night.

Proximal Neuropathy

Proximal neuropathy, sometimes called lumbosacral plexus neuropathy, femoral neuropathy, or diabetic amyotrophy, starts with pain in either the thighs, hips, buttocks, or legs, usually on one side of the body. This type of neuropathy is more common in those with type 2 diabetes and in older people. It causes weakness in the legs, manifested by an inability to go from a sitting to a standing position without help. Treatment for weakness or pain is usually needed. The length of the recovery period varies, depending on the type of nerve damage.

Focal Neuropathy

Occasionally, diabetic neuropathy appears suddenly and affects specific nerves, most often in the head, torso, or leg. Focal neuropathy may cause the following symptoms:

- Inability to focus the eye
- Double vision
- Aching behind one eye
- Paralysis on one side of the face (Bell's palsy)
- Severe pain in the lower back or pelvis
- Pain in the front of a thigh
- Pain in the chest, stomach, or flank
- Pain on the outside of the shin or inside the foot
- Chest or abdominal pain that is sometimes mistaken for heart disease, heart attack, or appendicitis

Focal neuropathy is painful and unpredictable and occurs most often in older people. However, it tends to improve by itself over weeks or months and does not cause long-term damage.

People with diabetes also tend to develop nerve compressions, also called entrapment syndromes. One of the most common is carpal tunnel syndrome, which causes numbness and tingling of the hand and sometimes muscle weakness or pain. Other nerves susceptible to entrapment may cause pain on the outside of the shin or the inside of the foot.

Preventing Diabetic Neuropathy

The best way to prevent neuropathy is to keep your blood glucose levels as close to the normal range as possible. Maintaining safe blood glucose levels protects nerves throughout your body.

For additional information on preventing diabetes complications, including neuropathy, see the Prevent Diabetes Problems series, available from the National Diabetes Information Clearinghouse at 800-860-8747.

Diagnosis

Neuropathy is diagnosed on the basis of symptoms and a physical exam. During the exam, the doctor may check blood pressure and heart rate, muscle strength, reflexes, and sensitivity to position, vibration, temperature, or a light touch.

The doctor may also do other tests to help determine the type and extent of nerve damage.

- A comprehensive foot exam assesses skin, circulation, and sensation. The test can be done during a routine office visit. To assess protective sensation or feeling in the foot, a nylon mono-filament (similar to a bristle on a hairbrush) attached to a wand is used to touch the foot. Those who cannot sense pressure from the monofilament have lost protective sensation and are at risk for developing foot sores that may not heal properly. Other tests include checking reflexes and assessing vibration perception, which is more sensitive than touch pressure.

- Nerve conduction studies check the transmission of electrical current through a nerve. With this test, an image of the nerve conducting an electrical signal is projected onto a screen. Nerve impulses that seem slower or weaker than usual indicate possible damage. This test allows the doctor to assess the condition of all the nerves in the arms and legs.

- Electromyography (EMG) shows how well muscles respond to electrical signals transmitted by nearby nerves. The electrical activity of the muscle is displayed on a screen. A response that is slower or weaker than usual suggests damage to the nerve or muscle. This test is often done at the same time as nerve conduction studies.

- Quantitative sensory testing (QST) uses the response to stimuli, such as pressure, vibration, and temperature, to check for neuropathy. QST is increasingly used to recognize sensation loss and excessive irritability of nerves.

- A check of heart rate variability shows how the heart responds to deep breathing and to changes in blood pressure and posture.

- Ultrasound uses sound waves to produce an image of internal organs. An ultrasound of the bladder and other parts of the urinary tract, for example, can show how these organs preserve a normal structure and whether the bladder empties completely after urination.

- Nerve or skin biopsy involves removing a sample of nerve or skin tissue for examination by microscope. This test is most often used in research settings.

Treatment

The first step is to bring blood glucose levels within the normal range to prevent further nerve damage. Blood glucose monitoring, meal planning, exercise, and oral drugs or insulin injections are needed to control blood glucose levels. Although symptoms may get worse when blood glucose is first brought under control, over time, maintaining lower blood glucose levels helps lessen neuropathic symptoms. Importantly, good blood glucose control may also help prevent or delay the onset of further problems.

Additional treatment depends on the type of nerve problem and symptom, as described in the following sections.

Foot Care

People with neuropathy need to take special care of their feet. The nerves to the feet are the longest in the body and are the ones most often affected by neuropathy. Loss of sensation in the feet means that sores or injuries may not be noticed and may become ulcerated or infected. Circulation problems also increase the risk of foot ulcers.

More than half of all lower limb amputations in the United States occur in people with diabetes—86,000 amputations per year. Doctors estimate that nearly half of the amputations caused by neuropathy and poor circulation could have been prevented by careful foot care. Here are the steps to follow:

- Clean your feet daily, using warm—not hot—water and a mild soap. Avoid soaking your feet. Dry them with a soft towel; dry carefully between your toes.

- Inspect your feet and toes every day for cuts, blisters, redness, swelling, calluses, or other problems. Use a mirror (laying a mirror on the floor works well) or get help from someone else if you cannot see the bottoms of your feet. Notify your health care provider of any problems.

- Moisturize your feet with lotion, but avoid getting it between your toes.

- After a bath or shower, file corns and calluses gently with a pumice stone.

- Each week or when needed, cut your toenails to the shape of your toes and file the edges with an emery board.

- Always wear shoes or slippers to protect your feet from injuries. Prevent skin irritation by wearing thick, soft, seamless socks.

- Wear shoes that fit well and allow your toes to move. Break in new shoes gradually by wearing them for only an hour at a time at first.

- Before putting your shoes on, look them over carefully and feel the insides with your hand to make sure they have no tears, sharp edges, or objects in them that might injure your feet.

- If you need help taking care of your feet, make an appointment to see a foot doctor, also called a podiatrist.

Pain Relief

To relieve pain, burning, tingling, or numbness, the doctor may suggest aspirin, acetaminophen, or nonsteroidal anti-inflammatory drugs (NSAIDs) such as ibuprofen. (People with renal disease should use NSAIDs only under a doctor's supervision.) A topical cream called capsaicin is another option. Tricyclic antidepressant medications such as amitriptyline, imipramine, and nortriptyline, or anticonvulsant medications such as carbamazepine or gabapentin may relieve pain in some people. Codeine may be prescribed for a short time to relieve severe pain. Also, mexiletine, used to regulate heartbeat, has been effective in treating pain in several clinical trials.[1]

Other pain treatments include transcutaneous electronic nerve stimulation (TENS), which uses small amounts of electricity to block pain signals, as well as hypnosis, relaxation training, biofeedback, and acupuncture. Walking regularly or using elastic stockings may also help leg pain.

Gastrointestinal Problems

To relieve mild symptoms of gastroparesis—indigestion, belching, nausea, or vomiting—doctors suggest eating small, frequent meals, avoiding fats, and eating less fiber. When symptoms are severe, the doctor may prescribe erythromycin to speed digestion, metoclopramide to speed digestion and help relieve nausea, or other drugs to help regulate digestion or reduce stomach acid secretion.

To relieve diarrhea or other bowel problems, the doctor may prescribe an antibiotic such as tetracycline, or other medications as appropriate.

Dizziness and Weakness

Sitting or standing slowly may help prevent the light-headedness, dizziness, or fainting associated with blood pressure and circulation problems. Raising the head of the bed or wearing elastic stockings may also help. Some people may benefit from increased salt in the diet and treatment with salt-retaining hormones. Others may benefit from high blood pressure medications. Physical therapy can help when muscle weakness or loss of coordination is a problem.

Urinary and Sexual Problems

To clear up a urinary tract infection, the doctor will probably prescribe an antibiotic. Drinking plenty of fluids will help prevent another infection. People who have incontinence should try to urinate at regular intervals (every three hours, for example) since they may not be able to tell when their bladder is full.

To treat erectile dysfunction in men, the doctor will first do tests to rule out a hormonal cause. Several methods are available to treat erectile dysfunction caused by neuropathy, including taking oral drugs, using a mechanical vacuum device, or injecting a drug called a vasodilator into the penis before sex. The vacuum and vasodilator raise blood flow to the penis, making it easier to have and maintain an erection. Another option is to surgically implant an inflatable or semirigid device in the penis. A constriction ring or penile sling may be helpful.[2]

Vaginal lubricants may be useful for women when neuropathy causes vaginal dryness. To treat problems with arousal and orgasm, the doctor may refer the woman to a gynecologist.

Editor's Notes:

1. Since this article was written, several additional medications have come into use for treatment of painful diabetic neuropathy. Two newer antidepressants, venlafaxine (Effexor™) and duloxetine (Cymbalta™) can be effective for nerve-related pain. In addition, two newer anti-seizure medications, pregabalin (Lyrica™) and topiramate (Topamax™) can also be effective for painful neuropathy. No single medication is clearly better for neuropathy pain than others; different patients respond differently to the various drugs. The additional medications expand the available options for treatment.

2. Newer oral medications such as sildenafil (Viagra™), vardenafil (Levitra™), and tadalafil (Cialis™) may be effective for sexual problems related to diabetic neuropathy, but this can vary considerably from patient to patient. For patients who do not respond to them, some patients may benefit from a medication called alprostadil (Muse™), which can be given as a small pellet inserted into the tip of the penis before sex.

Chapter 37

Gastroparesis

Gastroparesis, also called delayed gastric emptying, is a disorder in which the stomach takes too long to empty its contents. It often occurs in people with type 1 diabetes or type 2 diabetes.

Gastroparesis happens when nerves to the stomach are damaged or stop working. The vagus nerve controls the movement of food through the digestive tract. If the vagus nerve is damaged, the muscles of the stomach and intestines do not work normally, and the movement of food is slowed or stopped.

Diabetes can damage the vagus nerve if blood glucose levels remain high over a long period of time. High blood glucose causes chemical changes in nerves and damages the blood vessels that carry oxygen and nutrients to the nerves.

Signs and Symptoms

Signs and symptoms of gastroparesis are heartburn, nausea, vomiting of undigested food, an early feeling of fullness when eating, weight loss, abdominal bloating, erratic blood glucose levels, lack of appetite, gastroesophageal reflux, and spasms of the stomach wall. These symptoms may be mild or severe, depending on the person.

Excerpted from "Gastroparesis and Diabetes," National Digestive Diseases Information Clearinghouse, National Institute of Diabetes and Digestive and Kidney Diseases, NIH Pub. No. 04-4348, December 2003.

Complications of Gastroparesis

If food lingers too long in the stomach, it can cause problems like bacterial overgrowth from the fermentation of food. Also, the food can harden into solid masses called bezoars that may cause nausea, vomiting, and obstruction in the stomach. Bezoars can be dangerous if they block the passage of food into the small intestine.

Gastroparesis can make diabetes worse by adding to the difficulty of controlling blood glucose. When food that has been delayed in the stomach finally enters the small intestine and is absorbed, blood glucose levels rise. Since gastroparesis makes stomach emptying unpredictable, a person's blood glucose levels can be erratic and difficult to control.

Diagnosis

The diagnosis of gastroparesis is confirmed through one or more of the following tests.

Barium x-ray: After fasting for 12 hours, you will drink a thick liquid called barium, which coats the inside of the stomach, making it show up on the x-ray. Normally, the stomach will be empty of all food after 12 hours of fasting. If the x-ray shows food in the stomach, gastroparesis is likely. If the x-ray shows an empty stomach but the doctor still suspects that you have delayed emptying, you may need to repeat the test another day. On any one day, a person with gastroparesis may digest a meal normally, giving a falsely normal test result. If you have diabetes, your doctor may have special instructions about fasting.

Barium beefsteak meal: You will eat a meal that contains barium, thus allowing the radiologist to watch your stomach as it digests the meal. The amount of time it takes for the barium meal to be digested and leave the stomach gives the doctor an idea of how well the stomach is working. This test can help detect emptying problems that do not show up on the liquid barium x-ray. In fact, people who have diabetes-related gastroparesis often digest fluid normally, so the barium beefsteak meal can be more useful.

Radioisotope gastric-emptying scan: You will eat food that contains a radioisotope, a slightly radioactive substance that will show up on the scan. The dose of radiation from the radioisotope is small and not dangerous. After eating, you will lie under a machine that detects the radioisotope and shows an image of the food in the stomach and how quickly it leaves the stomach. Gastroparesis is diagnosed if more than half of the food remains in the stomach after two hours.

Gastric manometry: This test measures electrical and muscular activity in the stomach. The doctor passes a thin tube down the throat into the stomach. The tube contains a wire that takes measurements of the stomach's electrical and muscular activity as it digests liquids and solid food. The measurements show how the stomach is working and whether there is any delay in digestion.

Blood tests: The doctor may also order laboratory tests to check blood counts and to measure chemical and electrolyte levels.

Others: To rule out causes of gastroparesis other than diabetes, the doctor may do an upper endoscopy or an ultrasound.

- **Upper endoscopy:** After giving you a sedative, the doctor passes a long, thin tube called an endoscope through the mouth and gently guides it down the esophagus into the stomach. Through the endoscope, the doctor can look at the lining of the stomach to check for any abnormalities.

- **Ultrasound:** To rule out gallbladder disease or pancreatitis as a source of the problem, you may have an ultrasound test, which uses harmless sound waves to outline and define the shape of the gallbladder and pancreas.

Treatment

The primary treatment goal for gastroparesis related to diabetes is to regain control of blood glucose levels. Treatments include insulin, oral medications, changes in what and when you eat, and, in severe cases, feeding tubes and intravenous feeding.

It is important to note that in most cases treatment does not cure gastroparesis—it is usually a chronic condition. Treatment helps you manage the condition so that you can be as healthy and comfortable as possible.

Insulin for Blood Glucose Control

If you have gastroparesis, your food is being absorbed more slowly and at unpredictable times. To control blood glucose, you may need to take insulin more often, take your insulin after you eat instead of before, and check your blood glucose levels frequently after you eat and administer insulin whenever necessary. Your doctor will give you specific instructions based on your particular needs.

Medication

Several drugs are used to treat gastroparesis. Your doctor may try different drugs or combinations of drugs to find the most effective treatment.

Metoclopramide (Reglan): This drug stimulates stomach muscle contractions to help empty food. It also helps reduce nausea and vomiting. Metoclopramide is taken 20 to 30 minutes before meals and at bedtime. Side effects of this drug are fatigue, sleepiness, and sometimes depression, anxiety, and problems with physical movement.

Erythromycin: This antibiotic also improves stomach emptying. It works by increasing the contractions that move food through the stomach. Side effects are nausea, vomiting, and abdominal cramps.

Domperidone: The Food and Drug Administration is reviewing domperidone, which has been used elsewhere in the world to treat gastroparesis. It is a promotility agent like metoclopramide. Domperidone also helps with nausea.

Other medications: Other medications may be used to treat symptoms and problems related to gastroparesis. For example, an antiemetic can help with nausea and vomiting. Antibiotics will clear up a bacterial infection. If you have a bezoar, the doctor may use an endoscope to inject medication that will dissolve it.

Meal and Food Changes

Changing your eating habits can help control gastroparesis. Your doctor or dietitian will give you specific instructions, but you may be asked to eat six small meals a day instead of three large ones. If less food enters the stomach each time you eat, it may not become overly full. Or the doctor or dietitian may suggest that you try several liquid meals a day until your blood glucose levels are stable and the gastroparesis is corrected. Liquid meals provide all the nutrients found in solid foods, but can pass through the stomach more easily and quickly.

The doctor may also recommend that you avoid high-fat and high-fiber foods. Fat naturally slows digestion—a problem you do not need if you have gastroparesis—and fiber is difficult to digest. Some high-fiber foods like oranges and broccoli contain material that cannot be digested. Avoid these foods because the indigestible part will remain in the stomach too long and possibly form bezoars.

Feeding Tube

If other approaches do not work, you may need surgery to insert a feeding tube. The tube, called a jejunostomy tube, is inserted through the skin on your abdomen into the small intestine. The feeding tube allows you to put nutrients directly into the small intestine, bypassing the stomach altogether. You will receive special liquid food to use with the tube. A jejunostomy is particularly useful when gastroparesis prevents the nutrients and medication necessary to regulate blood glucose levels from reaching the bloodstream. By avoiding the source of the problem—the stomach—and putting nutrients and medication directly into the small intestine, you ensure that these products are digested and delivered to your bloodstream quickly. A jejunostomy tube can be temporary and is used only if necessary when gastroparesis is severe.

Parenteral Nutrition

Parenteral nutrition refers to delivering nutrients directly into the bloodstream, bypassing the digestive system. The doctor places a thin tube called a catheter in a chest vein, leaving an opening to it outside the skin. For feeding, you attach a bag containing liquid nutrients or medication to the catheter. The fluid enters your bloodstream through the vein. Your doctor will tell you what type of liquid nutrition to use.

This approach is an alternative to the jejunostomy tube and is usually a temporary method to get you through a difficult spell of gastroparesis. Parenteral nutrition is used only when gastroparesis is severe and is not helped by other methods.

New Treatments

A gastric neurostimulator has been developed to assist people with gastroparesis. The battery-operated device is surgically implanted and emits mild electrical pulses that help control nausea and vomiting associated with gastroparesis. This option is available to people whose nausea and vomiting do not improve with medications.

The use of botulinum toxin has been shown to improve stomach emptying and the symptoms of gastroparesis by decreasing the prolonged contractions of the muscle between the stomach and the small intestine (pyloric sphincter). The toxin is injected into the pyloric sphincter.

Chapter 38

Diabetic Retinopathy

Diabetic Retinopathy Defined

What is diabetic eye disease?

Diabetic eye disease refers to a group of eye problems that people with diabetes may face as a complication of diabetes. All can cause severe vision loss or even blindness. Diabetic eye disease may include the following:

- **Diabetic retinopathy:** Damage to the blood vessels in the retina.

- **Cataract:** Clouding of the eye's lens. Cataracts develop at an earlier age in people with diabetes.

- **Glaucoma:** Increase in fluid pressure inside the eye that leads to optic nerve damage and loss of vision. A person with diabetes is nearly twice as likely to get glaucoma as other adults.

What is diabetic retinopathy?

Diabetic retinopathy is the most common diabetic eye disease and a leading cause of blindness in American adults. It is caused by changes in the blood vessels of the retina.

"Diabetic Retinopathy," National Eye Institute (http://www.nei.nih.gov), December 2006.

In some people with diabetic retinopathy, blood vessels may swell and leak fluid. In other people, abnormal new blood vessels grow on the surface of the retina. The retina is the light-sensitive tissue at the back of the eye. A healthy retina is necessary for good vision.

If you have diabetic retinopathy, at first you may not notice changes to your vision. But over time, diabetic retinopathy can get worse and cause vision loss. Diabetic retinopathy usually affects both eyes.

What are the stages of diabetic retinopathy?

Diabetic retinopathy has four stages:

1. **Mild nonproliferative retinopathy:** At this earliest stage, microaneurysms occur. They are small areas of balloon-like swelling in the retina's tiny blood vessels.

2. **Moderate nonproliferative retinopathy:** As the disease progresses, some blood vessels that nourish the retina are blocked.

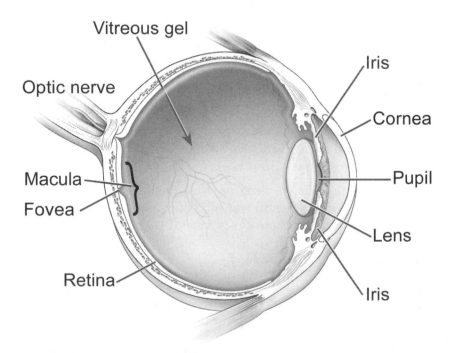

Figure 38.1. *The Human Eye.*

3. **Severe nonproliferative retinopathy:** Many more blood vessels are blocked, depriving several areas of the retina with their blood supply. These areas of the retina send signals to the body to grow new blood vessels for nourishment.

4. **Proliferative retinopathy:** At this advanced stage, the signals sent by the retina for nourishment trigger the growth of new blood vessels. This condition is called proliferative retinopathy. These new blood vessels are abnormal and fragile. They grow along the retina and along the surface of the clear, vitreous gel that fills the inside of the eye. By themselves, these blood vessels do not cause symptoms or vision loss. However, they have thin, fragile walls. If they leak blood, severe vision loss and even blindness can result.

Causes and Risk Factors

How does diabetic retinopathy cause vision loss?

Blood vessels damaged from diabetic retinopathy can cause vision loss in two ways:

1. Fragile, abnormal blood vessels can develop and leak blood into the center of the eye, blurring vision. This is proliferative retinopathy and is the fourth and most advanced stage of the disease.

2. Fluid can leak into the center of the macula, the part of the eye where sharp, straight-ahead vision occurs. The fluid makes the macula swell, blurring vision. This condition is called macular edema. It can occur at any stage of diabetic retinopathy, although it is more likely to occur as the disease progresses. About half of the people with proliferative retinopathy also have macular edema.

Who is at risk for diabetic retinopathy?

All people with diabetes—both type 1 and type 2—are at risk. That's why everyone with diabetes should get a comprehensive dilated eye exam at least once a year. The longer someone has diabetes, the more likely he or she will get diabetic retinopathy. Between 40 to 45 percent of Americans diagnosed with diabetes have some stage of diabetic retinopathy. If you have diabetic retinopathy, your doctor can recommend treatment to help prevent its progression.

During pregnancy, diabetic retinopathy may be a problem for women with diabetes. To protect vision, every pregnant woman with diabetes should have a comprehensive dilated eye exam as soon as possible. Your doctor may recommend additional exams during your pregnancy.

What can I do to protect my vision?

If you have diabetes get a comprehensive dilated eye exam at least once a year and remember these facts:

- Proliferative retinopathy can develop without symptoms. At this advanced stage, you are at high risk for vision loss.

- Macular edema can develop without symptoms at any of the four stages of diabetic retinopathy.

- You can develop both proliferative retinopathy and macular edema and still see fine. However, you are at high risk for vision loss.

- Your eye care professional can tell if you have macular edema or any stage of diabetic retinopathy. Whether or not you have

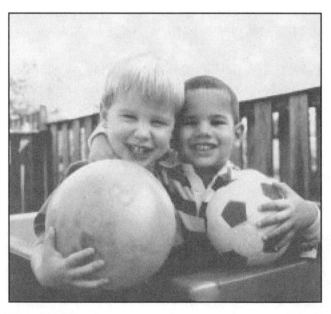

Figure 38.2. Normal Vision

symptoms, early detection and timely treatment can prevent vision loss.

If you have diabetic retinopathy, you may need an eye exam more often. People with proliferative retinopathy can reduce their risk of blindness by 95 percent with timely treatment and appropriate follow-up care.

The Diabetes Control and Complications Trial (DCCT) showed that better control of blood sugar levels slows the onset and progression of retinopathy. The people with diabetes who kept their blood sugar levels as close to normal as possible also had much less kidney and nerve disease. Better control also reduces the need for sight-saving laser surgery.

This level of blood sugar control may not be best for everyone, including some elderly patients, children under age 13, or people with heart disease. Be sure to ask your doctor if such a control program is right for you.

Other studies have shown that controlling elevated blood pressure and cholesterol can reduce the risk of vision loss. Controlling these will help your overall health as well as help protect your vision.

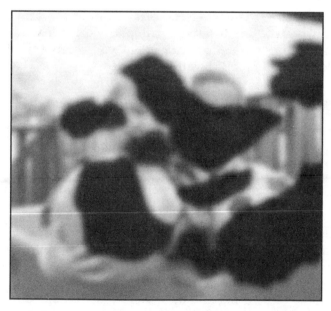

Figure 38.3. *The same scene as that shown in Figure 38.2, this time viewed by a person with diabetic retinopathy.*

Symptoms and Detection

Does diabetic retinopathy have any symptoms?

Often there are no symptoms in the early stages of the disease, nor is there any pain. Don't wait for symptoms. Be sure to have a comprehensive dilated eye exam at least once a year.

Blurred vision may occur when the macula—the part of the retina that provides sharp central vision—swells from leaking fluid. This condition is called macular edema.

If new blood vessels grow on the surface of the retina, they can bleed into the eye and block vision.

What are the symptoms of proliferative retinopathy if bleeding occurs?

At first, you will see a few specks of blood, or spots, "floating" in your vision. If spots occur, see your eye care professional as soon as possible. You may need treatment before more serious bleeding occurs. Hemorrhages tend to happen more than once, often during sleep.

Sometimes, without treatment, the spots clear, and you will see better. However, bleeding can reoccur and cause severely blurred vision. You need to be examined by your eye care professional at the first sign of blurred vision, before more bleeding occurs.

If left untreated, proliferative retinopathy can cause severe vision loss and even blindness. Also, the earlier you receive treatment, the more likely treatment will be effective.

How are diabetic retinopathy and macular edema detected?

Diabetic retinopathy and macular edema are detected during a comprehensive eye exam that includes the following:

1. **Visual acuity test:** This eye chart test measures how well you see at various distances.

2. **Dilated eye exam:** Drops are placed in your eyes to widen, or dilate, the pupils. This allows the eye care professional to see more of the inside of your eyes to check for signs of the disease. Your eye care professional uses a special magnifying lens to examine your retina and optic nerve for signs of damage and other eye problems. After the exam, your close-up vision may remain blurred for several hours.

3. **Tonometry:** An instrument measures the pressure inside the eye. Numbing drops may be applied to your eye for this test.

Your eye care professional checks your retina for early signs of the disease, including leaking blood vessels, retinal swelling (macular edema), pale, fatty deposits on the retina (signs of leaking blood vessels), damaged nerve tissue, and any changes to the blood vessels.

If your eye care professional believes you need treatment for macular edema, he or she may suggest a fluorescein angiogram. In this test, a special dye is injected into your arm. Pictures are taken as the dye passes through the blood vessels in your retina. The test allows your eye care professional to identify any leaking blood vessels and recommend treatment.

Treatment

How is diabetic retinopathy treated?

During the first three stages of diabetic retinopathy, no treatment is needed, unless you have macular edema. To prevent progression of diabetic retinopathy, people with diabetes should control their levels of blood sugar, blood pressure, and blood cholesterol.

Proliferative retinopathy is treated with laser surgery. This procedure is called scatter laser treatment. Scatter laser treatment helps to shrink the abnormal blood vessels. Your doctor places 1,000 to 2,000 laser burns in the areas of the retina away from the macula, causing the abnormal blood vessels to shrink. Because a high number of laser burns are necessary, two or more sessions usually are required to complete treatment. Although you may notice some loss of your side vision, scatter laser treatment can save the rest of your sight. Scatter laser treatment may slightly reduce your color vision and night vision.

Scatter laser treatment works better before the fragile, new blood vessels have started to bleed. That is why it is important to have regular, comprehensive dilated eye exams. Even if bleeding has started, scatter laser treatment may still be possible, depending on the amount of bleeding.

If the bleeding is severe, you may need a surgical procedure called a vitrectomy. During a vitrectomy, blood is removed from the center of your eye.

How is a macular edema treated?

Macular edema is treated with laser surgery. This procedure is called focal laser treatment. Your doctor places up to several hundred small laser burns in the areas of retinal leakage surrounding the macula. These burns slow the leakage of fluid and reduce the amount of fluid in the retina. The surgery is usually completed in one session. Further treatment may be needed.

A patient may need focal laser surgery more than once to control the leaking fluid. If you have macular edema in both eyes and require laser surgery, generally only one eye will be treated at a time, usually several weeks apart.

Focal laser treatment stabilizes vision. In fact, focal laser treatment reduces the risk of vision loss by 50 percent. In a small number of cases, if vision is lost, it can be improved. Contact your eye care professional if you have vision loss.

What happens during laser treatment?

Both focal and scatter laser treatment are performed in your doctor's office or eye clinic. Before the surgery, your doctor will dilate your pupil and apply drops to numb the eye. The area behind your eye also may be numbed to prevent discomfort.

The lights in the office will be dim. As you sit facing the laser machine, your doctor will hold a special lens to your eye. During the procedure, you may see flashes of light. These flashes eventually may create a stinging sensation that can be uncomfortable. You will need someone to drive you home after surgery. Because your pupil will remain dilated for a few hours, you should bring a pair of sunglasses.

For the rest of the day, your vision will probably be a little blurry. If your eye hurts, your doctor can suggest treatment.

Laser surgery and appropriate follow-up care can reduce the risk of blindness by 90 percent. However, laser surgery often cannot restore vision that has already been lost. That is why finding diabetic retinopathy early is the best way to prevent vision loss.

What is a vitrectomy?

If you have a lot of blood in the center of the eye (vitreous gel), you may need a vitrectomy to restore your sight. If you need vitrectomies in both eyes, they are usually done several weeks apart.

A vitrectomy is performed under either local or general anesthesia. Your doctor makes a tiny incision in your eye. Next, a small instrument is used to remove the vitreous gel that is clouded with blood. The vitreous gel is replaced with a salt solution. Because the vitreous gel is mostly water, you will notice no change between the salt solution and the original vitreous gel.

You will probably be able to return home after the vitrectomy. Some people stay in the hospital overnight. Your eye will be red and sensitive. You will need to wear an eye patch for a few days or weeks to protect your eye. You also will need to use medicated eyedrops to protect against infection.

Are scatter laser treatment and vitrectomy effective in treating proliferative retinopathy?

Yes. Both treatments are very effective in reducing vision loss. People with proliferative retinopathy have less than a five percent chance of becoming blind within five years when they get timely and appropriate treatment. Although both treatments have high success rates, they do not cure diabetic retinopathy.

Once you have proliferative retinopathy, you always will be at risk for new bleeding. You may need treatment more than once to protect your sight.

What can I do if I already have lost some vision from diabetic retinopathy?

If you have lost some sight from diabetic retinopathy, ask your eye care professional about low vision services and devices that may help you make the most of your remaining vision. Ask for a referral to a specialist in low vision. Many community organizations and agencies offer information about low vision counseling, training, and other special services for people with visual impairments. A nearby school of medicine or optometry may provide low vision services.

Chapter 39

Diabetes and Bone-Related Concerns

Renal Osteodystrophy

The medical term "renal" describes things related to the kidneys. Renal osteodystrophy is a bone disease that occurs when your kidneys fail to maintain the proper levels of calcium and phosphorus in your blood. It's a common problem in people with kidney disease and affects 90 percent of dialysis patients.

Renal osteodystrophy is most serious in children because their bones are still growing. The condition slows bone growth and causes deformities. One such deformity occurs when the legs bend inward toward each other or outward away from each other; this deformity is referred to as "renal rickets." Another important consequence is short stature. Symptoms can be seen in growing children with renal disease even before they start dialysis.

The bone changes from renal osteodystrophy can begin many years before symptoms appear in adults with kidney disease. For this reason, it's called the "silent crippler." The symptoms of renal osteodystrophy aren't usually seen in adults until they have been on dialysis for several years. Older patients and women who have gone through

This chapter includes: "Renal Osteodystrophy," National Kidney and Urologic Diseases Information Clearinghouse, National Institute of Diabetes and Digestive and Kidney Diseases, NIH Pub. No. 05-4630, January 2005; and excerpts from "What People with Diabetes Need to Know about Osteoporosis," National Institute of Arthritis and Musculoskeletal and Skin Diseases, November 2006.

menopause are at greater risk for this disease because they're already vulnerable to osteoporosis, another bone disease, even without kidney disease. If left untreated, the bones gradually become thin and weak, and a person with renal osteodystrophy may begin to feel bone and joint pain. There's also an increased risk of bone fractures.

Hormones and Minerals

In healthy adults, bone tissue is continually being remodeled and rebuilt. The kidneys play an important role in maintaining healthy bone mass and structure because one of their jobs is to balance calcium and phosphorus levels in the blood.

Calcium is a mineral that builds and strengthens bones. It's found in many foods, particularly milk and other dairy products. If calcium levels in the blood become too low, four small glands in the neck called the parathyroid glands release a hormone called parathyroid hormone (PTH). This hormone draws calcium from the bones to raise blood calcium levels. Too much PTH in the blood will remove too much calcium from the bones; over time, the constant removal of calcium weakens the bones.

Phosphorus, which is found in most foods, also helps regulate calcium levels in the bones. Healthy kidneys remove excess phosphorus from the blood. When the kidneys stop working normally, phosphorus levels in the blood can become too high, leading to lower levels of calcium in the blood and resulting in the loss of calcium from the bones.

Healthy kidneys produce calcitriol, a form of vitamin D, to help the body absorb dietary calcium into the blood and the bones. If calcitriol levels drop too low, PTH levels increase, and calcium is removed from the bones. Calcitriol and PTH work together to keep calcium balance normal and bones healthy. In a patient with kidney failure, the kidneys stop making calcitriol. The body then can't absorb calcium from food and starts removing it from the bones.

Diagnosis

To diagnose renal osteodystrophy, your doctor may take a sample of your blood to measure levels of calcium, phosphorus, PTH, and calcitriol. The doctor may perform a bone biopsy to see how dense your bones are. A bone biopsy is done under local anesthesia and involves removing a small sample of bone from the hip and analyzing it under a microscope. Determining the cause of renal osteodystrophy helps the doctor decide on a course of treatment.

Treatment

Controlling PTH levels prevents calcium from being withdrawn from the bones. Usually, overactive parathyroid glands are controllable with a change in diet, dialysis treatment, or medication. The drug cinacalcet hydrochloride (Sensipar), approved by the Food and Drug Administration in 2004, lowers PTH levels by imitating calcium. If PTH levels can't be controlled, the parathyroid glands may need to be removed surgically.

If your kidneys aren't making adequate amounts of calcitriol, you can take synthetic calcitriol as a pill or in an injectable form. Your doctor may prescribe a calcium supplement in addition to calcitriol.

Renal osteodystrophy can also be treated with changes in diet. Reducing dietary intake of phosphorus is one of the most important steps in preventing bone disease. Almost all foods contain phosphorus, but it's especially high in milk, cheese, dried beans, peas, nuts, and peanut butter. Limit drinks such as cocoa, dark sodas, and beer. Often, medications such as calcium carbonate (Tums), calcium acetate (PhosLo), sevelamer hydrochloride (Renagel), or lanthanum carbonate (Fosrenol) are prescribed with meals and snacks to bind phosphorus in the bowel. These decrease the absorption of phosphorus into the blood. Be sure your phosphate binder is aluminum-free because aluminum can be toxic and cause anemia. A renal dietitian can help develop a dietary plan to control phosphorus levels in the blood.

Exercise has been found to increase bone strength in some patients. It's important, however, to consult a doctor or health care professional before beginning any exercise program.

A good treatment program, including proper attention to dialysis, diet, and medications, can improve your body's ability to repair bones damaged by renal osteodystrophy.

What People with Diabetes Need to Know about Osteoporosis

What Is Osteoporosis?

Osteoporosis is a condition in which the bones become less dense and more likely to fracture. Fractures from osteoporosis can result in pain and disability. Osteoporosis is a major health threat for an estimated 44 million Americans, 68 percent of whom are women.

Risk factors for developing osteoporosis include the following:

• being thin or having a small frame

- having a family history of the disease

- for women, being postmenopausal, having an early menopause, or not having menstrual periods (amenorrhea)

- using certain medications, such as glucocorticoids

- not getting enough calcium

- not getting enough physical activity

- smoking

- drinking too much alcohol

Osteoporosis is a disease that often can be prevented. If undetected, it can progress for many years without symptoms until a fracture occurs.

The Diabetes—Osteoporosis Link

Type 1 diabetes is linked to low bone density, although researchers don't know exactly why. Insulin, which is deficient in type 1 diabetes, may promote bone growth and strength. The onset of type 1 diabetes typically occurs at a young age when bone mass is still increasing. It is possible that people with type 1 diabetes achieve lower peak bone mass, the maximum strength and density that bones reach. People usually reach their peak bone mass by age 30. Low peak bone mass increases one's risk of developing osteoporosis later in life. Some people with type 1 diabetes also have celiac disease which is associated with reduced bone mass. It is also possible that cytokines, substances produced by various cells in the body, play a role in the development of both type 1 diabetes and osteoporosis.

Recent research also suggests that women with type 1 diabetes may have an increased fracture risk, since vision problems and nerve damage associated with the disease have been linked to an increased risk of falls and related fractures. Hypoglycemia, or low blood sugar reactions, may also contribute to falls.

Increased body weight can reduce one's risk of developing osteoporosis. Since excessive weight is common in people with type 2 diabetes, affected people were long believed to be protected against osteoporosis. However, while bone density is increased in people with type 2 diabetes, fractures are increased. As with type 1 diabetes this may be due to increased falls because of vision problems and nerve damage. Moreover, the sedentary lifestyle common in many people with type 2 diabetes also interferes with bone health.

Managing Osteoporosis

Strategies to prevent and treat osteoporosis in people with diabetes are the same as for those without diabetes.

Nutrition: A diet rich in calcium and vitamin D is important for healthy bones. Good sources of calcium include low-fat dairy products; dark green, leafy vegetables; and calcium-fortified foods and beverages. Many low-fat and low-sugar sources of calcium are available. Also, supplements can help you meet the daily requirements of calcium and other important nutrients.

Vitamin D plays an important role in calcium absorption and bone health. It is synthesized in the skin through exposure to sunlight. While many people are able to obtain enough vitamin D naturally, older individuals are often deficient in this vitamin due, in part, to limited time spent outdoors. They may require vitamin D supplements to ensure an adequate daily intake.

Exercise: Like muscle, bone is living tissue that responds to exercise by becoming stronger. The best exercise for your bones is weight-bearing exercise that forces you to work against gravity. Some examples include walking, stair climbing, and dancing. Regular exercise can help prevent bone loss and, by enhancing balance and flexibility, reduce the likelihood of falling and breaking a bone. Exercise is especially important for people with diabetes since exercise helps insulin lower blood glucose levels.

Healthy lifestyle: Smoking is bad for bones as well as for the heart and lungs. Women who smoke tend to go through menopause earlier, triggering earlier bone loss. In addition, smokers may absorb less calcium from their diets. Alcohol can also negatively affect bone health. Heavy drinkers are more prone to bone loss and fracture because of poor nutrition as well as an increased risk of falling. Avoiding smoking and alcohol can also help with managing diabetes.

Bone density test: Specialized tests known as bone mineral density (BMD) tests measure bone density in various parts of the body. These tests can detect osteoporosis before a bone fracture occurs and predict one's chances of fracturing in the future. The most widely recognized bone mineral density test is called a dual-energy x-ray absorptiometry or DXA test. It is painless: a bit like having an x-ray, but with much less exposure to radiation. It can measure bone density at your

379

hip and spine. People with diabetes should talk to their doctors about whether they might be candidates for a bone density test.

Medication: Like diabetes, there is no cure for osteoporosis. However, there are medications available for preventing and treating osteoporosis. Several medications (alendronate, risedronate, ibandronate, raloxifene, calcitonin, teriparatide, and estrogen/hormone therapy) are approved by the Food and Drug Administration for the prevention and/ or treatment of osteoporosis in postmenopausal women. Alendronate and risedronate are also approved for use in men and in both women and men with glucocorticoid-induced osteoporosis. Teriparatide is approved for use in women and men with severe osteoporosis.

Resources

For additional information on osteoporosis, visit the NIH Resource Center's website at http://www.niams.nih.gov/bone/index.htm or call 800-624-2663.

For additional information on diabetes, visit the National Institute of Diabetes and Digestive and Kidney Diseases website at http://diabetes .niddk.nih.gov or call 800-860-8747.

For Your Information

This chapter contains information about medications used to treat the health condition discussed here. When this information was printed, it included the most up-to-date (accurate) information available. Occasionally, new information on medication is released.

For updates and for any questions about any medications you are taking, please contact the U.S. Food and Drug Administration at 888-INFO-FDA (888-463-6332, a toll-free call) or visit their website at http://www.fda.gov.

Chapter 40

Diabetes and Depression

Depression can strike anyone, but people with diabetes, a serious disorder that afflicts an estimated 18 million Americans, may be at greater risk. In addition, individuals with depression may be at greater risk for developing diabetes. Treatment for depression helps people manage symptoms of both diseases, thus improving the quality of their lives.

Several studies suggest that diabetes doubles the risk of depression compared to those without the disorder.[1] The chances of becoming depressed increase as diabetes complications worsen. Research shows that depression leads to poorer physical and mental functioning, so a person is less likely to follow a required diet or medication plan. Treating depression with psychotherapy, medication, or a combination of these treatments can improve a patient's well-being and ability to manage diabetes.

Causes underlying the association between depression and diabetes are unclear. Depression may develop because of stress but also may result from the metabolic effects of diabetes on the brain. Studies suggest that people with diabetes who have a history of depression are more likely to develop diabetic complications than those without depression. People who suffer from both diabetes and depression tend to have higher health care costs in primary care.[2]

Despite the enormous advances in brain research in the past 20 years, depression often goes undiagnosed and untreated. People with diabetes, their families and friends, and even their physicians may not distinguish the symptoms of depression. However, skilled health professionals will recognize these symptoms and inquire about their duration and severity, diagnose the disorder, and suggest appropriate treatment.

Treatment for Depression

Depression Facts

Depression is a serious medical condition that affects thoughts, feelings, and the ability to function in everyday life. Depression can occur at any age. National Institute of Mental Health (NIMH)-sponsored studies estimate that 6% of 9- to 17-year-olds in the U.S. and almost 10 percent of American adults, or about 19 million people age 18 and older, experience some form of depression every year. Although available therapies alleviate symptoms in over 80 percent of those treated, less than half of people with depression get the help they need.

Depression results from abnormal functioning of the brain. The causes of depression are currently a matter of intense research. An interaction between genetic predisposition and life history appear to determine a person's level of risk. Episodes of depression may then be triggered by stress, difficult life events, side effects of medications, or other environmental factors. Whatever its origins, depression can limit the energy needed to keep focused on treatment for other disorders, such as diabetes.

Symptoms of Depression

Symptoms of depression most commonly include:

- persistent sad, anxious, or "empty" mood;
- feelings of hopelessness, pessimism;
- feelings of guilt, worthlessness, helplessness;
- loss of interest or pleasure in hobbies and activities that were once enjoyed, including sex;
- decreased energy, fatigue, being "slowed down";
- difficulty concentrating, remembering, making decisions;
- insomnia, early-morning awakening, or oversleeping;
- appetite and/or weight changes;

- thoughts of death or suicide, or suicide attempts;
- restlessness, irritability.

If five or more of these symptoms are present every day for at least two weeks and interfere with routine daily activities such as work, self-care, and childcare or social life, seek an evaluation for depression.

Get Treatment for Depression

While there are many different treatments for depression, they must be carefully chosen by a trained professional based on the circumstances of the person and family. Prescription antidepressant medications are generally well-tolerated and safe for people with diabetes. Specific types of psychotherapy, or "talk" therapy, also can relieve depression. However, recovery from depression takes time. Antidepressant medications can take several weeks to work and may need to be combined with ongoing psychotherapy. Not everyone responds to treatment in the same way. Prescriptions and dosing may need to be adjusted.

In people who have diabetes and depression, scientists report that psychotherapy and antidepressant medications have positive effects on both mood and glycemic control. Additional trials will help us better understand the links between depression and diabetes and the behavioral and physiologic mechanisms by which improvement in depression fosters better adherence to diabetes treatment and healthier lives.

Treatment for depression in the context of diabetes should be managed by a mental health professional—for example, a psychiatrist, psychologist, or clinical social worker—who is in close communication with the physician providing the diabetes care. This is especially important when antidepressant medication is needed or prescribed, so that potentially harmful drug interactions can be avoided. In some cases, a mental health professional that specializes in treating individuals with depression and co-occurring physical illnesses such as diabetes may be available. People with diabetes who develop depression, as well as people in treatment for depression who subsequently develop diabetes, should make sure to tell any physician they visit about the full range of medications they are taking.

Use of herbal supplements of any kind should be discussed with a physician before they are tried. Recently, scientists have discovered that St. John's wort, an herbal remedy sold over-the-counter and promoted as a treatment for mild depression, can have harmful interactions with some other medications.

Other mental disorders, such as bipolar disorder (manic-depressive illness) and anxiety disorders, may occur in people with diabetes, and they too can be effectively treated. For more information about these and other mental illnesses, contact NIMH.

Remember, depression is a treatable disorder of the brain. Depression can be treated in addition to whatever other illnesses a person might have, including diabetes. If you think you may be depressed or know someone who is, don't lose hope. Seek help for depression.

1. Anderson RJ, Lustman PJ, Clouse RE, et al. Prevalence of depression in adults with diabetes: a systematic review. *Diabetes*, 2000; 49(Suppl 1): A64.

2. Ciechanowski PS, Katon WJ, Russo JE. Depression and diabetes: impact of depressive symptoms on adherence, function, and costs. *Archives of Internal Medicine*, 2000; 160(21): 3278–85.

Part Five

Diabetes and Kidney Failure

Chapter 41

Your Kidneys and How They Work

Your two kidneys are vital organs that perform many functions to keep your blood clean and chemically balanced. Understanding how your kidneys work can help you to keep them healthy.

What do my kidneys do?

Your kidneys are bean-shaped organs, each about the size of your fist. They are located near the middle of your back, just below the rib cage. The kidneys are sophisticated reprocessing machines. Every day, your kidneys process about 200 quarts of blood to sift out about two quarts of waste products and extra water. The waste and extra water become urine, which flows to your bladder through tubes called ureters. Your bladder stores urine until you go to the bathroom.

The wastes in your blood come from the normal breakdown of active tissues and from the food you eat. Your body uses the food for energy and self-repair. After your body has taken what it needs from the food, waste is sent to the blood. If your kidneys did not remove these wastes, the wastes would build up in the blood and damage your body.

The actual filtering occurs in tiny units inside your kidneys called nephrons. Every kidney has about a million nephrons. In the nephron, a glomerulus—which is a tiny blood vessel, or capillary—intertwines

National Kidney and Urologic Diseases Information Clearinghouse, National Institute of Diabetes and Digestive and Kidney Diseases, NIH Pub. No. 06-4241, November 2005.

with a tiny urine-collecting tube called a tubule. A complicated chemical exchange takes place, as waste materials and water leave your blood and enter your urinary system.

At first, the tubules receive a combination of waste materials and chemicals that your body can still use. Your kidneys measure out chemicals like sodium, phosphorus, and potassium and release them back to the blood to return to the body. In this way, your kidneys regulate the body's level of these substances. The right balance is necessary for life, but excess levels can be harmful.

In addition to removing wastes, your kidneys release three important hormones:

- Erythropoietin, or EPO, which stimulates the bone marrow to make red blood cells

- Renin, which regulates blood pressure

Figure 41.1. The kidneys remove wastes and extra water from the blood to form urine. Urine flows from the kidneys to the bladder through the ureters.

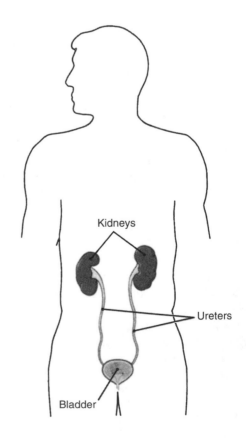

388

- Calcitriol, the active form of vitamin D, which helps maintain calcium for bones and for normal chemical balance in the body

What is renal function?

Your health care team may talk about the work your kidneys do as renal function. If you have two healthy kidneys, you have 100 percent of your renal function. This is more renal function than you really need. Some people are born with only one kidney, and these people are able to lead normal, healthy lives. Many people donate a kidney for transplantation to a family member or friend. Small declines in renal function may not cause a problem.

But many people with reduced renal function have a kidney disease that will get worse. You will have serious health problems if you have less than 25 percent of your renal function. If your renal function drops

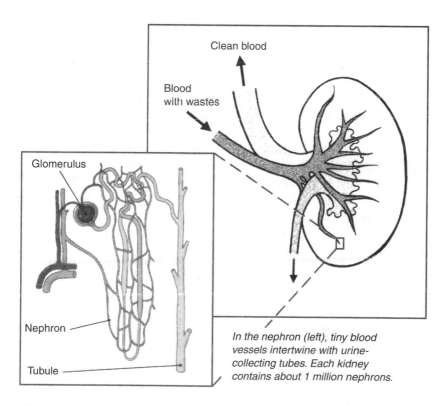

Clean blood

Blood with wastes

Glomerulus

Nephron

Tubule

In the nephron (left), tiny blood vessels intertwine with urine-collecting tubes. Each kidney contains about 1 million nephrons.

Figure 41.2. *Filtering occurs in nephrons, tiny units inside the kidneys.*

below 10 to 15 percent, you cannot live long without some form of renal replacement therapy—either dialysis or transplantation.

Why do kidneys fail?

Most kidney diseases attack the nephrons, causing them to lose their filtering capacity. Damage to the nephrons may happen quickly, often as the result of injury or poisoning. But most kidney diseases destroy the nephrons slowly and silently. Only after years or even decades will the damage become apparent. Most kidney diseases attack both kidneys simultaneously.

The two most common causes of kidney disease are diabetes and high blood pressure. If your family has a history of any kind of kidney problems, you may be at risk for kidney disease.

Diabetic nephropathy: Diabetes is a disease that keeps the body from using glucose (sugar) as it should. If glucose stays in your blood instead of breaking down, it can act like a poison. Damage to the nephrons from unused glucose in the blood is called diabetic nephropathy. If you keep your blood glucose levels down, you can delay or prevent diabetic nephropathy.

High blood pressure: High blood pressure can damage the small blood vessels in your kidneys. The damaged vessels cannot filter wastes from your blood as they are supposed to.

Your doctor may prescribe blood pressure medication. Blood pressure medicines called angiotensin-converting enzyme (ACE) inhibitors and angiotensin receptor blockers (ARBs) have been found to protect the kidneys even more than other medicines that lower blood pressure to similar levels. The National Heart, Lung, and Blood Institute (NHLBI), one of the National Institutes of Health, recommends that people with diabetes or reduced kidney function should keep their blood pressure below 130/80 mm Hg.

Glomerular diseases: Several different types of kidney disease are grouped together under this category, including autoimmune diseases, infection-related diseases, and sclerotic diseases. As the name indicates, glomerular diseases attack the tiny blood vessels (glomeruli) within the kidney. The most common primary glomerular diseases include membranous nephropathy, IgA nephropathy, and focal segmental glomerulosclerosis. Protein, blood, or both in the urine are often the first signs of these diseases. They can slowly destroy kidney function. Blood pressure control is important with any kidney disease.

390

Treatments for glomerular diseases may include immunosuppressive drugs or steroids to reduce inflammation and proteinuria, depending on the specific disease.

What are the signs of kidney disease?

People in the early stages of kidney disease usually do not feel sick at all.

If your kidney disease gets worse, you may need to urinate more often or less often. You may feel tired or itchy. You may lose your appetite or experience nausea and vomiting. Your hands or feet may swell or feel numb. You may get drowsy or have trouble concentrating. Your skin may darken. You may have muscle cramps.

What medical tests will my doctor use to detect kidney disease?

Since you can have kidney disease without any symptoms, your doctor may first detect the condition through routine blood and urine tests. The National Kidney Foundation recommends three simple tests to screen for kidney disease: a blood pressure measurement, a spot check for protein or albumin in the urine (proteinuria), and a calculation of glomerular filtration rate (GFR) based on a serum creatinine measurement. Measuring urea nitrogen in the blood provides additional information.

Blood pressure measurement: High blood pressure can lead to kidney disease. It can also be a sign that your kidneys are already impaired. The only way to know whether your blood pressure is high is to have a health professional measure it with a blood pressure cuff. The result is expressed as two numbers. The top number, which is called the systolic pressure, represents the pressure when your heart is beating. The bottom number, which is called the diastolic pressure, shows the pressure when your heart is resting between beats. Your blood pressure is considered normal if it stays below 120/80 (expressed as "120 over 80"). The NHLBI recommends that people with kidney disease use whatever therapy is necessary, including lifestyle changes and medicines, to keep their blood pressure below 130/80.

Microalbuminuria and proteinuria: Healthy kidneys take wastes out of the blood but leave protein. Impaired kidneys may fail to separate a blood protein called albumin from the wastes. At first, only small amounts of albumin may leak into the urine, a condition

391

known as microalbuminuria, a sign of deteriorating kidney function. As kidney function worsens, the amount of albumin and other proteins in the urine increases, and the condition is called proteinuria. Your doctor may test for protein using a dipstick in a small sample of your urine taken in the doctor's office. The color of the dipstick indicates the presence or absence of proteinuria.

A more sensitive test for protein or albumin in the urine involves laboratory measurement and calculation of the protein-to-creatinine or albumin-to-creatinine ratio. This test should be used to detect kidney disease in people at high risk, especially those with diabetes. If your first laboratory test shows high levels of protein, another test should be done one to two weeks later. If the second test also shows high levels of protein, you have persistent proteinuria and should have additional tests to evaluate your kidney function.

Glomerular filtration rate (GFR) based on creatinine measurement: GFR is a calculation of how efficiently the kidneys are filtering wastes from the blood. A traditional GFR calculation requires an injection into the bloodstream of a substance that is later measured in a 24-hour urine collection. Recently, scientists found they could calculate GFR without an injection or urine collection. The new calculation requires only a measurement of the creatinine in a blood sample.

Creatinine is a waste product in the blood created by the normal breakdown of muscle cells during activity. Healthy kidneys take creatinine out of the blood and put it into the urine to leave the body. When kidneys are not working well, creatinine builds up in the blood.

In the lab, your blood will be tested to see how many milligrams of creatinine are in one deciliter of blood (mg/dL). Creatinine levels in the blood can vary, and each laboratory has its own normal range, usually 0.6 to 1.2 mg/dL. If your creatinine level is only slightly above this range, you probably will not feel sick, but the elevation is a sign that your kidneys are not working at full strength. One formula for estimating kidney function equates a creatinine level of 1.7 mg/dL for most men and 1.4 mg/dL for most women to 50 percent of normal kidney function. But because creatinine values are so variable and can be affected by diet, a GFR calculation is more accurate for determining whether a person has reduced kidney function.

The new GFR calculation uses the patient's creatinine measurement along with weight, age, and values assigned for sex and race. Some medical laboratories may make the GFR calculation when a creatinine value is measured and include it on their lab report.

Blood urea nitrogen (BUN): Blood carries protein to cells throughout the body. After the cells use the protein, the remaining waste product is returned to the blood as urea, a compound that contains nitrogen. Healthy kidneys take urea out of the blood and put it in the urine. If your kidneys are not working well, the urea will stay in the blood.

A deciliter of normal blood contains 7 to 20 milligrams of urea. If your BUN is more than 20 mg/dL, your kidneys may not be working at full strength. Other possible causes of an elevated BUN include dehydration and heart failure.

Additional tests for kidney disease: If blood and urine tests indicate reduced kidney function, your doctor may recommend additional tests to help identify the cause of the problem.

Renal imaging: Methods of renal imaging (taking pictures of the kidneys) include ultrasound, computed tomography (CT scan), and magnetic resonance imaging (MRI). These tools are most helpful in finding unusual growths or blockages to the flow of urine.

Renal biopsy: Your doctor may want to see a tiny piece of your kidney tissue under a microscope. To obtain this tissue sample, the doctor will perform a renal biopsy—a hospital procedure in which the doctor inserts a needle through your skin into the back of the kidney. The needle retrieves a strand of tissue about 1/2 to 3/4 of an inch long. For the procedure, you will lie on your stomach on a table and receive local anesthetic to numb the skin. The sample tissue will help the doctor identify problems at the cellular level.

What are the stages of kidney disease?

Your GFR is the best indicator of how well your kidneys are working. In 2002, the National Kidney Foundation published treatment guidelines that identified five stages of chronic kidney disease (CKD) based on declining GFR measurements. The guidelines recommend different actions based on the stage of kidney disease.

- **Increased risk of CKD:** A GFR of 90 or above is considered normal. Even with a normal GFR, you may be at increased risk for developing CKD if you have diabetes, high blood pressure, or a family history of kidney disease. The risk increases with age: People over 65 are more than twice as likely to develop CKD as people between the ages of 45 and 65. African Americans also have a higher risk of developing CKD.

393

- **Stage 1:** Kidney damage with normal GFR (90 or above). Kidney damage may be detected before the GFR begins to decline. In this first stage of kidney disease, the goals of treatment are to slow the progression of CKD and reduce the risk of heart and blood vessel disease.

- **Stage 2:** Kidney damage with mild decrease in GFR (60 to 89). When kidney function starts to decline, your health care provider will estimate the progression of your CKD and continue treatment to reduce the risk of other health problems.

- **Stage 3:** Moderate decrease in GFR (30 to 59). When CKD has advanced to this stage, anemia and bone problems become more common. Work with your health care provider to prevent or treat these complications.

- **Stage 4:** Severe reduction in GFR (15 to 29). Continue following the treatment for complications of CKD and learn as much as you can about the treatments for kidney failure. Each treatment requires preparation. If you choose hemodialysis, you will need to have a procedure to make a vein in your arm larger and stronger for repeated needle insertions. For peritoneal dialysis, you will need to have a catheter placed in your abdomen. Or you may want to ask family or friends to consider donating a kidney for transplantation.

- **Stage 5:** Kidney failure (GFR less than 15). When the kidneys do not work well enough to maintain life, you will need dialysis or a kidney transplant.

In addition to tracking your GFR, blood tests can show when substances in your blood are out of balance. If phosphorus or potassium levels start to climb, a blood test will prompt your health care provider to address these issues before they permanently affect your health.

What can I do about kidney disease?

Unfortunately, chronic kidney disease often cannot be cured. But if you are in the early stages of a kidney disease, you may be able to make your kidneys last longer by taking certain steps. You will also want to be sure that risks for heart attack and stroke are minimized, since CKD patients are susceptible to these problems.

- If you have diabetes, watch your blood glucose closely to keep it under control. Consult your doctor for the latest in treatment.

- Avoid pain pills that may make your kidney disease worse. Check with your doctor before taking any medicine.

Blood pressure: People with reduced kidney function (a high creatinine level in the blood or a low creatinine clearance) should have their blood pressure controlled, and an ACE inhibitor or an ARB should be one of their medications. Many people will require two or more types of medication to keep their blood pressure below 130/80 mm Hg. A diuretic is an important addition to the ACE inhibitor or ARB.

Diet: People with reduced kidney function need to be aware that some parts of a normal diet may speed their kidney failure.

Protein: Protein is important to your body. It helps your body repair muscles and fight disease. Protein comes mostly from meat. As discussed in an earlier section, healthy kidneys take wastes out of the blood but leave protein. Impaired kidneys may fail to separate the protein from the wastes.

Some doctors tell their kidney patients to limit the amount of protein they eat so that the kidneys have less work to do. But you cannot avoid protein entirely. You may need to work with a dietitian to find the right food plan.

Cholesterol: Another problem that may be associated with kidney failure is too much cholesterol in your blood. High levels of cholesterol may result from a high-fat diet.

Cholesterol can build up on the inside walls of your blood vessels. The buildup makes pumping blood through the vessels harder for your heart and can cause heart attacks and strokes.

Smoking: Smoking not only increases the risk of kidney disease, it contributes to deaths from strokes and heart attacks in people with CKD. You should try your best to stop smoking.

Sodium: Sodium is a chemical found in salt and other foods. Sodium in your diet may raise your blood pressure, so you should limit foods that contain high levels of sodium. High-sodium foods include canned or processed foods like frozen dinners and hot dogs.

Potassium: Potassium is a mineral found naturally in many fruits and vegetables, like oranges, potatoes, bananas, dried fruits, dried beans and peas, and nuts. Healthy kidneys measure potassium in your blood and remove excess amounts. Diseased kidneys may fail to remove excess potassium, and with very poor kidney function, high potassium levels can affect the heart rhythm.

Treating anemia: Anemia is a condition in which the blood does not contain enough red blood cells. These cells are important because they carry oxygen throughout the body. If you are anemic, you will feel tired and look pale. Healthy kidneys make the hormone EPO, which stimulates the bones to make red blood cells. Diseased kidneys may not make enough EPO. You may need to take injections of a man-made form of EPO.

Preparing for end-stage renal disease: As your kidney disease progresses, you will need to make several decisions. You will need to learn about your options for treating ESRD so that you can make an informed choice between hemodialysis, peritoneal dialysis, and transplantation.

What happens if my kidneys fail completely?

Complete and irreversible kidney failure is sometimes called end-stage renal disease, or ESRD. If your kidneys stop working completely, your body fills with extra water and waste products. This condition is called uremia. Your hands or feet may swell. You will feel tired and weak because your body needs clean blood to function properly.

Untreated uremia may lead to seizures or coma and will ultimately result in death. If your kidneys stop working completely, you will need to undergo dialysis or kidney transplantation.

Dialysis: The two major forms of dialysis are hemodialysis and peritoneal dialysis. In hemodialysis, your blood is sent through a filter that removes waste products. The clean blood is returned to your body. Hemodialysis is usually performed at a dialysis center three times per week for three to four hours.

In peritoneal dialysis, a fluid is put into your abdomen. This fluid captures the waste products from your blood. After a few hours, the fluid containing your body's wastes is drained away. Then, a fresh bag of fluid is dripped into the abdomen. Patients can perform peritoneal dialysis themselves. Patients using continuous ambulatory peritoneal dialysis (CAPD) change fluid four times a day. Another form of peritoneal dialysis, called continuous cycling peritoneal dialysis (CCPD), can be performed at night with a machine that drains and refills the abdomen automatically.

Transplantation: A donated kidney may come from an anonymous donor who has recently died or from a living person, usually a relative. The kidney that you receive must be a good match for your body. The more the new kidney is like you, the less likely your immune system is to reject it. Your immune system protects you from disease by attacking anything that is not recognized as a normal part of your body. So your immune system will attack a kidney that appears too "foreign." You will take special drugs to help trick your immune system so it does not reject the transplanted kidney.

Chapter 42

Kidney Failure: Choosing a Treatment That's Right for You

Your kidneys filter wastes from your blood and regulate other functions of your body. When your kidneys fail, you need treatment to replace the work your kidneys normally perform.

Developing kidney failure means that you have some decisions to make about your treatment. If you choose to receive treatment, your choices are hemodialysis, which requires a machine used to filter your blood outside your body; peritoneal dialysis, which uses the lining of your belly to filter your blood inside the body; and kidney transplantation, in which a new kidney is placed in your body. Each of them has advantages and disadvantages. You may also choose to forgo treatment. By learning about your choices, you can work with your doctor to decide what's best for you. No matter which treatment you choose, you'll need to make some changes in your life, including how you eat and plan your activities. But with the help of your health care team, family, and friends, you can lead a full, active life.

When Your Kidneys Fail

Healthy kidneys clean your blood by removing excess fluid, minerals, and wastes. They also make hormones that keep your bones strong and your blood healthy. When your kidneys fail, harmful wastes

Excerpted from "Kidney Failure: Choosing a Treatment That's Right for You," National Kidney and Urologic Diseases Information Clearinghouse, National Institute of Diabetes and Digestive and Kidney Diseases, NIH Pub. No. 07-2412, March 2007.

build up in your body, your blood pressure may rise, and your body may retain excess fluid and not make enough red blood cells. When this happens, you need treatment to replace the work of your failed kidneys.

Treatment Choice: Hemodialysis

Purpose

Hemodialysis cleans and filters your blood using a machine to temporarily rid your body of harmful wastes, extra salt, and extra water. Hemodialysis helps control blood pressure and helps your body keep the proper balance of important chemicals such as potassium, sodium, calcium, and bicarbonate.

How It Works

Hemodialysis uses a special filter called a dialyzer that functions as an artificial kidney to clean your blood. During treatment, your blood travels through tubes into the dialyzer, which filters out wastes and extra water. Then the cleaned blood flows through another set of tubes back into your body. The dialyzer is connected to a machine that monitors blood flow and removes wastes from the blood.

Hemodialysis is usually needed three times a week. Each treatment lasts from three to five or more hours. During treatment, you can read, write, sleep, talk, or watch TV.

Who Performs It

Hemodialysis is usually done in a dialysis center by nurses and trained technicians. In some parts of the country, certain centers are available to offer the training and support for home hemodialysis, which requires the help of a partner, usually a family member or friend, and sufficient space and water supply in the home. If you decide to do home dialysis, you and your partner will receive special training. As home hemodialysis machines become more convenient and the support more available, home hemodialysis may be an option across the country.

Possible Complications

Vascular access problems are the most common reason for hospitalization among people on hemodialysis. Common problems include infection, blockage from clotting, and poor blood flow. These problems can keep your treatments from working. You may need to undergo repeated surgeries in order to get a properly functioning access.

Other problems can be caused by rapid changes in your body's water and chemical balance during treatment. Muscle cramps and hypotension—a sudden drop in blood pressure—are two common side effects. Hypotension can make you feel weak, dizzy, or sick to your stomach.

You'll probably need a few months to adjust to hemodialysis. Side effects can often be treated quickly and easily, so you should always report them to your doctor and dialysis staff. You can avoid many side effects if you follow a proper diet, limit your liquid intake, and take your medicines as directed.

Pros and Cons

Each person responds differently to similar situations. What may be a negative factor for one person may be positive for another. See a list of the general advantages and disadvantages of in-center and home hemodialysis below.

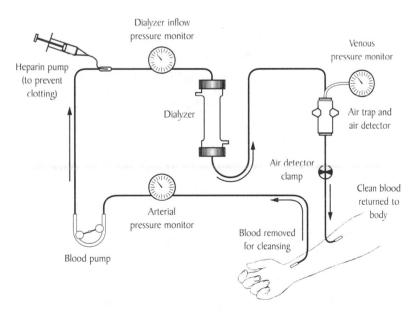

Figure 42.1. *Hemodialysis*

In-Center Hemodialysis, Pros

- Facilities are widely available.
- You have trained professionals with you at all times.
- You can get to know other patients.

In-Center Hemodialysis, Cons

- Treatments are scheduled by the center and are relatively fixed.
- You must travel to the center for treatment.

Home Hemodialysis, Pros

- You can do it at the times you choose—but you still must do it as often as your doctor orders.
- You don't have to travel to a center.
- You gain a sense of independence and control over your treatment.
- Newer machines require less space.

Home Hemodialysis, Cons

- You must have a helper.
- Helping with treatments may be stressful to your family.
- You and your helper need training.
- You need space for storing the machine and supplies at home.

Working with Your Health Care Team

Questions you may want to ask:

- Is hemodialysis the best treatment choice for me? Why?
- If I'm treated at a center, can I go to the center of my choice?
- What should I look for in a dialysis center?
- Will my kidney doctor see me at dialysis?
- What does hemodialysis feel like?
- What is self-care dialysis?
- Is home hemodialysis available in my area? How long does it take to learn? Who will train my partner and me?

- What kind of blood access is best for me?

- As a hemodialysis patient, will I be able to keep working? Can I have treatments at night?

- How much should I exercise?

- Who will be on my health care team? How can these people help me?

- With whom can I talk about finances, sexuality, or family concerns?

- How/where can I talk with other people who have faced this decision?

Treatment Choice: Peritoneal Dialysis

Purpose

Peritoneal dialysis is another procedure that removes extra water, wastes, and chemicals from your body. This type of dialysis uses the lining of your abdomen, or belly, to filter your blood. This lining is called the peritoneal membrane and acts as the artificial kidney.

How It Works

A mixture of minerals and sugar dissolved in water, called dialysis solution, travels through a soft tube into your belly. The sugar—called dextrose—draws wastes, chemicals, and extra water from the tiny blood vessels in your peritoneal membrane into the dialysis solution. After several hours, the used solution is drained from your abdomen through the tube, taking the wastes from your blood with it. Then you fill your abdomen with fresh dialysis solution, and the cycle is repeated. The process of draining and refilling is called an exchange.

Types of Peritoneal Dialysis

Three types of peritoneal dialysis are available.

Continuous ambulatory peritoneal dialysis (CAPD): CAPD requires no machine and can be done in any clean, well-lit place. With CAPD, your blood is always being cleaned. The dialysis solution passes from a plastic bag through the catheter and into your abdomen, where it stays for several hours with the catheter sealed. The time period that dialysis solution is in your abdomen is called the dwell time. Next, you drain the dialysis solution into an empty bag for disposal. You then refill your abdomen with fresh dialysis solution so the cleaning process can begin again. With CAPD, the dialysis solution stays in your abdomen for a dwell time of four to six hours, or more. The process of draining the used dialysis solution and replacing it with fresh solution takes about 30 to 40 minutes. Most people change the dialysis solution at least four times a day and sleep with solution in their abdomens at night. With CAPD, it's not necessary to wake up and perform dialysis tasks during the night.

Continuous cycler-assisted peritoneal dialysis (CCPD): CCPD uses a machine called a cycler to fill and empty your abdomen three to five times during the night while you sleep. In the morning, you begin one exchange with a dwell time that lasts the entire day. You may do an additional exchange in the middle of the afternoon without the cycler to increase the amount of waste removed and to reduce the amount of fluid left behind in your body.

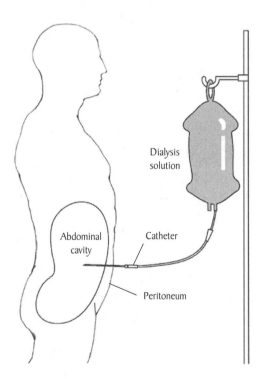

Figure 42.2. Peritoneal Dialysis

Combination of CAPD and CCPD: If you weigh more than 175 pounds or if your peritoneum filters wastes slowly, you may need a combination of CAPD and CCPD to get the right dialysis dose. For example, some people use a cycler at night but also perform one exchange during the day. Others do four exchanges during the day and use a minicycler to perform one or more exchanges during the night. You'll work with your health care team to determine the best schedule for you.

Who Performs It

Both types of peritoneal dialysis are usually performed by the patient without help from a partner. CAPD is a form of self-treatment that needs no machine. However, with CCPD, you need a machine to drain and refill your abdomen.

Possible Complications

The most common problem with peritoneal dialysis is peritonitis, a serious abdominal infection. This infection can occur if the opening where the catheter enters your body becomes infected or if contamination occurs as the catheter is connected or disconnected from the bags. Peritonitis requires antibiotic treatment by your doctor.

To avoid peritonitis, you must be careful to follow procedures exactly and learn to recognize the early signs of peritonitis, which include fever, unusual color or cloudiness of the used fluid, and redness or pain around the catheter. Report these signs to your doctor immediately so that peritonitis can be treated quickly to avoid serious problems.

Pros and Cons

Each type of peritoneal dialysis has advantages and disadvantages.

CAPD, Pros

- You can do it alone.
- You can do it at times you choose as long as you perform the required number of exchanges each day.
- You can do it in many locations.
- You don't need a machine.

405

CAPD, Cons

- It can disrupt your daily schedule.
- It is a continuous treatment, and all exchanges must be performed seven days a week.

CCPD, Pros

- You can do it at night, mainly while you sleep.
- You are free from exchanges during the day.

CCPD, Cons

- You need a machine.
- Your movement at night is limited by your connection to the cycler.

Working with Your Health Care Team

Questions you may want to ask:

- Is peritoneal dialysis the best treatment choice for me? Why? If yes, which type is best?
- How long will it take me to learn how to do peritoneal dialysis?
- What does peritoneal dialysis feel like?
- How will peritoneal dialysis affect my blood pressure?
- How will I know if I have peritonitis? How is it treated?
- As a peritoneal dialysis patient, will I be able to continue working?
- How much should I exercise?
- Where do I store supplies?
- How often do I see my doctor?
- Who will be on my health care team? How can these people help me?
- Whom do I contact with problems?
- With whom can I talk about finances, sexuality, or family concerns?
- How/where can I talk with other people who have faced this decision?

Dialysis Is Not a Cure

Hemodialysis and peritoneal dialysis are treatments that help replace the work your kidneys did. These treatments help you feel better and live longer, but they don't cure kidney failure. Although patients with kidney failure are now living longer than ever, over the years kidney disease can cause problems such as heart disease, bone disease, arthritis, nerve damage, infertility, and malnutrition. These problems won't go away with dialysis, but doctors now have new and better ways to prevent or treat them. You should discuss these complications and treatments with your doctor.

Treatment Choice: Kidney Transplantation

Purpose

Kidney transplantation surgically places a healthy kidney from another person into your body. The donated kidney does the work that your two failed kidneys used to do.

How It Works

A surgeon places the new kidney inside your lower abdomen and connects the artery and vein of the new kidney to your artery and vein. Your blood flows through the donated kidney, which makes urine, just like your own kidneys did when they were healthy. The new kidney may start working right away or may take up to a few weeks to make urine. Unless your own kidneys are causing infection or high blood pressure, they are left in place.

The Time It Takes

How long you'll have to wait for a kidney varies. Because there aren't enough deceased donors for every person who needs a transplant, you must be placed on a waiting list. However, if a voluntary donor gives you a kidney, the transplant can be scheduled as soon as you're both ready. Avoiding the long wait is a major advantage of living donation.

The surgery takes three to four hours. The usual hospital stay is about a week. After you leave the hospital, you'll have regular follow-up visits.

If someone has given you a kidney, the donor will probably stay in the hospital about the same amount of time. However, a new technique for removing a kidney for donation uses a smaller incision and may make it possible for the donor to leave the hospital in two to three days.

Between 85 and 90 percent of transplants from deceased donors are working one year after surgery. Transplants from living relatives often work better than transplants from deceased donors because they're usually a closer match.

Possible Complications

Transplantation is the closest thing to a cure. But no matter how good the match, your body may reject your new kidney. A common cause of rejection is not taking medication as prescribed.

Your doctor will give you drugs called immunosuppressants to help prevent your body's immune system from attacking the kidney, a process called rejection. You'll need to take immunosuppressants every day for as long as the transplanted kidney is functioning. Sometimes, however, even these drugs can't stop your body from rejecting the new kidney. If this happens, you'll go back to some form of dialysis and possibly wait for another transplant.

Immunosuppressants can weaken your immune system, which can lead to infections. Some drugs may also change your appearance. Your face may get fuller; you may gain weight or develop acne or facial hair. Not all patients have these problems, though, and diet and makeup can help.

Immunosuppressants work by diminishing the ability of immune cells to function. In some patients, over long periods of time, this diminished immunity can increase the risk of developing cancer. Some immunosuppressants can cause cataracts, diabetes, extra stomach acid, high blood pressure, and bone disease. When used over time, these drugs may also cause liver or kidney damage in a few patients.

Pros and Cons

Kidney transplantation has advantages and disadvantages.

Kidney Transplantation, Pros

- A transplanted kidney works like a normal kidney.
- You may feel healthier or "more normal."
- You have fewer diet restrictions.
- You won't need dialysis.

- Patients who successfully go through the selection process have a higher chance of living a longer life.

Kidney Transplantation, Cons

- It requires major surgery.
- You may need to wait for a donor.
- Your body may reject the new kidney, so one transplant may not last a lifetime.
- You'll need to take immunosuppressants, which may cause complications.

Working with Your Health Care Team

Questions you may want to ask:

- Is transplantation the best treatment choice for me? Why?
- What are my chances of having a successful transplant?
- How do I find out whether a family member or friend can donate?

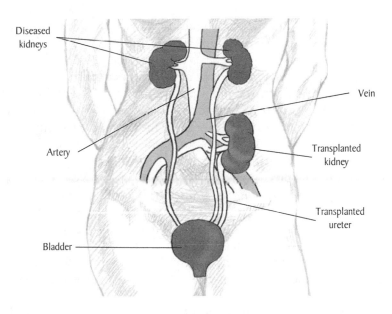

Figure 42.3. Kidney Transplantation

- What are the risks to a family member or friend who donates?

- If a family member or friend doesn't donate, how do I get placed on a waiting list for a kidney?

- How long will I have to wait?

- What symptoms does rejection cause?

- How long does a transplant work?

- What side effects do immunosuppressants cause?

- Who will be on my health care team? How can these people help me?

- With whom can I talk about finances, sexuality, or family concerns?

- How or where can I talk with other people who have faced this decision?

Treatment Choice: Refusing or Withdrawing from Treatment

For many people, dialysis and transplantation not only extend life but also improve quality of life. For others who have serious ailments in addition to kidney failure, dialysis may seem a burden that only prolongs suffering. You have the right to refuse or withdraw from dialysis if you feel you have no hope of leading a life with dignity and meaning. You may want to speak with your spouse, family, religious counselor, or social worker as you make this decision.

If you withdraw from dialysis treatments or refuse to begin them, you may live for a few days or for several weeks, depending on your health and your remaining kidney function. Your doctor can give you medicines to make you more comfortable during this time. Should you change your mind about refusing dialysis, you may start or resume your treatments at any time.

Even if you're satisfied with your quality of life on dialysis, you should think about circumstances that might make you want to stop dialysis treatments. At some point in a medical crisis, you might lose the ability to express your wishes to your doctor. An advance directive is a statement or document in which you give instructions either to withhold treatment or to provide it, depending on your wishes and the specific circumstances.

An advance directive may be a living will, a document that details the conditions under which you would want to refuse treatment. You may state that you want your health care team to use all available means to sustain your life. Or you may direct that you be withdrawn from dialysis if you become permanently unresponsive or fall into a coma from which you won't awake. In addition to dialysis, other life-sustaining treatments that you may choose or refuse include the following:

- cardiopulmonary resuscitation (CPR)
- tube feedings
- mechanical or artificial respiration
- antibiotics
- surgery
- blood transfusions

Another form of advance directive is called a durable power of attorney for health care decisions or a health care proxy. In this type of advance directive, you assign a person to make health care decisions for you if you become unable to make them for yourself. Make sure the person you name understands your values and is willing to follow through on your instructions.

Each state has its own laws governing advance directives. You can obtain a form for an advance medical directive that's valid in your state from the National Hospice and Palliative Care Organization.

Paying for Treatment

Treatment for kidney failure is expensive, but federal health insurance plans pay much of the cost, usually up to 80 percent. Often, private insurance or state programs pay the rest.

Conclusion

Deciding which type of treatment is best for you isn't easy. Your decision depends on your medical condition, lifestyle, and personal likes and dislikes. Discuss the pros and cons of each treatment with your health care team and family. You can switch between treatment methods during the course of your therapy. If you start one form of treatment and decide you'd like to try another, talk with your doctor. The key is to learn as much as you can about your choices first. With that knowledge, you and your doctor will choose the treatment that suits you best.

Chapter 43

Understanding Hemodialysis

Chapter Contents

Section 43.1—Hemodialysis for the Treatment of
  Kidney Failure 414
Section 43.2—Vascular Access for Hemodialysis 418
Section 43.3—Hemodialysis Dose and Adequacy 422
Section 43.4—Home Hemodialysis... 426
Section 43.5—Eat Right to Feel Right on Hemodialysis.......... 429

Section 43.1

Hemodialysis for the Treatment of Kidney Failure

Excerpted from "Treatment Methods for Kidney Failure: Hemodialysis," National Kidney and Urologic Diseases Information Clearinghouse, National Institute of Diabetes and Digestive and Kidney Diseases, NIH Pub. No. 07-4666, December 2006.

Hemodialysis is the most common method used to treat advanced and permanent kidney failure. Since the 1960s, when hemodialysis first became a practical treatment for kidney failure, we've learned much about how to make hemodialysis treatments more effective and minimize side effects. In recent years, more compact and simpler dialysis machines have made home dialysis increasingly attractive. But even with better procedures and equipment, hemodialysis is still a complicated and inconvenient therapy that requires a coordinated effort from your whole health care team, including your nephrologist, dialysis nurse, dialysis technician, dietitian, and social worker. The most important members of your health care team are you and your family. By learning about your treatment, you can work with your health care team to give yourself the best possible results, and you can lead a full, active life.

How Hemodialysis Works

In hemodialysis, your blood is allowed to flow, a few ounces at a time, through a special filter that removes wastes and extra fluids. The clean blood is then returned to your body. Removing the harmful wastes and extra salt and fluids helps control your blood pressure and keep the proper balance of chemicals like potassium and sodium in your body.

One of the biggest adjustments you must make when you start hemodialysis treatments is following a strict schedule. Most patients go to a clinic—a dialysis center—three times a week for three to five or more hours each visit. For example, you may be on a Monday-Wednesday-Friday schedule or a Tuesday-Thursday-Saturday schedule. You may

414

be asked to choose a morning, afternoon, or evening shift, depending on availability and capacity at the dialysis unit. Your dialysis center will explain your options for scheduling regular treatments.

Researchers are exploring whether shorter daily sessions, or longer sessions performed overnight while the patient sleeps, are more effective in removing wastes. Newer dialysis machines make these alternatives more practical with home dialysis. But the federal government has not yet established a policy to pay for more than three hemodialysis sessions a week.

Several centers around the country teach people how to perform their own hemodialysis treatments at home. A family member or friend who will be your helper must also take the training, which usually takes at least four to six weeks. Home dialysis gives you more flexibility in your dialysis schedule. With home hemodialysis, the time for each session and the number of sessions per week may vary, but you must maintain a regular schedule by giving yourself dialysis treatments as often as you would receive them in a dialysis unit.

Adjusting to Changes

Even in the best situations, adjusting to the effects of kidney failure and the time you spend on dialysis can be difficult. Aside from the "lost time," you may have less energy. You may need to make changes in your work or home life, giving up some activities and responsibilities. Keeping the same schedule you kept when your kidneys were working can be very difficult now that your kidneys have failed. Accepting this new reality can be very hard on you and your family. A counselor or social worker can answer your questions and help you cope.

Many patients feel depressed when starting dialysis, or after several months of treatment. If you feel depressed, you should talk with your social worker, nurse, or doctor because this is a common problem that can often be treated effectively.

Getting Your Vascular Access Ready

One important step before starting hemodialysis is preparing a vascular access, a site on your body from which your blood is removed and returned. A vascular access should be prepared weeks or months before you start dialysis. It will allow easier and more efficient removal and replacement of your blood with fewer complications.

Equipment and Procedures

When you first visit a hemodialysis center, it may seem like a complicated mix of machines and people. But once you learn how the procedure works and become familiar with the equipment, you'll be more comfortable.

Dialysis Machine

The dialysis machine is about the size of a dishwasher. This machine has three main jobs:

- Pump blood and watch flow for safety

- Clean wastes from blood

- Watch your blood pressure and the rate of fluid removal from your body

Dialyzer

The dialyzer is a large canister containing thousands of small fibers through which your blood is passed. Dialysis solution, the cleansing

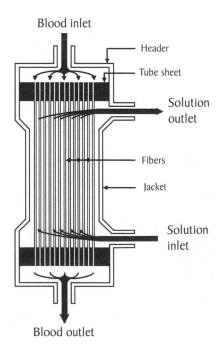

Figure 43.1. Structure of a typical hollow fiber dialyzer.

fluid, is pumped around these fibers. The fibers allow wastes and extra fluids to pass from your blood into the solution, which carries them away. The dialyzer is sometimes called an artificial kidney.

Reuse. Your dialysis center may use the same dialyzer more than once for your treatments. Reuse is considered safe as long as the dialyzer is cleaned before each use. The dialyzer is tested each time to make sure it's still working, and it should never be used for anyone but you. Before each session, you should be sure that the dialyzer is labeled with your name and check to see that it has been cleaned, disinfected, and tested.

Dialysis Solution

Dialysis solution, also known as dialysate, is the fluid in the dialyzer that helps remove wastes and extra fluid from your blood. It contains chemicals that make it act like a sponge. Your doctor will give you a specific dialysis solution for your treatments. This formula can be adjusted based on how well you handle the treatments and on your blood tests.

Needles

Many people find the needle sticks to be one of the hardest parts of hemodialysis treatments. Most people, however, report getting used to them after a few sessions. If you find the needle insertion painful, an anesthetic cream or spray can be applied to the skin. The cream or spray will numb your skin briefly so you won't feel the needle.

Most dialysis centers use two needles—one to carry blood to the dialyzer and one to return the cleaned blood to your body. Some specialized needles are designed with two openings for two-way flow of blood, but these needles are less efficient and require longer sessions. Needles for high-flux or high-efficiency dialysis need to be a little larger than those used with regular dialyzers.

Some people prefer to insert their own needles. You'll need training on inserting needles properly to prevent infection and protect your vascular access. You may also learn a "ladder" strategy for needle placement in which you "climb" up the entire length of the access session by session so that you don't weaken an area with a grouping of needle sticks. A different approach is the "buttonhole" strategy in which you use a limited number of sites but insert the needle back into the same hole made by the previous needle stick. Whether you insert your own needles or not, you should know these techniques to better care for your access.

417

Tests to See How Well Your Dialysis Is Working

About once a month, your dialysis care team will test your blood by using one of two formulas [described in Section 43.3] to see whether your treatments are removing enough wastes. Both tests look at one specific waste product, called blood urea nitrogen (BUN), as an indicator for the overall level of waste products in your system.

Financial Issues

Treatment for kidney failure is expensive, but federal health insurance plans pay much of the cost, usually up to 80 percent. Often, private insurance or State programs pay the rest. Your social worker can help you locate resources for financial assistance.

Section 43.2

Vascular Access for Hemodialysis

Excerpted from "Vascular Access for Hemodialysis," National Kidney and Urologic Diseases Information Clearinghouse, National Institute of Diabetes and Digestive and Kidney Diseases, NIH Pub. No. 05-4554, January 2005.

If you will be starting hemodialysis treatments in the next several months, you will need to work with your health care team to learn how the treatments work and what you can do to get the most from them. One important step before starting regular hemodialysis sessions is preparing a vascular access, which is the site on your body where blood will be removed and returned during dialysis. To maximize the amount of blood cleansed during hemodialysis, the vascular access should provide high volumes of blood flow continuously during treatments.

A vascular access should be prepared weeks or months before you start dialysis. It will allow easier and more efficient removal and replacement of your blood with fewer complications. There are three basic kinds of vascular accesses for hemodialysis: an arteriovenous (AV) fistula, an AV graft, and a venous catheter. A fistula is an opening or connection between any two parts of the body that are usually separate, for example, a hole in the tissue that normally separates the bladder from the bowel. While most kinds of fistula are a problem, an AV fistula is useful because it causes the vein to grow large and strong for easy access to the blood system. The AV fistula is considered the best long-term vascular access for hemodialysis because it provides adequate blood flow for dialysis, lasts a long time, and has a complication rate lower than the other access types. If an AV fistula cannot be created, an AV graft or venous catheter may be needed.

Arteriovenous Fistula

An AV fistula requires advance planning because a fistula takes a while after surgery to develop (in rare cases, as long as 24 months). But a properly formed fistula is less likely than other kinds of vascular accesses to form clots or become infected. Also, fistulas tend to last many years, longer than any other kind of vascular access.

A surgeon creates an AV fistula by connecting an artery directly to a vein, usually in the forearm. Connecting the artery to the vein causes more blood to flow into the vein. As a result, the vein grows larger and stronger, making repeated insertions for hemodialysis treatments easier. For the surgery, you'll be given a local anesthetic. In most cases, the procedure can be performed on an outpatient basis.

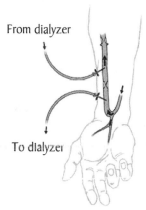

Figure 43.2. *Forearm arteriovenous fistula.*

From dialyzer

To dialyzer

Arteriovenous Graft

If you have small veins that won't develop properly into a fistula, you can get a vascular access that uses a synthetic tube implanted under the skin in your arm. The tube becomes an artificial vein that can be used repeatedly for needle placement and blood access during hemodialysis. A graft doesn't need to develop as a fistula does, so it can be used sooner after placement, often within two or three weeks.

Compared with fistulas, grafts tend to have more problems with clotting or infection and need replacement sooner, but a well-cared-for graft can last for several years.

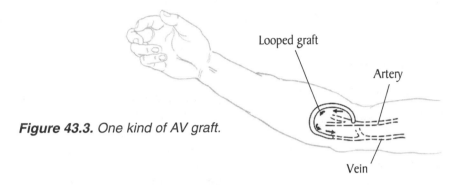

Figure 43.3. *One kind of AV graft.*

Venous Catheter for Temporary Access

If your kidney disease has progressed quickly, you may not have time to get a permanent vascular access before you start hemodialysis treatments. You may need to use a venous catheter as a temporary access.

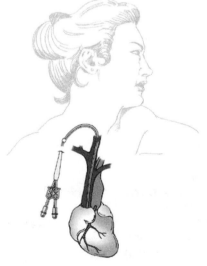

Figure 43.4. *Venous catheter for temporary hemodialysis access.*

A catheter is a tube inserted into a vein in either your neck, chest, or leg near the groin. It has two chambers to allow two-way flow of blood. Once a catheter is placed, needle insertion is not necessary.

Catheters are not ideal for permanent access. They can clog, become infected, or cause narrowing of the veins in which they are placed. But if you need to start hemodialysis immediately, a catheter will suffice for several weeks or months while your permanent access develops.

For some patients, fistula or graft surgery is not successful, and a long-term catheter access must be used. Catheters that will be needed for more than about three weeks are designed to be tunneled under the skin to increase comfort and reduce complications.

Possible Complications

All three types of vascular access—AV fistula, AV graft, and venous catheter—can have complications that require further treatment or surgery. The most common complications are access infection and low blood flow due to blood clotting in the access.

Venous catheters are most likely to develop infection and clotting problems that may require medications and catheter removal or replacement.

AV grafts may also develop low blood flows, an indication of clotting or narrowing of the access. In this situation, the AV graft may require angioplasty, a procedure to widen the small segment that is narrowed. Another option is to perform surgery on the AV graft and replace the narrow segment.

Infection and low blood flow are much less common in AV fistulas than in AV grafts and venous catheters. Still, having an AV fistula is not a guarantee against complications.

Taking Care of Your Access

You can do several things to protect your access.

- Make sure your nurse or technician checks your access before each treatment.

- Keep your access clean at all times.

- Use your access site only for dialysis.

- Be careful not to bump or cut your access.

- Don't let anyone put a blood pressure cuff on your access arm.

421

- Don't wear jewelry or tight clothes over your access site.
- Don't sleep with your access arm under your head or body.
- Don't lift heavy objects or put pressure on your access arm.
- Check the pulse in your access every day.

Section 43.3

Hemodialysis Dose and Adequacy

Excerpted from "Hemodialysis Dose and Adequacy," National Kidney and Urologic Diseases Information Clearinghouse, National Institute of Diabetes and Digestive and Kidney Diseases, NIH Pub. No. 06-4556, December 2005.

When kidneys fail, dialysis is necessary to remove waste products such as urea from the blood. By itself, urea is not very toxic, but its level represents the levels of many other waste products that build up in the blood when the kidneys fail.

To see whether dialysis is removing enough urea, the clinic should periodically—normally once a month—test a patient's blood to measure dialysis adequacy. Blood is sampled at the start of dialysis and at the end. The levels of urea in the two blood samples are then compared. Two methods are generally used to assess dialysis adequacy, URR and Kt/V.

What is the URR?

The reduction in urea as a result of dialysis, or the URR, is one measure of how effectively a dialysis treatment removed waste products from the body. URR stands for urea reduction ratio, but it is commonly expressed as a percentage.

Example: If the initial (predialysis) urea level was 50 mg/dL and the postdialysis urea level was 15 mg/dL, the amount of urea removed is 35 mg/dL.

- 50 mg/dL – 15 mg/dL = 35 mg/dL

The amount of urea removed (35 mg/dL) is expressed as a percentage of the predialysis urea level (50 mg/dL).

- 35/50 = 70/100 = 70%

Although no fixed number can be said to represent an adequate dialysis, it has been shown that patients generally live longer and have fewer hospitalizations if the URR is at least 60 percent. For this reason, some groups advising on national standards have recommended a minimum URR of 65 percent.

The URR is usually measured only once every 12 to 14 treatments, which is once a month. It may vary considerably from treatment to treatment. For this reason, a single value below 65 percent should not be of great concern, but on average the URR should exceed 65 percent.

What is the Kt/V?

Another way of measuring dialysis adequacy is the Kt/V. In this measurement:

- K stands for the dialyzer clearance, expressed in milliliters per minute (mL/min);

- t stands for time;

- Kt, the top part of the fraction, is clearance multiplied by time, representing the volume of fluid completely cleared of urea during a single treatment;

- V, the bottom part of the fraction, is the volume of water a patient's body contains.

Example: If the dialyzer's clearance is 300 mL/min and a dialysis session lasts for 180 minutes (3 hours), Kt will be 300 mL/min x 180 min. This equals 54,000 mL, or 54 liters.

- Kt = 300 mL/min x 180 min

- Kt = 54,000 mL = 54 liters

The body is about 60 percent water by weight. If a patient weighs 70 kilograms (154 lbs.), V will be 42 liters.

- V = 70 kg x .60 = 42 liters

So the ratio (K x t) to V, or Kt/V, compares the amount of fluid that passes through the dialyzer with the amount of fluid in the patient's body. The Kt/V for this patient would be 1.3.

- Kt/V = 54/42 = 1.3

The Kt/V is mathematically related to the URR and is in fact derived from it, except that the Kt/V also takes into account two additional factors:

- Urea generated by the body during dialysis
- Extra urea removed during dialysis along with excess fluid

The Kt/V is more accurate than the URR in measuring how much urea is removed during dialysis, primarily because the Kt/V also considers the amount of urea removed with excess fluid. Consider two patients with the same URR and the same postdialysis weight, one with a weight loss of 1 kg during the treatment and the other with a weight loss of 3 kg. The patient who loses 3 kg will have a higher Kt/V, even though both have the same URR.

This does not mean that it is better to gain more water weight between dialysis sessions so that more fluid has to be removed, since this has bad effects on the heart and circulation. However, patients who lose more weight during dialysis will have a higher Kt/V for the same level of URR.

How does the Kt/V compare with the URR?

On average, a Kt/V of 1.2 is roughly equivalent to a URR of about 63 percent. For this reason, another standard of adequate dialysis is a minimum Kt/V of 1.2. This is the standard adopted by the Dialysis Outcomes Quality Initiative (DOQI) group. Like the URR, the Kt/V may vary considerably from treatment to treatment because of measurement error and other factors. So while a single low value is not always of concern, the average Kt/V should be at least 1.2. In some patients with large fluid losses during dialysis, the Kt/V can be greater than 1.2 with a URR slightly below 65 percent (in the range of 58 percent to 65 percent). In such cases, the DOQI guidelines consider the Kt/V to be the primary measure of adequacy.

Is a Kt/V of 1.2 good enough?

These numbers—a URR of 65 percent and a Kt/V of 1.2—have been determined to be benchmarks of dialysis adequacy on the basis of studies in large groups of patients. These studies generally showed that patients with lower Kt/V and/or URR numbers had more health problems and a greater risk of death. However, the HEMO clinical trial showed that a Kt/V greater than 1.2 did not result in improved outcomes.

What should you do if your Kt/V is below 1.2 or if your URR is below 65 percent?

1. If your Kt/V is always above 1.2 and your URR is close to 65 percent (it may be a few points lower if you have large fluid losses during dialysis), then your treatment is meeting adequacy guidelines.

2. If your average Kt/V (usually the average of three measurements) is consistently below 1.2, then you and your nephrologist need to discuss ways to improve it. Since the V value is fixed (it represents the total volume of water in your body), Kt/V can be improved either by increasing K (clearance) or t (session length). To increase t, you need to dialyze for a longer period. For example, if your Kt/V is 0.9 and you want to go up to 1.2, then you need 1.2/0.9 = 1.33 times more Kt. If K is not changed, this means that the length of your session needs to increase by 33 percent. If your session lasts three hours, it should be increased to four hours.

    The other way to improve the Kt in Kt/V is to increase K, the dialyzer clearance, which depends primarily on the rate of blood flow through the dialyzer. No matter how good a dialyzer you have, how well it works depends primarily on moving blood through it. In many patients, a good rate is difficult to achieve because of access problems.

    If your blood flow rate is good, you can get further improvements in clearance by making sure that you use a big dialyzer or, in some cases, by increasing the flow rate for dialysis solution from the usual 500 mL/min to 600 or 800 mL/min. A good flow rate for adult patients is 350 mL/min and higher. A few centers are even using two dialyzers at the same time to increase K in large patients.

    However, the rate of blood flow through the dialyzer is key, and a good vascular access is very important to make sure you are getting good clearance.

3. If during any given month your Kt/V is very low, the measurement should be repeated, unless there was an obvious reason for the low Kt/V. Obvious reasons include treatment interruption, problems with blood or solution flow, and some problem in sampling either the pre- or postdialysis blood. If there is no clear-cut reason for the sudden drop, then a problem with needle placement, like accidental needle reversal, or with the vascular access, like recirculation, should be suspected.

Section 43.4

Home Hemodialysis

Home hemodialysis is carried out in the patient's home by the patient or with assistance from a family member or other helper. First developed in Boston, London, and Seattle in the early 1960s, home hemodialysis was soon found to be a safe, effective, and economical way of providing dialysis. By 1972, of the 10,000 or so patients on dialysis in the United States, more than 4,000 were being treated at home.

Why is home hemodialysis good for patients? First, evidence from research studies show that home hemodialysis patients live longer than patients treated in a dialysis center. There is also good evidence that the quality of life for these patients is better. These benefits are important, but there are others. In Seattle, it was first noticed in the 1960s that home hemodialysis patients became more independent and self-sufficient. It was also observed that the more patients knew about their disease and the more responsibility they took for their own treatment, the better their quality of life resulted. These factors apply not only to end-stage renal disease (ESRD) patients, but also to those with any chronic disease—a concept that is being researched today.

Other advantages of home hemodialysis include:

- A greater opportunity for rehabilitation, including work or education;

- The opportunity to perform longer dialysis, even overnight dialysis;

- Access sticking by one person, either by patient or assistant;

- The flexibility to dialyze at times convenient for the patients, saving in travel time and hassle;

- Not having to dialyze in the center with sick patients and with risk of exposure to infections, such as hepatitis C;

- And finally, the feeling of accomplishment.

What are the disadvantages of home hemodialysis? These are primarily psychological rather than medical. The most common is "burn out" of the family member or assistant. This is why it is crucial to emphasize the importance of patients taking care of themselves. The home program can also arrange for patients to dialyze in-center to allow time-off or vacation for the assistant. Although there may be individual disadvantages, there are many patients who have carried out home hemodialysis successfully for years.

What is needed for home hemodialysis? First and most obvious is a willing patient with a home having adequate space for the equipment and storage of supplies. There must be suitable electrical outlets and plumbing to make the dialysate and to drain the machine. The home hemodialysis training program will check these requirements before accepting the patient. It is important that the patient be trained to stick themselves and to dialyze themselves. However, in many cases when using standard dialysis equipment, a family member or other aide may be required.

What about home hemodialysis training? This takes anywhere from three weeks to three months, depending on the training program and the abilities of the patient. The training is usually carried out in the outpatient setting. Patient and helper are tested throughout the training process to ensure that they can perform safe dialysis, have knowledge of how to handle problems with equipment and during emergency situations and how to get support by telephone or modem in order to deal with questions and non-emergency situations.

427

Is it difficult to learn to do your own dialysis? Not particularly. Do not be overwhelmed by the complicated looking machine. If you can drive a car safely, you can certainly learn to operate a dialysis machine equally well. In neither case do you need to know the details of what is under the hood or in the machine. Rather, you have to learn how to use the device safely. Remember, most ordinary people can learn to drive with appropriate training and the same applies to dialysis.

What happens after the patient goes home? The patient will be expected to send information about each dialysis session to the training unit either by filling out a form or by direct electronic connection. Once a month, the patient will be expected to provide a blood sample for the usual tests. The patient is expected to see the nephrologist at least monthly in the physician's office. There will be a training nurse available by telephone at all times who can answer questions, assist the patient in dealing with problems, arrange for technical support for the machine if needed and advise the patient to contact their nephrologist if necessary or to go to the emergency room for acute problems. It is also likely that a training nurse will visit you at home at least once a year to advise and observe dialysis sessions. You will be expected to give your own erythropoietin (EPO) injections, but you will have to come in to the center or the physician's office for other intravenous (IV) injections.

Who pays for home hemodialysis? Medicare pays in just the same way that it pays for center dialysis. Private insurance, Medicaid, or state programs will usually pick up most of the co-insurance costs. The primary individual costs will be for additional electricity and water required for dialysis, and in some areas these costs may be subsidized by a city or utility company.

What does the future hold for home hemodialysis? There will be more of it! There is good evidence that longer dialysis and/or more frequent dialysis is better. In the United States, the average in-center patient dialyzes less than four hours for three times a week and, despite lots of efforts over the last ten years, patient survival has not improved. A few programs provide six to eight hours of dialysis overnight three times a week, but there is still a great lack of home hemodialysis programs in this country.

Studies have shown that dialyzing five, six, and even seven times a week improves patient well-being remarkably, minimizes symptoms both during and between dialyses and reduces the frequency of complications and of days in a hospital. More frequent dialysis can be done by short daily dialysis for two to three hours or long nightly dialysis for six to eight hours—and the most convenient place to perform either of these treatments is at home. Currently, home hemodialysis at least three times a week remains the best treatment for patients who are willing to do this.

What should you do? Hopefully this information has raised your interest in home hemodialysis. Talk to the American Association of Kidney Patients (AAKP), your local patient organization, or the ESRD [End State Renal Disorder] Network in your region and ask to be put in touch with patients who are on home hemodialysis. Talk to them about their experience. It will require interested patients like you to ask your doctor and your unit how you could get home hemodialysis. Home dialysis could become a reality for many more patients over the next few years. Currently, dialyzing overnight provides the best treatment available for dialyzing three times a week. For nightly dialysis, every other night might be better. Remember, regardless of which treatment you choose, you have the option to take charge of your healthcare.

Section 43.5

Eat Right to Feel Right on Hemodialysis

Excerpted from "Eat Right to Feel Right on Hemodialysis," National Kidney and Urologic Diseases Information Clearinghouse, National Institute of Diabetes and Digestive and Kidney Diseases, NIH Pub. No. 07-4274, December 2007.

When you start hemodialysis, you must make many changes in your life. Watching the foods you eat will make you healthier. This publication will help you choose the right foods.

Use this information with a dietitian to help you learn how to eat right to feel right on hemodialysis. Read each section, then go through the exercise for that section with your dietitian.

Once you have completed every exercise, keep a copy of them to remind yourself of foods you can eat and foods you need to avoid.

How does food affect my hemodialysis?

Food gives you energy and helps your body repair itself. Food is broken down in your stomach and intestines. Your blood picks up nutrients from the digested food and carries them to all your body cells. These cells take nutrients from your blood and put waste products back into the bloodstream. When your kidneys were healthy, they worked around the clock to remove wastes from your blood. The wastes left your body when you urinated. Other wastes are removed in bowel movements.

Now that your kidneys have stopped working, hemodialysis removes wastes from your blood. But between dialysis sessions, wastes can build up in your blood and make you sick. You can reduce the amount of wastes by watching what you eat and drink. A good meal plan can improve your dialysis and your health.

Your clinic has a dietitian to help you plan meals. A dietitian specializes in food and nutrition. A dietitian with special training in care for kidney health is called a renal dietitian.

What do I need to know about fluids?

You already know you need to watch how much you drink. Any food that is liquid at room temperature also contains water. These foods include soup, Jell-O, and ice cream. Many fruits and vegetables contain lots of water, too. They include melons, grapes, apples, oranges, tomatoes, lettuce, and celery. All these foods add to your fluid intake.

Fluid can build up between dialysis sessions, causing swelling and weight gain. The extra fluid affects your blood pressure and can make your heart work harder. You could have serious heart trouble from overloading your system with fluid.

Your dry weight is your weight after a dialysis session when all of the extra fluid in your body has been removed. If you let too much fluid build up between sessions, it is harder to get down to your proper dry weight. Your dry weight may change over a period of three to six weeks. Talk with your doctor regularly about what your dry weight should be.

Control your thirst: The best way to reduce fluid intake is to reduce thirst caused by the salt you eat. Avoid salty foods like chips and pretzels. Choose low-sodium products.

You can keep your fluids down by drinking from smaller cups or glasses. Freeze juice in an ice cube tray and eat it like a popsicle. (Remember to count the popsicle in your fluid allowance.) The dietitian will be able to give you other tips for managing your thirst.

Talk with a dietitian: Even though you are on hemodialysis, your kidneys may still be able to remove some fluid. Or your kidneys may not remove any fluid at all. That is why every patient has a different daily allowance for fluid. Talk with your dietitian about how much fluid you can have each day.

What do I need to know about potassium?

Potassium is a mineral found in many foods, especially milk, fruits, and vegetables. It affects how steadily your heart beats. Healthy kidneys keep the right amount of potassium in the blood to keep the heart beating at a steady pace. Potassium levels can rise between dialysis sessions and affect your heartbeat. Eating too much potassium can be very dangerous to your heart. It may even cause death.

To control potassium levels in your blood, avoid foods like avocados, bananas, kiwis, and dried fruit, which are very high in potassium. Also, eat smaller portions of other high-potassium foods. For example, eat half a pear instead of a whole pear. Eat only very small portions of oranges and melons.

Potatoes and other vegetables: You can remove some of the potassium from potatoes and other vegetables by peeling them, then soaking them in a large amount of water for several hours. Drain and rinse the vegetables before cooking them. Your dietitian will give you more specific information about the potassium content of foods.

High-Potassium Foods

- Apricots
- Avocados
- Bananas
- Beets
- Brussels sprouts
- Cantaloupe
- Clams
- Dates
- Figs kiwi fruit
- Lima beans
- Melons
- Milk
- Nectarines

- Orange juice
- Oranges
- Peanuts
- Pears (fresh)
- Potatoes
- Prune juice
- Prunes
- Raisins
- Sardines
- Spinach
- Tomatoes
- Winter squash
- Yogurt

431

What do I need to know about phosphorus?

Phosphorus is a mineral found in many foods. If you have too much phosphorus in your blood, it pulls calcium from your bones. Losing calcium will make your bones weak and likely to break. Also, too much phosphorus may make your skin itch. Foods like milk and cheese, dried beans, peas, colas, nuts, and peanut butter are high in phosphorus. Usually, people on dialysis are limited to ½ cup of milk per day. The renal dietitian will give you more specific information regarding phosphorus.

You probably will need to take a phosphate binder like Renagel, PhosLo, Tums, or calcium carbonate to control the phosphorus in your blood between dialysis sessions. These medications act like sponges to soak up, or bind, phosphorus while it is in the stomach. Because it is bound, the phosphorus does not get into the blood. Instead, it is passed out of the body in the stool.

What do I need to know about protein?

Before you were on dialysis, your doctor may have told you to follow a low-protein diet. Being on dialysis changes this. Most people on dialysis are encouraged to eat as much high-quality protein as they can. Protein helps you keep muscle and repair tissue. The better nourished you are, the healthier you will be. You will also have greater resistance to infection and recover from surgery more quickly.

Your body breaks protein down into a waste product called urea. If urea builds up in your blood, it's a sign you have become very sick. Eating mostly high-quality proteins is important because they produce less waste than others. High-quality proteins come from meat, fish, poultry, and eggs (especially egg whites).

What do I need to know about sodium?

Sodium is found in salt and other foods. Most canned foods and frozen dinners contain large amounts of sodium. Too much sodium makes you thirsty. But if you drink more fluid, your heart has to work harder to pump the fluid through your body. Over time, this can cause high blood pressure and congestive heart failure.

Try to eat fresh foods that are naturally low in sodium. Look for products labeled low sodium.

Do not use salt substitutes because they contain potassium. Talk with a dietitian about spices you can use to flavor your food. The dietitian can help you find spice blends without sodium or potassium.

What do I need to know about calories?

Calories provide energy for your body. If your doctor recommends it, you may need to cut down on the calories you eat. A dietitian can help you plan ways to cut calories in the best possible way.

Some people on dialysis need to gain weight. You may need to find ways to add calories to your diet. Vegetable oils—like olive oil, canola oil, and safflower oil—are good sources of calories. Use them generously on breads, rice, and noodles.

Butter and margarines are rich in calories. But these fatty foods can also clog your arteries. Use them less often. Soft margarine that comes in a tub is better than stick margarine. Vegetable oils are the healthiest way to add fat to your diet if you need to gain weight.

Hard candy, sugar, honey, jam, and jelly provide calories and energy without clogging arteries or adding other things that your body does not need. If you have diabetes, be very careful about eating sweets. A dietitian's guidance is very important for people with diabetes.

Should I take vitamins and minerals?

Vitamins and minerals may be missing from your diet because you have to avoid so many foods. Your doctor may prescribe a vitamin and mineral supplement like Nephrocaps.

Warning: Do not take vitamin supplements that you can buy off the store shelf. They may contain vitamins or minerals that are harmful to you.

Chapter 44

Understanding Peritoneal Dialysis

Chapter Contents

Section 44.1—Peritoneal Dialysis for the Treatment
of Kidney Failure 436

Section 44.2—Peritoneal Dialysis Dose
and Adequacy 444

435

Section 44.1

Peritoneal Dialysis for the Treatment of Kidney Failure

Excerpted from "Treatment Methods for Kidney Failure: Peritoneal Dialysis," National Kidney and Urologic Diseases Information Clearinghouse, National Institute of Diabetes and Digestive and Kidney Diseases, NIH Pub. No. 06-4688, December 2006.

With peritoneal dialysis (PD), you have some choices in treating advanced and permanent kidney failure. Since the 1980s, when PD first became a practical and widespread treatment for kidney failure, much has been learned about how to make PD more effective and minimize side effects. Since you don't have to schedule dialysis sessions at a center, PD gives you more control. You can give yourself treatments at home, at work, or on trips. But this independence makes it especially important that you work closely with your health care team: your nephrologist, dialysis nurse, dialysis technician, dietitian, and social worker. But the most important members of your health care team are you and your family. By learning about your treatment, you can work with your health care team to give yourself the best possible results, and you can lead a full, active life.

How PD Works

In PD, a soft tube called a catheter is used to fill your abdomen with a cleansing liquid called dialysis solution. The walls of your abdominal cavity are lined with a membrane called the peritoneum, which allows waste products and extra fluid to pass from your blood into the dialysis solution. The solution contains a sugar called dextrose that will pull wastes and extra fluid into the abdominal cavity. These wastes and fluid then leave your body when the dialysis solution is drained. The used solution, containing wastes and extra fluid, is then thrown away. The process of draining and filling is called an exchange and takes about 30 to 40 minutes. The period the dialysis solution is in your abdomen is called the dwell time. A typical schedule calls for four exchanges a day, each with a dwell time of four to six hours. Different types of PD have different schedules of daily exchanges.

One form of PD, continuous ambulatory peritoneal dialysis (CAPD), doesn't require a machine. As the word ambulatory suggests, you can walk around with the dialysis solution in your abdomen. Another form of PD, continuous cycler-assisted peritoneal dialysis (CCPD), requires a machine called a cycler to fill and drain your abdomen, usually while you sleep. CCPD is also sometimes called automated peritoneal dialysis (APD).

Getting Ready for PD

Whether you choose an ambulatory or automated form of PD, you'll need to have a soft catheter placed in your abdomen. The catheter is the tube that carries the dialysis solution into and out of your abdomen. If your doctor uses open surgery to insert your catheter, you will be placed under general anesthesia. Another technique requires only local anesthetic. Your doctor will make a small cut, often below and a little to the side of your navel (belly button), and then guide the catheter through the slit into the peritoneal cavity. As soon as the catheter is in place, you can start to receive solution through it, although you probably won't begin a full schedule of exchanges for two to three weeks. This break-in period lets you build up scar tissue that will hold the catheter in place.

The standard catheter for PD is made of soft tubing for comfort. It has cuffs made of a polyester material, called Dacron, that merge with your scar tissue to keep it in place. The end of the tubing that is inside your abdomen has many holes to allow the free flow of solution in and out.

Types of PD

The type of PD you choose will depend on the schedule of exchanges you would like to follow, as well as other factors. You may start with one type of PD and switch to another, or you may find that a combination of automated and nonautomated exchanges suits you best. Work with your health care team to find the best schedule and techniques to meet your lifestyle and health needs.

Continuous ambulatory peritoneal dialysis (CAPD): If you choose CAPD, you'll drain a fresh bag of dialysis solution into your abdomen. After four to six or more hours of dwell time, you'll drain the solution, which now contains wastes, into the bag. You then repeat the

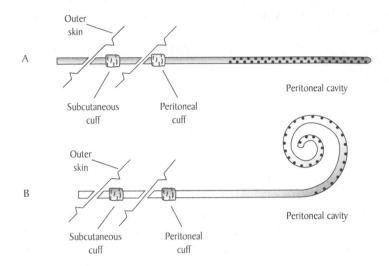

Figure 44.1. Two double-cuff Tenckhoff peritoneal catheters: standard (A), curled (B).

cycle with a fresh bag of solution. You don't need a machine for CAPD; all you need is gravity to fill and empty your abdomen. Your doctor will prescribe the number of exchanges you'll need, typically three or four exchanges during the day and one evening exchange with a long overnight dwell time while you sleep.

Continuous cycler-assisted peritoneal dialysis (CCPD): CCPD uses an automated cycler to perform three to five exchanges during the night while you sleep. In the morning, you begin one exchange with a dwell time that lasts the entire day.

Customizing Your PD

If you've chosen CAPD, you may have a problem with the long overnight dwell time. It's normal for some of the dextrose in the solution to cross into your body and become glucose. The absorbed dextrose doesn't create a problem during short dwell times. But overnight, some people absorb so much dextrose that it starts to draw fluid from the peritoneal cavity back into the body, reducing the efficiency of the exchange. If you have this problem, you may be able to use a minicycler (a small version of a machine that automatically fills and drains your abdomen) to exchange your solution once or several times overnight while you sleep. These additional, shorter exchanges will minimize solution absorption and give you added clearance of wastes and excess fluid.

If you've chosen CCPD, you may have a solution absorption problem with the daytime exchange, which has a long dwell time. You may find you need an additional exchange in the mid-afternoon to increase the amount of waste removed and to prevent excessive absorption of solution.

Preventing Problems

Infection is the most common problem for people on PD. Your health care team will show you how to keep your catheter bacteria-free to avoid peritonitis, which is an infection of the peritoneum. Improved catheter designs protect against the spread of bacteria, but peritonitis is still a common problem that sometimes makes continuing PD impossible. You should follow your health care team's instructions carefully, but here are some general rules:

- Store supplies in a cool, clean, dry place.
- Inspect each bag of solution for signs of contamination before you use it.
- Find a clean, dry, well-lit space to perform your exchanges.
- Wash your hands every time you need to handle your catheter.
- Clean the exit site with antiseptic every day.
- Wear a surgical mask when performing exchanges.

Keep a close watch for any signs of infection and report them so they can be treated promptly. Here are some signs to watch for:

- Fever
- Nausea or vomiting
- Redness or pain around the catheter
- Unusual color or cloudiness in used dialysis solution
- A catheter cuff that has been pushed out

Equipment and Supplies for PD

Transfer Set

A transfer set is tubing that connects the bag of dialysis solution to the catheter. When your catheter is first placed, the exposed end of the tube will be securely capped to prevent infection. Under the cap is a universal connector.

When you start dialysis training, your dialysis nurse will provide a transfer set. The type of transfer set you receive depends on the company that supplies your dialysis solution. Different companies have different systems for connecting to your catheter.

Connecting the transfer set requires sterile technique. You and your nurse will wear surgical masks. Your nurse will soak the transfer set and the end of your catheter in an antiseptic solution for five minutes before making the connection. The nurse will wear rubber gloves while making the connection.

Depending on the company that supplies your solution, your transfer set may require a new cap each time you disconnect from the bag after an exchange. With a different system, the tubing that connects to the transfer set includes a piece that can be clamped at the end of an exchange and then broken off from the tubing so that it stays on the transfer set as a cap until it is removed for the next exchange. Your dialysis nurse will train you in the aseptic (germ-free) technique for connecting at the beginning of an exchange and disconnecting at the end. Follow instructions carefully to avoid infection.

Dialysis Solution

Dialysis solution comes in 1.5-, 2-, 2.5-, or 3-liter bags. A liter is slightly more than 1 quart. The dialysis dose can be increased by using a larger bag, but only within the limit of the amount your abdomen can hold. The solution contains a sugar called dextrose, which pulls extra fluid from your blood. Your doctor will prescribe a formula that fits your needs.

You'll need a clean space to store your bags of solution and other supplies. You may also need a special heating device to warm each bag of solution to body temperature before use. Most solution bags come in a protective outer wrapper that allows for microwave heating. Do not microwave a bag of solution after it has been removed from its wrapper because microwaving can change the chemical makeup of the solution.

Cycler

The cycler—which automatically fills and drains your abdomen, usually at night while you sleep—can be programmed to deliver specified volumes of dialysis solution on a specified schedule. Most systems include the following components:

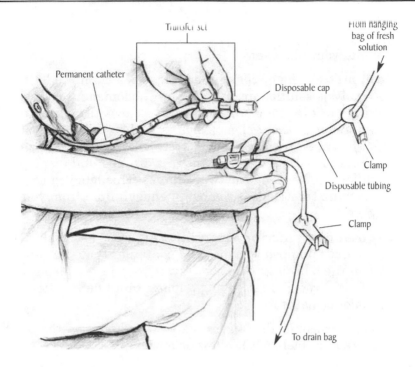

Figure 44.2. Transfer set. Between exchanges, you can keep your catheter and transfer set hidden inside your clothing. At the beginning of an exchange, you will remove the disposable cap from the transfer set and connect it to a Y-tube. The branches of the Y-tube connect to the drain bag and the bag of fresh dialysis solution. Always wash your hands before handling your catheter and transfer set, and wear a surgical mask whenever you connect or disconnect.

- **Solution storage:** At the beginning of the session, you connect bags of dialysis solution to tubing that feeds the cycler. Most systems include a separate tube for the last bag because this solution may have a higher dextrose content so that it can work for a day-long dwell time.

- **Pump:** The pump sends the solution from the storage bags to the heater bag before it enters the body and then sends it to the disposal container or drain line after it's been used. The pump doesn't fill and drain your abdomen; gravity performs that job more safely.

- **Heater bag:** Before the solution enters your abdomen, a measured dose is warmed to body temperature. Once the solution is

441

the right temperature and the previous exchange has been drained, a clamp is released to allow the warmed solution to flow into your abdomen.

- **Fluid meter:** The cycler's timer releases a clamp to let the used dialysis solution drain from your abdomen into a disposal container or drain line. As the solution flows through the tube, a fluid meter in the cycler measures and records how much solution has been removed. Some systems compare the amount of solution inserted with the amount drained and display the net difference between the two volumes. This lets you know whether the treatment is removing enough fluid from your body.

- **Disposal container or drain line:** After the used solution is weighed, it's pumped to a disposal container that you can throw away in the morning. With some systems, you can dispose of the used fluid directly by stringing a long drain line from the cycler to a toilet or bathtub.

- **Alarms:** Sensors will trigger an alarm and shut off the machine if there's a problem with inflow or outflow.

Compliance

One of the big problems with PD is that patients sometimes don't perform all of the exchanges prescribed by their medical team. They either skip exchanges or sometimes skip entire treatment days when using CCPD. Skipping PD treatments has been shown to increase the risk of hospitalization and death.

Remaining Kidney Function

Normally the PD prescription factors in the amount of residual, or remaining, kidney function. Residual kidney function typically falls, although slowly, over months or even years of PD. This means that more often than not, the number of exchanges prescribed, or the volume of exchanges, needs to increase as residual kidney function falls.

The doctor should determine your PD dose on the basis of practice standards established by the National Kidney Foundation Dialysis Outcomes Quality Initiative (NKF-DOQI). Work closely with your health care team to ensure that you get the proper dose, and follow instructions carefully to make sure you get the most out of your dialysis exchanges.

Adjusting to Changes

You can do your exchanges in any clean space, and you can take part in many activities with solution in your abdomen. Even though PD gives you more flexibility and freedom than hemodialysis, which requires being connected to a machine for three to five hours three times a week, you must still stick to a strict schedule of exchanges and keep track of supplies. You may have to cut back on some responsibilities at work or in your home life. Accepting this new reality can be very hard on you and your family. A counselor or social worker can help you cope.

Many patients feel depressed when starting dialysis, or after several months of treatment. Some people can't get used to the fact that the solution makes their body look larger. If you feel depressed, you should talk with your social worker, nurse, or doctor because depression is a common problem that can often be treated effectively.

How Diet Can Help

Eating the right foods can help improve your dialysis and your health. You may have chosen PD over hemodialysis because the diet is less restrictive. With PD, you're removing wastes from your body slowly but constantly, while in hemodialysis, wastes may build up for two or three days between treatments. You still need to be very careful about the foods you eat, however, because PD is much less efficient than working kidneys. Your clinic has a dietitian to help you plan meals. Follow the dietitian's advice closely to get the most from your dialysis treatments. You can also ask your dietitian for recipes and titles of cookbooks for patients with kidney disease. Following the restrictions of a diet for kidney failure might be hard at first, but with a little creativity, you can make tasty and satisfying meals.

Financial Issues

Treatment for kidney failure is expensive, but federal health insurance programs pay much of the cost, usually up to 80 percent. Often, private insurance or state programs pay the rest. Your social worker can help you locate resources for financial assistance.

443

Section 44.2

Peritoneal Dialysis Dose and Adequacy

Excerpted from "Peritoneal Dialysis Dose and Adequacy," National Kidney and Urologic Diseases Information Clearinghouse, National Institute of Diabetes and Digestive and Kidney Diseases, NIH Pub. No. 07-4578, December 2006.

When kidneys fail, waste products such as urea and creatinine build up in the blood. One way to remove these wastes is a process called peritoneal dialysis (PD). The walls of the abdominal cavity are lined with a membrane called the peritoneum. During PD, a mixture of dextrose (sugar), salt, and other minerals dissolved in water, called dialysis solution, is placed in a person's abdominal cavity through a catheter. The body's peritoneal membrane enclosing the digestive organs allows waste products and extra body fluid to pass from the blood into the dialysis solution. These wastes then leave the body when the used solution is drained from the abdomen. Each cycle of draining and refilling is called an exchange. The time the solution remains in the abdomen between exchanges is called the dwell time. During this dwell time, some of the dextrose in the solution crosses the membrane and is absorbed by the body.

Many factors affect how much waste and extra fluid are removed from the blood. Some factors—such as the patient's size and the permeability, or speed of diffusion, of the peritoneum—cannot be controlled. Dialysis solution comes in 1.5-, 2-, 2.5-, or 3-liter bags for manual exchanges and 5- or 6-liter bags for automated exchanges. The dialysis dose can be increased by using a larger fill volume, but only within the limits of the person's abdominal capacity. Everyone's peritoneum filters wastes at a different rate. In some people, the peritoneum does not allow wastes to enter the dialysis solution efficiently enough to make PD feasible.

Other factors that determine how efficiently a person's blood is filtered can be controlled. Controllable factors include the number of daily exchanges and the dwell times. When fresh solution is first placed in the abdomen, it draws in wastes rapidly. As wastes fill the solution, it cleans the blood less efficiently. For example, a patient may perform one exchange with a 6-hour dwell time, during which the solution pulls in nearly as much urea as it can hold. But in the second half of that dwell time, urea is being removed from the blood very slowly. If the patient performed two exchanges with 3-hour dwell times instead, the amount of urea removed would be substantially greater than that removed in one 6-hour dwell time.

Another way to increase the amount of fluid and waste drawn into the peritoneal cavity is to use dialysis solution with a higher concentration of dextrose. Dialysis solution comes in 1.5 percent, 2.5 percent, and 4.25 percent dextrose concentrations. A higher dextrose concentration moves fluid and more wastes into the abdominal cavity, increasing both early and long-dwell exchange efficiency. Eventually, however, the body absorbs dextrose from the solution. As the concentration of dextrose in the body comes closer to that in the solution, dialysis becomes less effective, and fluid is slowly absorbed from the abdominal cavity.

Testing for Efficiency

The tests to see whether the exchanges are removing enough urea are especially important during the first weeks of dialysis, when the health care team needs to determine whether the patient is receiving an adequate amount, or dose, of dialysis.

The peritoneal equilibration test—often called the PET—measures how much dextrose has been absorbed from a bag of infused dialysis solution and how much urea and creatinine have entered into the solution during a 4-hour dwell. The peritoneal transport rate varies from person to person. People who have a high rate of transport absorb dextrose from the dialysis solution quickly, and they should be given a dialysis schedule that avoids exchanges with a long dwell time because they tend to absorb too much dextrose and dialysis solution from such exchanges.

In the clearance test, samples of used solution drained over a 24-hour period are collected, and a blood sample is obtained during the day when the solution is collected. The amount of urea in the solution is compared with the amount in the blood to see how effective the current PD schedule is in clearing the blood of urea. If the patient has more than a few ounces of urine output per day, the urine should also be collected during this period to measure its urea concentration.

From the used solution, urine, and blood measurements, one can compute a urea clearance, called Kt/V, and a creatinine clearance rate—normalized to body surface area. The residual clearance of the kidneys is also considered. Based on these measurements, one can determine whether the PD dose is adequate.

If the laboratory results show that the dialysis schedule is not removing enough urea and creatinine, the doctor may change the prescription by:

- increasing the number of exchanges per day for patients treated with CAPD or per night for patients treated with CCPD;

- increasing the volume—amount of solution in the bag—of each exchange in CAPD;

- adding an extra, automated middle-of-the-night exchange to the CAPD schedule;

- adding an extra middle-of-the-day exchange to the CCPD schedule;

- using a dialysis solution with a higher dextrose concentration.

Chapter 45

Skin and Hair Problems on Dialysis

How does dialysis affect my skin?

Many people on dialysis have skin changes. The skin may seem more fragile—it may bruise or even tear easily. Dry, itching, or cracking skin is common.

Some skin problems can be small. Others can make you feel bad about yourself or even cause you to not want to be seen by others. The good news is, many skin problems can be helped.

Why do I bruise more easily?

You may bruise easily if your dose of blood thinner (heparin) is too high. Or, easy bruising can occur if your blood level of platelets—clotting cells—is too low. With too few platelets, you might also have bleeding gums. Some drugs, like prednisone or Coumadin, can increase bruising.

Why does my skin itch all the time?

Itching has many causes, so you will need to be a detective. Often, itching is caused by high blood levels of phosphorus. In your body, extra phosphorus can bind with calcium to form sharp, itchy crystals. Taking your phosphate binders with food can help. Other causes of

"Just the Facts: Skin and Hair Problems on Dialysis," © 2005 Life Options Rehabilitation Program (www.lifeoptions.org). Reprinted with permission.

itching include not enough dialysis or dry skin. Long, hot baths that strip skin oils and alcohol-based products may dry the skin as well.

Why do I itch only at dialysis?

If you only itch on dialysis, an allergy may be the cause. One type of heparin (for example, pork) might make you itch, while another does not. Or bleach used to clean the chair may be to blame. Try putting a towel on the chair, or alert the dialysis staff.

Why is my skin so fragile?

Skin that rips at the slightest bump with purple or brown, itchy blisters can be a sign of a skin disease called "porphyria" (por-feer'-ee-a). This problem can be treated by a skin specialist.

Why is my hair falling out?

Hair is made of protein. If you become malnourished, a few months later your hair may break more easily and fall out. Eating enough good protein will help, but it takes a couple of months to see a change. Ask your dietitian about good protein sources. Hair loss can also be caused by thyroid problems, zinc deficiency, drug reactions, and other problems. Some patients have had hair loss when the unit changes the type of dialyzer (kidney) used. Talk with your doctor about this, or ask for a referral to a skin doctor.

How can I treat my skin and hair problems?

Problem: Every time I bump into something, I get a big bruise.

How can I prevent it?

- Make sure you know how much heparin you should get to be sure you receive the right dose.
- Ask your doctor about your platelet count or Coumadin level (called INR [international normalized ratio]) if you are on Coumadin.

What should I ask?

- Do you think my heparin dose is causing me to bruise easily?
- Is my platelet level (or INR) what it should be?

Problem: This itching is driving me crazy!

How can I prevent it?

- Try to figure out what is causing the itching. Is it better at some times than others? What helps or makes it worse? Does your skin look normal or different?

- Try a few over-the-counter lotions to see if one works for you. Some patients find that coconut oil is soothing.

- Ask your doctor about lotions that might help.

- Ask your doctor if an antihistamine would help.

What should I ask?

- Can you suggest some things I could try to help stop the itching?

- Are there any prescription lotions that you think would help?

- Do you have samples I could try, so I can find one that works before I have to pay for it?

Problem: I feel too ugly to go out. My skin is cracked and blistered.

How can I prevent it?

- Talk to your doctor as soon as you notice a skin problem that affects how you feel about yourself.

- Ask for a referral to a skin doctor.

What should I ask?

- I don't think my skin problem is normal, even for dialysis patients. Can you write me a referral to a skin doctor?

Problem: What can I do while I wait for my hair to grow back in?

How can I prevent it?

- Treat your hair gently—avoid harsh perms or colors.

- Don't use tight rubber bands.

- Ask a stylist for tips to hide thinning hair.

- Be sure to eat the right amount of protein—talk to your dietitian.

449

- Try to figure out what is causing the problem for you.

What should I ask?

- Could you please check my thyroid levels?

- What is my protein (albumin) level? (It should be at least 4.0g/dL.)

Chapter 46

Kidney Transplantation

If you have advanced and permanent kidney failure, kidney transplantation may be the treatment option that allows you to live much like you lived before your kidneys failed. Since the 1950s, when the first kidney transplants were performed, much has been learned about how to prevent rejection and minimize the side effects of medicines.

But transplantation is not a cure; it's an ongoing treatment that requires you to take medicines for the rest of your life. And the wait for a donated kidney can be years long.

A successful transplant takes a coordinated effort from your whole health care team, including your nephrologist, transplant surgeon, transplant coordinator, pharmacist, dietitian, and social worker. But the most important members of your health care team are you and your family. By learning about your treatment, you can work with your health care team to give yourself the best possible results, and you can lead a full, active life.

How Transplantation Works

Kidney transplantation is a procedure that places a healthy kidney from another person into your body. This one new kidney takes over the work of your two failed kidneys.

Excerpted from "Treatment Methods for Kidney Failure: Transplantation," National Kidney and Urologic Diseases Information Clearinghouse, National Institute of Diabetes and Digestive and Kidney Diseases, NIH Pub. No. 06-4687, May 2006.

A surgeon places the new kidney inside your lower abdomen and connects the artery and vein of the new kidney to your artery and vein. Your blood flows through the new kidney, which makes urine, just like your own kidneys did when they were healthy. Unless they are causing infection or high blood pressure, your own kidneys are left in place.

The Transplant Process

Your Doctor's Recommendation

The transplantation process begins when you learn that your kidneys are failing, and you must start to consider your treatment options. Whether transplantation is to be among your options will depend on your specific situation. Transplantation isn't for everyone. Your doctor may tell you that you have a condition that would make transplantation dangerous or unlikely to succeed.

Medical Evaluation at a Transplant Center

If your doctor sees transplantation as an option, the next step is a thorough medical evaluation at a transplant hospital. The pre-transplant evaluation may require several visits over the course of several weeks or even months. You'll need to have blood drawn and x-rays taken. You'll be tested for blood type and other matching factors that determine whether your body will accept an available kidney.

The medical team will want to see whether you're healthy enough for surgery. Cancer, a serious infection, or significant cardiovascular disease would make transplantation unlikely to succeed. In addition, the medical team will want to make sure that you can understand and follow the schedule for taking medicines.

If a family member or friend wants to donate a kidney, he or she will need to be evaluated for general health and to see whether the kidney is a good match.

Placement on the Waiting List

If the medical evaluation shows that you're a good candidate for a transplant but you don't have a family member or friend who can donate a kidney, you'll be put on the transplant program's waiting list to receive a kidney from a deceased donor—someone who has just died.

Waiting Period

How long you'll have to wait depends on many things but is primarily determined by the degree of matching between you and the donor. Some people wait several years for a good match, while others get matched within a few months.

While you're on the waiting list, notify the transplant center of changes in your health. Also, let the transplant center know if you move or change telephone numbers. The center will need to find you immediately when a kidney becomes available.

Organ procurement organizations (OPOs) are responsible for identifying potential organs for transplant and coordinating with the national network. The 69 regional OPOs are all United Network for Organ Sharing (UNOS) members. When a deceased donor kidney becomes available, the OPO notifies UNOS, and a computer-generated list of suitable recipients is created. Suitability is initially based on two factors:

- **Blood type:** Your blood type (A, B, AB, or O) must be compatible with the donor's blood type.

- **HLA factors:** HLA stands for human leukocyte antigen, a genetic marker located on the surface of your white blood cells. You inherit a set of three antigens from your mother and three from your father. A higher number of matching antigens increases the chance that your kidney will last for a long time.

If you're selected on the basis of the first two factors, a third is evaluated:

- **Antibodies:** Your immune system may produce antibodies that act specifically against something in the donor's tissues. To see whether this is the case, a small sample of your blood will be mixed with a small sample of the donor's blood in a tube. If no reaction occurs, you should be able to accept the kidney. Your transplant team might use the term negative cross-match to describe this lack of reaction.

Transplant Operation

If you have a living donor, you'll schedule the operation in advance. You and your donor will be operated on at the same time, usually in side-by-side rooms. One team of surgeons will perform the nephrectomy—that is, the removal of the kidney from the donor—while another prepares the recipient for placement of the donated kidney.

You'll be given a general anesthetic to make you sleep during the operation, which usually takes three or four hours. The surgeon will make a small cut in your lower abdomen. The artery and vein from the new kidney will be attached to your artery and vein. The ureter from the new kidney will be connected to your bladder.

Often, the new kidney will start making urine as soon as your blood starts flowing through it, but sometimes a few weeks pass before it starts working.

Recovery from Surgery

As after any major surgery, you'll probably feel sore and groggy when you wake up. However, many transplant recipients report feeling much better immediately after surgery. Even if you wake up feeling great, you'll need to stay in the hospital for about a week to recover from surgery, and longer if you have any complications.

Posttransplant Care

Your body's immune system is designed to keep you healthy by sensing "foreign invaders," such as bacteria, and rejecting them. But your immune system will also sense that your new kidney is foreign. To keep your body from rejecting it, you'll have to take drugs that turn off, or suppress, your immune response. You may have to take two or more of these immunosuppressant medicines, as well as medications to treat other health problems. Your health care team will help you learn what each pill is for and when to take it. Be sure that you understand the instructions for taking your medicines before you leave the hospital.

Rejection

You can help prevent rejection by taking your medicines and following your diet, but watching for signs of rejection—like fever or soreness in the area of the new kidney or a change in the amount of urine you make—is important. Report any such changes to your health care team.

Even if you do everything you're supposed to do, your body may still reject the new kidney and you may need to go back on dialysis. Unless your health care team determines that you're no longer a good candidate for transplantation, you can go back on the waiting list for another kidney.

Side Effects of Immunosuppressants

Immunosuppressants can weaken your immune system, which can lead to infections. Some drugs may also change your appearance. Your face may get fuller; you may gain weight or develop acne or facial hair. Not all patients have these problems, though, and diet and makeup can help.

Immunosuppressants work by diminishing the ability of immune cells to function. In some patients, over long periods of time, this diminished immunity can increase the risk of developing cancer. Some immunosuppressants cause cataracts, diabetes, extra stomach acid, high blood pressure, and bone disease. When used over time, these drugs may also cause liver or kidney damage in a few patients.

Organ Donation

Deceased Donor

Most transplanted kidneys come from people who have died. However, the number of people waiting for kidneys has increased in recent years, while the number of kidneys available from deceased donors has remained constant. The result is a shortage of kidneys and a longer waiting time for people with kidney failure.

Many suitable kidneys go unused because family members of potential donors don't know their loved one's wishes. People who wish to donate their organs should talk about this issue with their families. Several organizations, including UNOS and the National Kidney Foundation, provide organ donor cards for people who wish to make this life-preserving gift when they die. A properly completed organ donor card notifies medical officials that you've decided to donate your organs. In most states, you can indicate your desire to be an organ donor on your driver's license.

Living Donor

A growing number of transplanted kidneys are donated by living family members or friends. Potential donors need to be tested to make sure that donating a kidney won't endanger their health, as well as for matching factors. Most people, however, can donate a kidney with little risk.

A kidney from a living donor often has advantages over a deceased donor kidney:

- People who receive a kidney from a family member or friend don't have to wait until a kidney becomes available. Living donation allows for greater preparation and for the operation to be scheduled at a convenient time.

- Kidneys from family members are more likely to be good matches, although there's no guarantee.

- Kidneys from living donors don't need to be transported from one site to another, so the kidney is in better condition when it's transplanted.

- Living donation helps people waiting for kidneys from deceased donors by lowering the number of people on the waiting list.

Minority Donation

Diseases of the kidney are found more frequently in racial and ethnic minority populations in the United States than in the general population. African Americans, Asian Americans, Hispanics/Latinos, and Pacific Islander Americans are three times more likely to suffer from kidney failure than Americans of European descent. Successful transplantation is often enhanced if organs are matched between members of the same ethnic and racial group. A shortage of organs donated by minorities can contribute to longer waiting periods for transplants for minorities.

The National Minority Organ/Tissue Transplant Education Program (MOTTEP), with the support of the National Institutes of Health's Office of Research on Minority Health and the National Institute of Diabetes and Digestive and Kidney Diseases (NIDDK), is the first national program to empower minority communities to promote minority donation and transplantation, as well as good health habits. In turn, this effort should improve the chances for a well-matched organ among all those waiting for a transplant.

Chapter 47

Kidney and Pancreas Transplantation

What is a kidney pancreas transplant?

Combined transplantation of the kidney and pancreas is performed for those who have kidney failure as a complication of insulin-dependent diabetes mellitus (also called type 1 diabetes). Kidney and pancreas transplant candidates might be currently on dialysis or might require dialysis in the near future.

After combined transplantation of the kidney and pancreas, the kidney will be able to filter and excrete wastes so dialysis will not be needed. The transplanted pancreas will produce insulin to control the diabetes.

Am I a candidate for the double transplant?

If you have type 1 diabetes and you have kidney failure, or if your doctor thinks that kidney failure is beginning, the double transplant (combined kidney and pancreas) can be considered as a treatment option. Your doctor and transplant surgeon can determine if the double transplant is needed based on your medical condition, your overall health, and the results of a pre-transplant evaluation. A pre-transplant evaluation includes a complete physical, consultations with a transplant coordinator and surgeon, and a series of tests, including heart and bladder evaluations.

Where does my new kidney and pancreas come from?

Kidneys for transplantation come from two sources: living donors and deceased (non-living) donors. Living donors are usually immediate family members or sometimes spouses. Deceased donor kidneys come from people whose families give permission for organ donation at the time of death. Three out of four kidney transplants are performed with deceased donor kidneys.

Combined kidney and pancreas transplants and single pancreas transplants are only performed with deceased donor organs.

All donors are carefully screened to prevent any transmissible diseases or other complications. The donor is also carefully evaluated to make sure there is a suitable match to your tissue and blood type.

What is the procedure for receiving a deceased donor transplant?

After your doctor and transplant surgeon have determined the double transplant is needed, you will be placed on a waiting list to receive a deceased donor kidney and pancreas. Your name and blood test results will be placed on the United Network for Organ Sharing's (UNOS) national list.

When a deceased donor kidney and pancreas become available for transplantation, they are given to the best possible match, based on blood type, tissue (HLA) type, cross-match compatibility, and the length of time the recipient has been waiting. If a perfect match (six antigen match) is identified through the national list, the recipient matching the donor will be notified.

How long will I have to wait before I receive my transplant?

It is impossible to predict how long a wait there will be before a deceased donor kidney and pancreas become available. The average wait is about 24 to 36 months; however, it's possible the wait could be from a few days to many years. Some people might have to wait longer than others for their transplants because their blood and tissue types might be less common, so it takes longer to find a compatible match.

What happens during the kidney and pancreas transplant surgery?

Kidney and pancreas transplantation involves placing a healthy kidney and pancreas into the body where they can perform all of the functions that a failing kidney and pancreas cannot.

The new kidney is placed on the lower left side of the abdomen where it is surgically connected to nearby blood vessels. Placing the kidney in this position allows it to be easily connected to blood vessels and the bladder. The vein and artery of the new kidney are attached to your vein and artery. The new kidney's ureter is attached to your bladder to allow urine to pass out of your body.

The new pancreas is placed on the lower right side of your abdomen where it is surgically connected to nearby blood vessels. The vein and artery of the new pancreas are attached to your vein and artery.

The kidney and pancreas transplant surgery takes from five to seven hours. Transplant patients generally stay in the hospital about eight to 12 days.

What is the success rate of the double transplant?

After the double transplant is performed, there is an 80 percent to 85 percent chance that the patient will require no insulin and no dialysis for one year. In addition, there is a 70 percent chance that this success will continue over the next five years.

What are the benefits of double organ transplantation?

A successful kidney and pancreas transplant gives you increased strength, stamina, and energy. After transplantation, you should be able to return to a more normal lifestyle and have more control over your daily living. You can have a normal diet and more normal fluid intake.

If you were dependent on dialysis before the transplant, you'll have more freedom because you won't be bound to your dialysis schedule. The pancreas transplant will keep your blood sugar normal. Frequently after transplantation, your blood sugar level before eating will be 90 or less. After a meal, it might reach 140—all without insulin. Further complications of diabetes might be delayed with better blood sugar control.

What are the risks of double organ transplantation?

Since two organs are transplanted, the risk of surgical complications is about twice that of a single organ transplant (such as a kidney-only transplant). Since the pancreas is joined to the bladder during the operation, some loss of fluids occurs. You might need to drink more than usual after the transplant surgery in order to prevent dehydration.

There is also a risk of rejection after any type of transplant surgery. Rejection is your body's way of not accepting the new kidney and pancreas. Since your body recognizes the new organs as foreign objects, it will normally try to get rid of them or "reject" them. However, you are given medicines to prevent rejection. You will need to take these medicines for life and have your blood work drawn as scheduled to prevent rejection episodes.

Are pancreas transplants performed without kidney transplants?

In some circumstances, a pancreas transplant can be performed without a kidney transplant. The pancreas transplant might be performed for patients who have already had a kidney transplant or for patients who do not have kidney failure, but who have complications of type 1 diabetes.

The rate of pancreas transplant complications is similar to that of a kidney and pancreas transplant, but the chances of long-term success are not as good. However, newer drugs and better tissue-matching procedures can offer a reasonable success rate. Your doctor and transplant surgeon can determine if the pancreas transplant is needed without the kidney transplant, based on your medical condition.

Chapter 48

Pancreatic Islet Transplantation

What are pancreatic islets?

The pancreas, an organ about the size of a hand, is located behind the lower part of the stomach. It makes insulin and enzymes that help the body digest and use food. Throughout the pancreas are clusters of cells called the islets of Langerhans. Islets are made up of several types of cells, including beta cells that make insulin.

Insulin is a hormone that helps the body use glucose for energy. Diabetes develops when the body doesn't make enough insulin, cannot use insulin properly, or both, causing glucose to build up in the blood. In type 1 diabetes—an autoimmune disease—the beta cells of the pancreas no longer make insulin because the body's immune system has attacked and destroyed them. A person who has type 1 diabetes must take insulin daily to live. Type 2 diabetes usually begins with a condition called insulin resistance, in which the body has difficulty using insulin effectively. Over time, insulin production declines as well, so many people with type 2 diabetes eventually need to take insulin.

What is pancreatic islet transplantation?

In an experimental procedure called islet transplantation, islets are taken from the pancreas of a deceased organ donor. The islets are

Excerpted from "Pancreatic Islet Transplantation," National Diabetes Information Clearinghouse, National Institute of Diabetes and Digestive and Kidney Diseases, NIH Pub. No 07-4693, March 2007.

461

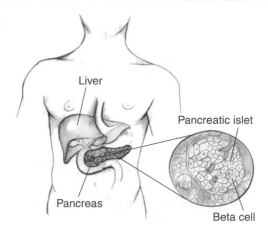

Figure 48.1. *The pancreas is located in the abdomen behind the stomach. Islets within the pancreas contain beta cells, which produce insulin.*

purified, processed, and transferred into another person. Once implanted, the beta cells in these islets begin to make and release insulin. Researchers hope that islet transplantation will help people with type 1 diabetes live without daily injections of insulin.

Research developments: Scientists have made many advances in islet transplantation in recent years. Since reporting their findings in the June 2000 issue of the *New England Journal of Medicine*, researchers at the University of Alberta in Edmonton, Canada, have continued to use and refine a procedure called the Edmonton protocol to transplant pancreatic islets into selected patients with type 1 diabetes that is difficult to control. In 2005, the researchers published 5-year follow-up results for 65 patients who received transplants at their center and reported that about 10 percent of the patients remained free of the need for insulin injections at 5-year follow-up. Most recipients returned to using insulin because the transplanted islets lost their ability to function over time. The researchers noted, however, that many transplant recipients were able to reduce their need for insulin, achieve better glucose stability, and reduce problems with hypoglycemia, also called low blood sugar.

In its 2006 annual report, the Collaborative Islet Transplant Registry, which is funded by the National Institute of Diabetes and Digestive and Kidney Diseases, presented data from 23 islet transplant programs on 225 patients who received islet transplants between 1999 and 2005. According to the report, nearly two-thirds of recipients achieved "insulin independence"—defined as being able to stop insulin injections for at least 14 days—during the year following transplantation. However, other data from the report showed that insulin independence is difficult to maintain over time. Six months after their last infusion of islets, more than half of recipients were free of the need for insulin injections, but at 2-year follow-up, the proportion dropped to about one-third of recipients. The report described other benefits of islet transplantation, including reduced need for insulin among recipients who still needed insulin, improved blood glucose control, and greatly reduced risk of episodes of severe hypoglycemia.

In a 2006 report of the Immune Tolerance Network's international islet transplantation study, researchers emphasized the value of transplantation in reversing a condition known as hypoglycemia unawareness. People with hypoglycemia unawareness are vulnerable to dangerous episodes of severe hypoglycemia because they are not able to recognize that their blood glucose levels are too low. The study showed that even partial islet function after transplant can eliminate hypoglycemia unawareness.

Transplant procedure: Researchers use specialized enzymes to remove islets from the pancreas of a deceased donor. Because the islets

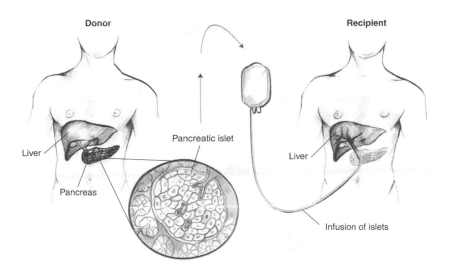

Figure 48.2. Islets extracted from a donor pancreas are infused into the liver. Once implanted, the beta cells in the islets begin to make and release insulin.

are fragile, transplantation occurs soon after they are removed. Typically a patient receives at least 10,000 islet "equivalents" per kilogram of body weight, extracted from two donor pancreases. Patients often require two transplants to achieve insulin independence. Some transplants have used fewer islet equivalents taken from a single donated pancreas.

Transplants are often performed by a radiologist, who uses x-rays and ultrasound to guide placement of a catheter—a small plastic tube—through the upper abdomen and into the portal vein of the liver. The islets are then infused slowly through the catheter into the liver. The patient receives a local anesthetic and a sedative. In some cases, a surgeon may perform the transplant through a small incision, using general anesthesia.

Islets begin to release insulin soon after transplantation. However, full islet function and new blood vessel growth associated with the islets take time. The doctor will order many tests to check blood glucose levels after the transplant, and insulin is usually given until the islets are fully functional.

What are the benefits and risks of islet transplantation?

The goal of islet transplantation is to infuse enough islets to control the blood glucose level without insulin injections. Other benefits may include improved glucose control and prevention of potentially dangerous episodes of hypoglycemia. Because good control of blood glucose can slow or prevent the progression of complications associated with diabetes, such as heart disease, kidney disease, and nerve or eye damage, a successful transplant may reduce the risk of these complications.

Risks of islet transplantation include the risks associated with the transplant procedure—particularly bleeding and blood clots—and side effects from the immunosuppressive drugs that transplant recipients must take to stop the immune system from rejecting the transplanted islets.

Immunosuppressive drugs: Rejection is the biggest problem with any transplant. The immune system is programmed to destroy bacteria, viruses, and tissue it recognizes as "foreign," including transplanted islets. In addition, the autoimmune response that destroyed transplant recipients' own islets in the first place can recur and attack the transplanted islets. Immunosuppressive drugs are needed to keep the transplanted islets functioning.

The Edmonton protocol introduced the use of a new combination of immunosuppressive drugs, also called anti-rejection drugs, including daclizumab (Zenapax), sirolimus (Rapamune), and tacrolimus (Prograf).

Daclizumab is given intravenously right after the transplant and then discontinued. Sirolimus and tacrolimus, the two main drugs that keep the immune system from destroying the transplanted islets, must be taken for life or for as long as the islets continue to function. These drugs have significant side effects and their long-term effects are still not fully known. Immediate side effects of immunosuppressive drugs may include mouth sores and gastrointestinal problems, such as stomach upset and diarrhea. Patients may also have increased blood cholesterol levels, hypertension, anemia, fatigue, decreased white blood cell counts, decreased kidney function, and increased susceptibility to bacterial and viral infections. Taking immunosuppressive drugs also increases the risk of tumors and cancer.

Researchers continue to develop and study modifications to the Edmonton protocol drug regimen, including the use of new drugs and new combinations of drugs designed to help reduce destruction of transplanted islets and promote their successful implantation. These therapies may help transplant recipients achieve better function and durability of transplanted islets with fewer side effects. The ultimate goal is to achieve immune tolerance of the transplanted islets, where the patient's immune system no longer recognizes the islets as foreign. If achieved, immune tolerance would allow patients to maintain transplanted islets without long-term immunosuppression.

Researchers are also trying to find new approaches that will allow successful transplantation without the use of immunosuppressive drugs. For example, one study is testing the transplantation of islets that are encapsulated with a special coating designed to prevent rejection.

Is there a shortage of islets?

A major obstacle to widespread use of islet transplantation is the shortage of islets. Although organs from about 7,000 deceased donors become available each year in the United States, fewer than half of the donated pancreases are suitable for whole organ pancreas transplantation or for harvesting of islets—enough for only a small percentage of those with type 1 diabetes. However, researchers are pursuing various approaches to solve this problem, such as transplanting islets from a single donated pancreas, from a portion of the pancreas of a living donor, or from pigs. Researchers have transplanted pig islets into other animals, including monkeys, by encapsulating the islets or by using drugs to prevent rejection. Another approach is creating islets from other types of cells, such as stem cells. New technologies could then be employed to grow islets in the laboratory.

465

Part VI

Diabetes-Related Research

Chapter 49

Diabetes Knowledge: Yesterday, Today, and Tomorrow

Diabetes Care Better Than Ten Years Ago, But More Improvement Needed

A published 2006 study conducted by the Centers for Disease Control (CDC) indicates improvement in diabetes care over the past 10 years; however, there is still a great need to focus on additional improvements. A summary presented here looks at changes in glucose and cholesterol control, along with blood pressure; yearly eye and foot examinations; new national initiatives on quality care, and why we need to continually focus on effective treatment and preventive measures.

Main Findings of the Study

1. Between the mid-1990s and now, there have been encouraging improvements in the quality of diabetes care. Gains have been identified in control of cholesterol and somewhat in glucose control; in the use of aspirin, influenza, and pneumococcal vaccines; and regular exams of eyes, feet, and teeth.

2. However, blood pressure (BP) control has not changed at all.

This chapter includes "News and Information: Diabetes Care Better Than 10 Years Ago, But More Improvement Needed," National Center for Chronic Disease Prevention and Health Promotion, June 2006; "Fact Sheet: Type 1 Diabetes," National Institutes of Health, nd; and "Fact Sheet: Type 2 Diabetes," National Institutes of Health, nd.

3. Despite the many improvements, two in five people with diabetes still have poor cholesterol control, one in three have poor BP control, one in five have poor glucose control.

4. Study results show that there are good treatments to prevent diabetes complications, and quality of care can be improved for the 14.6 million people in the United States who have diagnosed diabetes. Therefore, it is important that we not become complacent, but rather continue in our efforts to achieve further progress.

Why Have Improvements Occurred?

This study did not specifically look at "why," but a number of important developments have occurred during the last five to ten years that together could account for the improvements.

1. Good science has become available to support and promote tight glucose, blood pressure, and lipid control for people with diabetes. CDC and National Institute of Health (NIH) have invested in applied research aimed at promoting improvements in quality of care. More science is needed.

2. Several national initiatives to promote quality of diabetes care have been implemented.

   - The Alliance is a large coalition of government, managed care, and other players that has developed ways to measure and track quality of care, and has emphasized quality of care.

   - The CDC's Diabetes Prevention and Control Programs in all states has strongly emphasized and influenced improvements in diabetes quality of care.

   - The CDC and NIH have worked together in the National Diabetes Education Program to change the way diabetes is treated.

   - The Veteran's Administration (VA) has undergone major re-engineering aimed at improving quality of care.

Final Messages

Twenty-one million people in the United States have diagnosed and undiagnosed diabetes. There are several good treatments for preventing diabetes complications. As this study shows, it is possible to improve the quality of care, but we still have a long way to go.

Forty-one million people in the United States have pre-diabetes, and can develop diabetes in the future. Preventing diabetes in these people is very important to reducing the pain and suffering from its devastating complications.

Type 1 Diabetes

Thirty Years Ago

- Twenty percent of people born in the 1950s died within 20 years of a type 1 diabetes diagnosis. Over 30 percent died within 25 years.

- About one in four people developed kidney failure within 25 years of a type 1 diabetes diagnosis. Doctors could not detect early kidney disease and had no tools for slowing the progression to kidney failure.

- About 90 percent of people with type 1 diabetes developed diabetic retinopathy within 25 years of diagnosis. Blindness from diabetic retinopathy was responsible for about 20 percent of new cases of blindness between the ages of 45 and 74.

- Major birth defects in the offspring of mothers with type 1 diabetes were three times higher than the rate in the general population.

- Patients relied on injections of animal-derived insulin. The insulin pump would soon be introduced but would not become widely used for years.

- Researchers did not yet recognize the need for intensive glucose control to delay or prevent the debilitating eye, nerve, kidney, heart, and blood vessel complications of diabetes. Also, the importance of blood pressure control in preventing complications was not established yet.

- Patients monitored their glucose levels with urine tests, which recognized high but not dangerously low glucose levels and reflected past, not current, glucose levels. More reliable methods for testing blood glucose levels were not developed yet.

- Researchers had just discovered autoimmunity as the underlying cause of type 1 diabetes. However, they couldn't assess an

471

individual's level of risk for developing the disease, and they didn't know enough to even consider ways to prevent it.

Today

- For people born between 1975 and 1980, about 3.5 percent died within 20 years of diagnosis, and 7 percent died within 25 years of diagnosis. These death rates were much lower than those of patients born in the 1950s but still significantly increased compared to the general population.

- After 20 years of annual increases from 5 to 10 percent, rates for new kidney failure cases have leveled off. The most encouraging trend is in diabetes, where rates for new cases in whites under age 40 are the lowest in 20 years. Improved control of glucose and blood pressure and the use of specific antihypertensive drugs called ACE (angiotensin-converting enzyme) inhibitors and ARBs (angiotensin receptor blockers) prevent or delay the progression of kidney disease to kidney failure. With good care, fewer than 10 percent of people with diabetes develop kidney failure.

- With timely laser surgery and appropriate follow-up care, people with advanced diabetic retinopathy can reduce their risk of blindness by 90 percent.

- For expectant mothers with type 1 diabetes, tight control of glucose that begins before conception lowers the risk of birth defects, miscarriage, and newborn death to a range that is close to that of the general population.

- Patients now use a variety of insulin formulations, for example, rapid-acting, intermediate acting, and long-acting insulin, to control their blood glucose. Insulin pumps are widely used, and inhaled insulin is available. Components of an artificial pancreas are being tested in clinical studies.

- A major clinical trial, the Diabetes Control and Complications Trial, showed that intensive glucose control dramatically delays or prevents the eye, nerve, kidney, and heart complications of type 1 diabetes. This finding caused a paradigm shift in the way type 1 diabetes is controlled.

- Patients monitor their blood glucose with precise, less painful methods. The widely used hemoglobin A1C test (HbA1c) shows average blood glucose over the past three months.

- Scientists found a region of the human genome that accounts for half the increased risk of developing autoimmune diabetes. This key region houses genes that encode proteins involved in the immune response. Changes in other genes, such as the insulin gene and genes that regulate T cell activation also increase susceptibility.

- Researchers have learned a great deal about the underlying biology of autoimmune diabetes and can now predict who is at high, moderate, and low risk for developing type 1 diabetes. Exploiting this knowledge and advances in immunology, researchers seek to prevent type 1 diabetes and preserve insulin-producing cells in newly diagnosed patients. This new understanding allows diagnosis and treatment of type 1 diabetes before the development of life-threatening complications.

- Many people who received islet transplants for poorly controlled type 1 diabetes are free of the need for insulin administration a year later, and episodes of dangerously low blood glucose are greatly reduced for as long as five years after transplant, according to studies at 19 medical centers in the U.S. and Canada. However, transplanted islets' function is lost over time, and patients have side effects from immunosuppressive drugs.

Tomorrow

- By finding all the genes and environmental factors (for example, viruses, toxins, dietary factors) that contribute to type 1 diabetes, researchers will develop ways to safely prevent or reverse the autoimmune destruction of insulin-producing cells.

- Methods for safely imaging the insulin-producing beta cells will help scientists better understand the disease process and assess the benefits of treatments and preventions that are under study.

- Toxic suppression of the immune system to prevent rejection of transplanted organs and tissues will be replaced with safer, more targeted methods of immune modulation.

- New technologies, such as a closed loop system that automatically senses blood glucose and adjusts insulin dosage precisely, will become available. Patients will more easily control their blood glucose levels and develop fewer complications.

- Increased understanding of the molecular pathways by which blood glucose causes cell injury will allow scientists to develop novel therapies that prevent and repair the damage.

- Some of the most important progress in type 1 diabetes has been gained from clinical studies in patients with diabetes and those at risk for the disease. To maintain the rapid pace of discovery, it is critical for individuals to take part in well designed clinical studies. As one leading researcher put it, "The patient is the most important member of the research team."

Type 2 Diabetes

Thirty Years Ago

- No proven disease prevention strategies existed.

- The only ways to treat diabetes were the now obsolete forms of insulin from cows and pigs, and drugs that stimulate insulin release from the beta cells of the pancreas (sulfonylureas). Both of these therapies caused dangerous low blood sugar reactions and weight gain.

- No proven strategies existed to prevent disease complications, such as blindness, kidney disease, nerve damage, and heart disease.

- No proven tests were available for assessing patient control of blood sugar levels.

- While scientists knew that genes played a role (that is, the disease often runs in families), they had not identified any specific culprit genes.

- National efforts were not being made to combat obesity, a serious risk factor for the disease. Fewer people developed type 2 diabetes compared to today because overweight, obesity, and physical inactivity were not pervasive.

- Patients were almost exclusively adults—the reason that the disease was formerly called "adult onset diabetes." It was rare in children or young adults.

Today

- Type 2 diabetes can be prevented or delayed. The NIH-funded Diabetes Prevention Program (DPP) clinical trial studied over 3,000 adults at high risk for developing type 2 diabetes due to elevated blood sugar levels and overweight. The lifestyle intervention reduced by 58 percent the risk of getting type 2 diabetes. This dramatic result was achieved through modest weight loss (five to seven percent of body weight) and 30 minutes of exercise five times weekly. In another arm of the study, the drug metformin reduced development of diabetes by 31 percent. Both Caucasian and minority populations benefited from the interventions.

- Based on the DPP findings, the NIH developed the education campaign, *Small Steps, Big Rewards, Prevent Type 2 Diabetes,* to help people at high risk take the necessary action to prevent the disease (www.ndep.nih.gov). The CDC and over 200 private partners have joined this effort. Moreover, the NIH launched translation research initiatives to determine the best ways to promote adoption of the DPP prevention-oriented findings in real-world settings.

- Vigorous research continues to combat type 2 diabetes, which—even with proven prevention strategies—is escalating in the U.S. The escalation appears linked to the rising rate of obesity. Approximately 19–20 million Americans have type 2 diabetes, and about 1/3 of them don't even know it. Diabetes prevalence in this country has increased by 49 percent from 1990 to 2000. Diabetes is conservatively estimated to be the sixth leading cause of death in the U.S.

- Minority populations are disproportionately affected (African Americans, Hispanics, American Indians, Alaska Natives, Asian Americans, and Pacific Islanders).

- Increased diagnosis of type 2 diabetes in children is also associated with rising rates of obesity. This trend is especially alarming because, as younger people develop the disease, the complications, morbidity, and mortality associated with diabetes are all likely to occur earlier. Furthermore, offspring of women with type 2 diabetes are more likely to develop the disease. Therefore, the burgeoning of diabetes in younger populations could lead to a vicious cycle of ever-growing rates of diabetes.

- The NIH is launching a major clinical trial, called HEALTHY, which will examine whether an intervention given to middle schoolers will prevent development of risk factors. For youngsters who already have the disease, the TODAY clinical trial is determining the best treatment strategies.

- Research has vastly expanded understanding of the molecular underpinnings leading to diabetes and its complications and has laid the foundation for improvements in the survival and quality-of-life for people with the disease.

- Progress has been achieved in identifying some genes that predispose individuals to developing type 2 diabetes, and the NIH is supporting a major genetics consortium to pool data for the gene hunt.

- New drug development has been aided by NIH-supported clinical trials that validated a marker, called hemoglobin A1C (HbA1c). This marker reflects average blood sugar control over a three month period. Thus, a simple lab test can tell patients whether they are achieving good control of blood sugar levels.

- Tight control of blood sugar has become a standard of treatment based on results from NIH clinical trials demonstrating that tight control (that is, HbA1c less than 7) can prevent or delay the development of devastating complications. Unfortunately, few patients currently achieve the close control needed for preventing complications. Researchers are urgently seeking improved methods of achieving tight blood sugar control.

- New and more effective treatments have become available through research. New oral agents targeting the specific metabolic abnormalities of type 2 diabetes are available. Patients are now benefiting from improved forms of insulin, a range of oral medications to control blood sugar and reduce the need for insulin, and new drugs that may not only control blood sugar, but also strengthen the activity of patients' own insulin-producing cells.

- New technologies are emerging, such as the recently approved continuous glucose monitors. These devices have the potential to dramatically improve patients' ability to control their sugar levels—key for preventing complications—and to improve their quality-of-life by eliminating the need for invasive finger sticks.

- As a result of research, kidney disease can be detected earlier by standardized blood tests to estimate renal function and monitor urine protein excretion. Therefore, patients can be treated earlier to slow the rate of kidney damage. Improved control of glucose and blood pressure and the use of antihypertensive drugs called ACE inhibitors and ARBs prevent or delay the progression of kidney disease to kidney failure. With good care, fewer than 10 percent of patients develop kidney failure.

- Clinical trials have shown that blood pressure and lipid control reduce diabetes complications by up to 50 percent. Physicians are now much better equipped to control hypertension and unhealthy blood fats, which often accompany diabetes and raise the risk of heart disease, the leading cause of death of people with diabetes.

- With timely laser surgery and appropriate follow-up care, people with advanced diabetic retinopathy can reduce their risk of blindness by 90 percent.

- Currently, the NIH spends $1.055 billion on diabetes research. In 2002, total medical expenditures attributable to diabetes for all Americans was estimated at $132 billion. Approximately one-third of Medicare expenses are associated with treating diabetes and its complications.

Tomorrow

The NIH is poised to make major discoveries in the prediction of who will develop type 2 diabetes and its complications, to personalize individual treatments, and to use this information to preempt disease onset and development of complications. This knowledge will have a major impact on reducing the human and economic toll that type 2 diabetes places on the U.S.

- Researchers are pursuing earlier and more aggressive treatment approaches that would help to preempt complications. Clinical trials currently under way will provide information about preventing diabetes complications with intensified control of glucose, blood pressure, and lipids, with improvements in lifestyle to achieve weight loss, and through use of specific glucose control strategies and revascularization interventions.

- New understanding of the molecular links between obesity and insulin resistance will inform the development of new therapeutic targets for preventing and treating type 2 diabetes.

- Identification of susceptibility genes for diabetes and its complications will enable earlier implementation of prevention measures targeted to those at highest risk. Identification of genes

477

- Preempting the disease before it starts will eliminate the life-threatening complications, which will mean that people will live longer, healthier lives without fear—such as the fear of going blind or losing a lower limb.

- Research on the effect of maternal diabetes on offspring will help to uncover ways to break the vicious intergenerational cycle.

- Continued research on the mechanisms underlying the development and progression of disease complications will result in the ability to predict who is likely to develop them. With this knowledge, personalized treatments could then be developed to pre-empt complications. This strategy would dramatically improve the health and well being of patients.

- Results from NIH clinical trials will help to identify strategies to preempt type 2 diabetes in children, thereby stemming the alarming trend of increased rates of this disease in youth.

Chapter 50

Diabetes Research: An Update

Study Tests Oral Insulin to Prevent Type 1 Diabetes

A network of researchers funded by the National Institutes of Health is testing whether oral insulin can prevent or delay type 1 diabetes in a specific group of people at risk for the disease.

The network, known as Type 1 Diabetes TrialNet, is conducting the study in more than 100 medical centers across the United States, Canada, Europe, and Australia. An earlier trial suggested that oral insulin might delay type 1 diabetes for about four years in some people with insulin autoantibodies in their blood. Animal studies have also suggested that oral insulin may prevent type 1 diabetes.

Some scientists think introducing insulin through the digestive tract induces tolerance, or a quieting of the immune system. Insulin taken orally has no side effects because the digestive system breaks it down quickly. To lower blood glucose, people with diabetes must take insulin through an injection or pump.

This chapter includes excerpts from "Study Tests Oral Insulin to Prevent Type 1 Diabetes," *Diabetes Dateline*, Spring/Summer 2007; "Studies Test New Approaches to Islet Transplantation," *Diabetes Dateline*, Winter 2007; "For Safety, NHLBI Changes Intensive Blood Sugar Treatment Strategy in Clinical Trial of Diabetes and Cardiovascular Disease," *NIH News*, a press release dated February 6, 2008; and "Research Programs: Diabetes," an undated document produced by the National Institute of Diabetes and Digestive and Kidney Disease; website addresses were verified in March 2008.

"Our goal is to prevent type 1 diabetes or to delay it as long as possible," said TrialNet Study Chair Jay Skyler, MD, of the University of Miami. "If diabetes can be delayed, even for several years, those at risk will be spared the difficult challenges of controlling glucose and the development of complications for that much longer."

Other TrialNet Studies

Studies for those newly diagnosed: TrialNet studies are also aimed at safely preserving insulin production in people recently diagnosed with type 1 diabetes. In the few months after diagnosis, most people with diabetes still have a supply of functioning beta cells that, with the help of insulin injections, contribute to good blood glucose control. If beta cells could be protected, more people with type 1 diabetes would be able to tightly control their blood glucose, which prevents or delays damage to the eyes, nerves, kidneys, heart, and blood vessels.

One TrialNet study seeks to turn off the immune attack on beta cells with rituximab, a monoclonal antibody that binds to and temporarily destroys a specific class of immune cells. The rituximab trial is recruiting participants with type 1 diabetes diagnosed within the previous three months. Rituximab is approved by the U.S. Food and Drug Administration (FDA) to treat specific forms of lymphoma and moderate to severe rheumatoid arthritis but not to prevent type 1 diabetes.

Also underway is a study to test whether mycophenolate mofetil (MMF), or MMF plus Daclizumab (DZB), can slow or arrest the autoimmunity of type 1 diabetes. The FDA has approved MMF and DZB to prevent organ rejection after transplant. The study has recruited the necessary number of participants.

Newborn study: The Nutritional Intervention to Prevent Type 1 Diabetes (NIP) Trial is a pilot study of docosahexaenoic acid, an omega-3 fatty acid that may have anti-inflammatory benefits that prevent development of the autoimmunity that leads to type 1 diabetes.

The study is being conducted in babies less than five months old who have immediate family members with type 1 diabetes and pregnant mothers in their third trimester whose babies are at risk for type 1 diabetes, either because the mothers or other immediate relatives have the disease.

Studies Test New Approaches to Islet Transplantation

Researchers from six medical centers in the United States and Canada have begun testing new approaches to islet transplantation in adults with hard-to-control type 1 diabetes. The clinical studies, funded by the National Institutes of Health (NIH), will determine whether changes to current methods of islet transplantation lead to improved, long-lasting control of blood glucose with fewer side effects.

In islet transplantation, clusters of insulin-producing cells, called islets, are extracted from a donor pancreas and infused into the portal vein of a recipient's liver. In a successful transplant, the islets become embedded in the liver and begin producing insulin.

Currently, islet transplantation is appropriate only for people who already had a kidney transplant or who have severe hypoglycemia. As the procedure becomes safer and new sources of beta cells are developed, more people will benefit from transplantation.

For Safety, NHLBI Changes Intensive Blood Sugar Treatment Strategy in Clinical Trial of Diabetes and Cardiovascular Disease

The National Heart, Lung, and Blood Institute (NHLBI) of the National Institutes of Health has stopped one treatment within a large, ongoing North American clinical trial of diabetes and cardiovascular disease 18 months early due to safety concerns after review of available data, although the study will continue.

In this trial of adults with type 2 diabetes at especially high risk for heart attack and stroke, the medical strategy to intensively lower blood glucose (sugar) below current recommendations increased the risk of death compared with a less-intensive standard treatment strategy. Study participants receiving intensive blood glucose lowering treatment will now receive the less-intensive standard treatment.

The ACCORD (Action to Control Cardiovascular Risk in Diabetes) study enrolled 10,251 participants. Of these, 257 in the intensive treatment group have died, compared with 203 within the standard treatment group. This is a difference of 54 deaths, or 3 per 1,000 participants each year, over an average of almost four years of treatment. The death rates in both groups were lower than seen in similar populations in other studies.

"A thorough review of the data shows that the medical treatment strategy of intensively reducing blood sugar below current clinical guidelines causes harm in these especially high-risk patients with type 2 diabetes," said Elizabeth G. Nabel, MD, director, NHLBI. "Though we have stopped this part of the trial, we will continue to care for these participants, who now will receive the less-intensive standard treatment. In addition, we will continue to monitor the health of all participants, seek the underlying causes for this finding, and carry on with other important research within ACCORD."

Extensive analyses by ACCORD researchers have not determined a specific cause for the increased deaths among the intensive treatment group. Based on analyses conducted to date, there is no evidence that any medication or combination of medications is responsible.

Most participants in the intensive treatment group achieved their lower blood sugar goals with combinations of Food and Drug Administration–approved diabetes medications. For both the intensive and standard treatment groups, study clinicians could use all major classes of diabetes medications available: metformin, thiazolidinediones (TZDs, primarily rosiglitazone), insulins, sulfonylureas, exenatide, and acarbose.

"Because of the recent concerns with rosiglitazone, our extensive analysis included a specific review to determine whether there was any link between this particular medication and the increased deaths. We found no link," said William T. Friedewald, MD, ACCORD Steering Committee Chair and Clinical Professor of Medicine and Public Health at Columbia University.

ACCORD researchers will continue to monitor participants and conduct additional analyses to try and explain the findings.

Research Programs: Diabetes

Action for Health in Diabetes (Look AHEAD)
https://www.lookaheadtrial.org

Look AHEAD (Action For Health in Diabetes) is a multi-center randomized clinical trial to examine the effects of a lifestyle intervention designed to achieve and maintain weight loss over the long term through decreased caloric intake and exercise. Look AHEAD is focusing on the disease most affected by overweight and obesity, type 2 diabetes, and on the outcome that causes the greatest morbidity and mortality, cardiovascular disease.

Beta Cell Biology Consortium (BCBC)
http://www.betacell.org

The mission of the BCBC is to facilitate interdisciplinary approaches that will advance our understanding of pancreatic islet cell development, regenerative capacity and function. The long-term goal is to develop a cell-based therapy, or treatments leading to controlled beta-cell renewal, in order to restore normal insulin production to diabetic patients.

Bypass Angioplasty Revascularization Investigation (BARI) 2 Diabetes
http://www.bari2d.org

The BARI-2D study aims to determine the best therapies for people with type 2 diabetes and moderately severe cardiovascular disease.

Center for Inherited Disease Research (CIDR)
http://www.cidr.jhmi.edu

CIDR is a centralized facility established to provide genotyping and statistical genetics services for investigators seeking to identify genes that contribute to human disease. CIDR concentrates primarily on multifactorial hereditary disease although linage analysis of single gene disorders can also be accommodated.

Collaborative Islet Transplant Registry (CITR)
http://www.citregistry.org

The mission of CITR is to expedite progress and promote safety in islet/beta cell transplantation through the collection, analysis, and communication of comprehensive and current data on all islet/beta cell transplants performed in North America and soon some transplants in Europe and Australia. An annual report is available on the public website.

Diabetes Autoantibody Standardization Program (DASP)
http://www.idsoc.org/committees/antibody/dasphome.html

The fundamental aim of DASP is to improve the measurements of the autoantibodies predictive of type 1 diabetes.

Diabetes Control and Complications Trial (DCCT)
http://diabetes.niddk.nih.gov/dm/pubs/control/index.htm

The DCCT is a clinical study conducted from 1983 to 1993 by the National Institute of Diabetes and Digestive and Kidney Diseases (NIDDK). The study showed that keeping blood glucose levels as close to normal as possible slows the onset and progression of eye, kidney, and nerve diseases caused by diabetes. The Epidemiology of Diabetes Interventions and Complications (EDIC) is a follow-up study of people who participated in DCCT.

Diabetes Genome Anatomy Project (DGAP)
http://www.diabetesgenome.org

The Diabetes Genome Anatomy Project (DGAP) represents a unique, multidimensional initiative whose goal is to unravel the interface between insulin action, insulin resistance and the genetics of type 2 diabetes. The overall goal of the project is to identify the sets of the genes involved in insulin action and the predisposition to type 2 diabetes, as well as the secondary changes in gene expression that occur in response to the metabolic abnormalities present in diabetes.

Diabetes in America
http://diabetes.niddk.nih.gov/dm/pubs/america

Diabetes in America is a compilation and assessment of epidemiologic, public health, and clinical data on diabetes and its complications in the United States.

Diabetes Prevention Program (DPP)
http://www.bsc.gwu.edu/dpp/index.htmlvdoc

The DPP showed that lifestyle change or metformin delay the development of type 2 diabetes. The DPPOS is a long-term follow-up study of the DPP participants.

Diabetes Prevention Program Outcomes Study (DPPOS)
http://www.bsc.gwu.edu/dpp/protocol.htmlvdoc

The Diabetes Prevention Program Outcomes Study is studying the long term effect of diet and exercise and the diabetes medication, metformin, on the delay of type 2 diabetes in participants of the Diabetes Prevention Program (DPP).

Diabetes Prevention Trial—Type 1 (DPT-1)
http://www.niddk.nih.gov/patient/dpt_1/dpt_1.htm

The Diabetes Prevention Trial—Type 1 (DPT-1) consisted of two clinical trials that sought to delay or prevent type 1 diabetes, also known as insulin-dependent diabetes. These efforts are being continued by the Type 1 Diabetes TrialNet consortium.

Diabetes Research in Children Network (DirecNet)
http://public.direc.net

The mission of DirecNet is to investigate the potential use of glucose monitoring technology and its impact on the management of type 1 diabetes in children.

Diabetic Retinopathy Clinical Research Network (DRCR.net)
http://www.drcr.net

The Diabetic Retinopathy Clinical Research Network (DRCR.net) is a collaborative network dedicated to facilitating multicenter clinical research of diabetic retinopathy, diabetic macular edema and associated conditions. The DRCR.net supports the identification, design, and implementation of multicenter clinical research initiatives focused on diabetes-induced retinal disorders. Principal emphasis is placed on clinical trials, but epidemiologic outcomes and other research may be supported as well.

The Environmental Determinant of Diabetes in the Young (TEDDY)
http://teddy.epi.usf.edu

This consortium is organizing international efforts to identify infectious agents, dietary factors, or other environmental factors that trigger type 1 diabetes in genetically susceptible people.

Epidemiology of Diabetes Interventions and Complications (EDIC)
http://www.niddk.nih.gov/patient/edic/edic-public.htm; http://www.bsc.gwu.edu/bsc/studies/edic.html

An observational study examining the risk factors associated with the long-term complications of type 1 diabetes. The study began in 1994 and follows the 1,441 participants previously enrolled in the Diabetes Control and Complications Trial (DCCT).

Family Investigation of Nephropathy of Diabetes (FIND)
http://darwin.cwru.edu/FIND

The overall goal of FIND is to identify genetic pathways that may be critical for the development of nephropathy and lead to candidates amenable to therapeutic strategies to prevent the onset or progression of nephropathy. Such data might aid identification of people at risk for the development of progressive renal disease.

Islet Cell Resource Centers (ICR)
http://icr.coh.org

The three major goals of the ICRs are: 1) to provide pancreatic islets of cGMP-quality to eligible investigators for use in FDA approved, IRB-approved transplantation protocols; 2) to optimize the harvest, purification, function, storage, and shipment of islets while developing tests that characterize the quality and predict the effectiveness of islets transplanted into patients with diabetes mellitus; and 3) to provide pancreatic islets for basic science studies.

Islet Transplantation Trials for Type 1 Diabetes
http://www.isletstudy.org

A network of centers will conduct studies of islet transplantation in patients with type 1 diabetes to improve the safety and long-term success of methods for transplanting islets.

Non-Human Primate Transplantation Tolerance Cooperative Study Group (NHPCSG)
http://www.niddk.nih.gov/fund/diabetesspecialfunds/consortia/NHP.pdf

The NHPCSG, a multi-institution consortium, was established to evaluate the safety and efficacy of novel donor-specific, tolerance induction therapies in non-human primate (NHP) models of kidney and islet transplantation. The program also supports research into the immunological mechanisms of tolerance induction and development of surrogate markers for the induction, maintenance, and loss of tolerance.

SEARCH for Diabetes in Youth
http://www.searchfordiabetes.org

SEARCH is a multi-center study that identifies cases of diabetes in children/youth less than 20 years of age in six geographically dispersed populations that encompass the ethnic diversity of the United States.

Targeting Inflammation Using Salsalate for Type 2 Diabetes (TINSAL-T2D)
http://www.tinsal-t2d.org

The TINSAL-T2D study is a multi-center, randomized, double-blinded, placebo-controlled, parallel-group clinical trial. The primary objective of the study is to determine whether salicylates represent a new pharmacological option for glycemic control in patients with type 2 diabetes.

TODAY Trial
http://todaystudy.org/index.cgi

The TODAY (Treatment Options for type 2 Diabetes in Adolescents and Youth) study seeks to identify the best treatment of type 2 diabetes in children and teens.

Trial to Reduce IDDM in the Genetically at Risk (TRIGR)
http://trigr.epi.usf.edu

The primary objective of this multi-center, international study is to determine whether weaning to a casein hydrolysate formula during the first 6–8 months of life in place of cow's milk based formula reduces the incidence of autoimmunity and type 1 diabetes in genetically susceptible newborn infants.

Type 1 Diabetes Genetics Consortium (T1DGC)
http://www.t1dgc.org

T1DGC was established with the primary goal of organizing international efforts to identify genes that determine an individual's risk of type 1 diabetes.

Type 1 Diabetes TrialNet
http://www.diabetestrialnet.org

This clinical network seeks to prevent type 1 diabetes in high-risk people and to preserve insulin production in those newly diagnosed.

Chapter 51

Researching Diabetes Risk Factors

Section 51.1—Diabetes Risk Factors Develop
              Earlier in Women 490

Section 51.2—Androgen Deprivation Therapy May
              Increase Risk of Diabetes 492

Section 51.3—Researchers Identify New Genetic Risk
              Factors for Type 2 Diabetes 494

Section 51.4—Long-Term Use of Selenium Supplements
              and Risk for Type 2 Diabetes 496

Section 51.5—Does Prenatal Exposure to Viruses Place
              Children at Risk for Diabetes? 498

Section 51.6—Does Hepatitis C Infection Increase Risks
              for Diabetes? 501

Section 51.7—Greater Diabetes Risk in Patients Taking
              High Blood Pressure Medications 504

Section 51.1

Diabetes Risk Factors Develop Earlier in Women

"Diabetes Clock Ticking for Women," by Lois Baker, *University at Buffalo Reporter*, February 22, 2007. © University at Buffalo. Reprinted with permission.

The "diabetes clock" may start ticking in women years in advance of a medical diagnosis of the disease, new research has shown.

University at Buffalo (UB) epidemiologists have found that newly identified risk factors for diabetes found in the blood, such as markers of endothelial dysfunction, chronic sub-acute inflammation and blood clotting factors, are present early on in women who eventually progress from normal glucose status to the pre-diabetic condition.

Pre-diabetes is diagnosed when blood sugar levels are higher than normal (between 100–125 mg/deciliter of blood), but not high enough to indicate full-blown diabetes (over 125 mg/deciliter of blood). The markers weren't associated with progression from normal to pre-diabetic status in men.

Results of the study appear in the February 2007 issue of *Diabetes Care*.

"This is one of the first reports to show that otherwise healthy women are more likely than men to show elevated levels of endothelial factors and other markers of progression to pre-diabetes," said lead author Richard Donahue, professor of social and preventive medicine and associate dean for research in the School of Public Health and Health Professions.

"Because these pre-diabetic markers are not routinely assessed, and because diabetes is strongly linked with coronary heart disease, the study may help explain why the decline in death rates for heart disease in diabetic women lags behind that of diabetic men," he said.

"Previous research had shown that hypertension and cholesterol were elevated among women who later developed diabetes. However, current findings that these novel risk factors [markers of endothelial dysfunction, chronic sub-acute inflammation and blood clotting factors] are elevated among women even earlier than previously recognized does suggest that the 'diabetes clock' starts ticking sooner for women than for men."

The study involved 1,455 healthy participants originally enrolled in the Western New York Study, a case-control investigation of patterns of alcohol consumption and risk of cardiovascular disease conducted from 1996–2001. In the current study, all participants were free of pre-diabetes, type 2 diabetes and known cardiovascular disease. They received a physical examination when they entered the study and again for this six-year follow-up.

Standard measures—height, weight, waist girth, blood pressure—were taken, plus blood samples to determine concentrations of fasting glucose and insulin, specific proinflammatory markers, C-reactive protein and markers of dysfunction in the endothelial tissue, the tissue lining blood vessels.

Results showed that 52 women and 39 men had progressed from normal blood glucose levels to pre-diabetic status during the previous six years.

Donahue said the question of what explains the sex difference remains to be determined, and he plans to study this in the future. Meanwhile, he suggested that women whose blood glucose increases over time, even if it doesn't reach diabetic levels, should be screened more intensively for cardiovascular disease.

Karol Rejman, Lisa Rafalson, Jacek Dmochowski, Saverio Stranges and Maurizio Trevisan, all from the Department of Social and Preventive Medicine, contributed to the study. Dmochowski also is affiliated with the University of North Carolina-Charlotte.

The research was supported by a grant from the National Institutes of Health.

Section 51.2

Androgen Deprivation Therapy May Increase Risk of Diabetes

According to the results of a study published in the *Journal of Clinical Oncology*, use of a gonadotropin-releasing hormone (GnRH) agonist for the treatment of non-metastatic prostate cancer may increase the risk of diabetes and cardiovascular disease.

The prostate is a gland of the male reproductive system. It produces some of the fluid that transports sperm during ejaculation. After skin cancer, prostate cancer is the most common form of cancer diagnosed in men.

Androgen deprivation therapy, also known as hormonal therapy, is designed to block testosterone from stimulating the growth of hormone-dependent types of prostate cancer.

Among men with metastatic prostate cancer (cancer that has spread beyond the prostate to distant sites in the body), androgen deprivation therapy is often used to relieve symptoms. Androgen deprivation therapy may also improve survival for some men with earlier stage prostate cancer.

Androgen deprivation can be achieved through the use of medications such as gonadotropin-releasing hormone agonists, or by surgically removing the testicles (bilateral orchiectomy).

Men with early-stage prostate cancer generally have a favorable prognosis, and understanding the frequency of serious treatment-related side effects is an important part of treatment planning. Because androgen deprivation may increase fat mass and insulin resistance, it's possible that it could increase the risk of diabetes and cardiovascular disease.

To explore the risks of diabetes and cardiovascular disease in men with localized or regional prostate cancer (cancer that has not spread to distant sites in the body), researchers conducted a study among more than 70,000 Medicare enrollees with prostate cancer. Information about

492

medication use and health outcomes was collected from medical claims data.

Overall, 36% of the men had received a GnRH agonist and 7% underwent surgical removal of the testicles.

During four-and-a-half years of follow-up, 5.4% of study partici-pants had a heart attack and 4.5% experienced sudden cardiac death. Among the men who were initially free of diabetes, 10.9% developed diabetes. Among the men who were initially free of coronary heart disease, 25.3% developed coronary heart disease.

- Compared to men who did not receive androgen deprivation therapy, men who were treated with a GnRH agonist were 44% more likely to develop diabetes, 16% more likely to develop coro-nary heart disease, 11% more likely to have a heart attack, and 16% more likely to experience sudden cardiac death.

- Compared to men who did not receive androgen deprivation therapy, men who underwent surgical removal of their testicles were more 34% more likely to develop diabetes. Risks of coronary heart disease, heart attack, or sudden cardiac death were not increased. The researchers note that it's unclear why the risks of bilateral orchiectomy would differ from the risks of GnRH agonists. It's possible that the relatively small number of men who underwent orchiectomy may have produced some uncertainty in these results, but the researchers note that additional studies are needed to clarify this question.

The researchers conclude that use of GnRH agonists in the treat-ment of localized or regional prostate cancer may increase the risk of diabetes and cardiovascular disease. The researchers note that "De-cisions about GnRH agonist treatment for locoregional prostate can-cer should weigh improvements in cancer-specific outcomes against potential increased risks of diabetes and cardiovascular disease."

Reference: Keating NL, O'Malley J, Smith MR. Diabetes and Cardio-vascular Disease during Androgen Deprivation Therapy for Prostate Cancer. *Journal of Clinical Oncology*. 2006;24:4448-4456.

Section 51.3

Researchers Identify New Genetic Risk Factors for Type 2 Diabetes

From *Diabetes Dateline*, National Diabetes Information
Clearinghouse, National Institute of Diabetes and Digestive and
Kidney Diseases, Fall 2007.

In the most comprehensive look at genetic risk factors for type 2 diabetes to date, a U.S.-Finnish team, along with two consortia—the Diabetes Genetics Initiative at the Broad Institute and the Wellcome Trust Case Control Consortium/U.K. Type 2 Diabetes Genetics Consortium—has identified at least four new genetic variants associated with increased diabetes risk and confirmed the existence of another six. The groups' findings boost the number of genetic variants linked to increased susceptibility to type 2 diabetes to at least 10.

The U.S.-Finnish team received major support from the National Institute of Diabetes and Digestive and Kidney Diseases (NIDDK) and the National Human Genome Research Institute's (NHGRI) Division of Intramural Research, both part of the National Institutes of Health (NIH). The laboratory analysis of genetic variants in the first stage of the study was conducted by the Center for Inherited Disease Research with funding from the NIH and Johns Hopkins University.

"It has been a formidable challenge to identify the complex genetic factors involved in common diseases, such as type 2 diabetes," said NHGRI Director Francis Collins, M.D., Ph.D. "Now, thanks to the tools and technologies generated by the sequencing of the human genome and subsequent mapping of common human genetic variations, we finally are making significant progress."

In addition to lifestyle factors like obesity, poor diet, and lack of exercise, doctors have long known that heredity is a significant risk factor for developing type 2 diabetes—people who have a parent or sibling with type 2 diabetes face a 3.5 times greater risk of developing the disease than people with no family history. However, researchers have only just begun to zero in on particular genetic variants that increase or decrease disease susceptibility.

To make their discoveries, researchers used a relatively new, comprehensive strategy known as a genome-wide association study. For this kind of study, researchers use two groups of participants: a large group of people with the disease being studied and a large group of otherwise similar people without the disease. Using DNA purified from blood cells, researchers quickly survey each participant's complete set of DNA, or genome, for strategically selected markers of genetic variation.

If certain genetic variations are found more frequently in people with the disease compared with healthy people, the variations are said to be associated with the disease. The associated genetic variations can serve as a strong pointer to the region of the genome where the genetic risk factor resides. However, the first variants detected may not themselves directly influence disease susceptibility, and the actual causative variant may lie nearby. This means researchers often need to take additional steps, such as sequencing every DNA base pair in that particular region of the genome, to identify the exact genetic variant that affects disease risk.

Major Effort

The genomes of more than 32,000 people were tested for the study, making it one of the largest genome-wide association efforts conducted to date. The newly identified diabetes-associated variations lie in or near these genes:

- **IGF2BP2:** This gene codes for a protein called insulin-like growth factor 2 mRNA binding protein 2. Insulin-like growth factor 2 is thought to play a role in regulating insulin action.

- **CDKAL1:** This gene codes for a protein called CDK5 regulatory subunit associated protein1-like1. The protein may affect the activity of the cyclin-dependent kinase 5 (CDK5) protein, which stimulates insulin production and may influence other processes in the pancreas' insulin-producing, or beta, cells.

- **CDKN2A and CDKN2B:** The proteins produced by these genes inhibit the activity of cyclin-dependent protein kinases, including one that has been shown to influence the growth of beta cells in mice.

- **Chromosome 1:** One association is located in a region of chromosome 11 not known to contain any genes. Researchers speculate that the variant sequences may regulate the activity of

495

genes located elsewhere in the genome, but more work is needed to determine the exact relationships to pathways involved in type 2 diabetes.

Genetic variants associated with diabetes that were confidently confirmed by the new research are TCF7L2, SLC30A8, HHEX, PPARG, and KCNJ11.

"These genetic findings are exciting news for diabetes research," said NIDDK Director Griffin P. Rodgers, M.D. "While more work remains to be done, the newly identified genetic variants may point us in the direction of valuable new drug targets for the prevention or treatment of type 2 diabetes."

Section 51.4

Long-Term Use of Selenium Supplements and Risk for Type 2 Diabetes

What is the problem and what is known about it so far?

Selenium is a mineral that is required in very low doses for the body to function normally. It is an antioxidant, meaning that it prevents oxygen from damaging cells. Although most people get enough selenium in their diet, selenium is included in many multivitamins and is sold as a supplement itself. Many people take selenium supplements to stay healthy. Some research suggests that selenium supplements can improve the way the body handles sugar and might prevent some complications of diabetes. However, other research suggests that selenium supplementation has no effect on diabetes or health.

Why did the researchers do this particular study?

To see whether taking selenium supplements prevents diabetes.

Who was studied?

1202 people with skin cancer other than melanoma who were seen in dermatology clinics in areas of the United States where people tend to have low blood levels of selenium. None of the participants had diabetes.

How was the study done?

The researchers measured participants' blood selenium levels. They then randomly assigned the participants to take selenium supplements (200 micrograms) or placebo pills. They followed the participants over an average of seven years to see who developed diabetes. They then compared the number of people with diabetes in the two groups.

What did the researchers find?

More people who took selenium developed diabetes than those who took placebo pills. The risk for diabetes seemed to be higher in people who had higher blood selenium levels at the start of the study.

What were the limitations of the study?

The researchers relied on participants' reports that they developed diabetes and did not confirm those reports with measures of blood sugar. The findings apply to the specific dose of selenium used in the study. Participants tended to be older and white, so the findings might not apply to younger people and those of other races.

What are the implications of the study?

Selenium supplements appear to increase the risk for diabetes. Although the findings need to be confirmed, long-term selenium supplementation should not be viewed as harmless and a possibly healthy way to prevent illness.

Section 51.5

Does Prenatal Exposure to Viruses Place Children at Risk for Diabetes?

Type 1 diabetes is an autoimmune disease. The immune system attacks and destroys the beta cells of the pancreas. Beta cells make insulin, and once they are destroyed, they aren't replaced. The result is type 1 diabetes.

The big question is: Why does this happen?

Genetics is thought to play a role, but Åke Lernmark, PhD, professor at the University of Washington's School of Medicine, has another idea. He believes that women who are exposed to certain viruses when they are pregnant may be more likely to have children who develop type 1. Lernmark and his team of researchers are using funds from an American Diabetes Association Terry and Louise Gregg Diabetes in Pregnancy Research Award to test his theory.

Antibodies and Antigens

Your immune system is geared to protect you from a host of foreign invaders or "antigens," such as viruses and bacteria. It monitors your system 24/7. If it senses invader antigens, it releases proteins called antibodies to seek and destroy them. In such cases, your immune system is a real lifesaver.

Lernmark suspects that the immune system is occasionally tricked during pregnancy and makes a serious mistake; it incorrectly views certain substances that naturally occur in the body of the mother-to-be as antigens and makes antibodies to attack them.

The substances that may trigger a mistaken immune response include GAD, IA-2, and incomplete forms of insulin. GAD and IA-2 are proteins that normally reside in the beta cells, but in certain circumstances—which we'll get to in a moment—they may leak out into the blood and prompt an immune attack. Insulin normally circulates in the blood to help process glucose, but when the beta cells are damaged, insulin that is still being made leaks out before it's in the proper form, and the body sees it as foreign.

According to Lernmark, the more antibodies created in response to these antigens, the greater the diabetes risk to the child.

"Today we know that if a child has antibodies to all three, that child will definitely develop diabetes within two to five years," Lernmark says. "We can actually predict diabetes."

Lernmark's team will examine blood samples both from women who gave birth in a hospital in Sweden in the 1970s and from their children. The purpose is to determine if the mothers and children had these antibodies present in their blood when the children were born. Then they will look at the records and see which children later developed diabetes.

The idea to look back in the records came from Lernmark's colleague, Sten Ivarsson, MD, PhD, a pediatrician at the hospital in Sweden where the women gave birth. Early in Ivarsson's career, it was the hospital's practice to test women and their newborns for cytomegalovirus, a virus in the herpes family that can cause hearing impairment and deafness. It can be passed from an infected mother to her child during pregnancy. Over the years, the hospital collected more than 100,000 blood samples.

Ivarsson eventually became head of the pediatric diabetes unit. One day he treated a child for diabetes whose mother he remembered as having been tested for cytomegalovirus years before. Thinking of the blood samples still in storage, he approached Lernmark, and they came up with an idea: Why not go back and look at the samples to see if mother and child had the antibodies when the mother gave birth?

From there, the idea blossomed into the study it is now—"which means that if you're a scientist, you should never throw anything out, because you never know what you'll discover," Lernmark says.

The team has identified about 150 people with type 1 who were part of the original blood sample study. The next step is to look at the samples and see if either mother or child had the antibodies, and see which mothers also had diabetes themselves.

If the mothers had diabetes themselves, that might indicate a genetic risk. It's the mothers who did not have diabetes during pregnancy who hold special interest for Lernmark, because chances are something other than genetic programming triggered their immune systems, something temporary—like a virus.

A Virus

Lernmark believes that when a particular kind of virus strikes a pregnant woman, it may affect the developing immune system of her unborn child and make the child susceptible to the same virus later in life.

"When the mother is hit by the virus during pregnancy, the virus attacks the beta cells, the beta cells get sick and break apart, and GAD, IA-2, and unfinished insulin leak out into the blood," he says. "Antibodies attack because these things should not be in the blood. The virus, antibodies, and antigens leak over into the fetus.

"Meanwhile, the immune system of the child thinks the virus and the mother's antibodies and antigens are okay. The child's immune system sees them as part of the mother, so the child's immune system doesn't react," he explains. "The child is then born with an immunological disability. Years later, the virus comes along and the door is wide open for it. The child has no protection from infection. So, we think the children get hit twice, once from the mother, and once from the virus itself."

According to Lernmark's theory, once the child is infected, his or her own beta cells break apart and leak GAD, IA-2, and unfinished insulin into the blood. Then the immune system kicks in, the way the mother's immune system kicked in when she was pregnant and she was infected with the virus. Only for the child, whose immune system developed abnormally in the womb, the reaction goes one step further. T-cells, which are specialized attack cells in the immune system, recognize not only GAD, IA-2, and insulin, but also the beta cells where these antigens are coming from. Then the T-cells attack the beta cells. No beta cells means no insulin, and no insulin means diabetes.

What virus could be so dastardly? There are a number of suspects, but the Coxsackie family of viruses stands out.

There are some severe forms of Coxsackie virus, but the more common viruses in this family have mild symptoms, says Lernmark. They cause diarrhea, fever, and stomach upset, and they are passed by person-to-person contact either through unwashed hands or droplets in the air from sneezing or coughing. Also, these viruses change much like the flu. Because Coxsackie viruses are so common, their symptoms are so mild, and they change so frequently, there are no vaccines for them.

The next step, then, would be to find out who among the mothers and children were exposed to a Coxsackie virus. Lernmark's team may be able to determine this by looking at the blood samples, because Coxsackie viruses trigger antibodies of their own.

Working Backward

If it turns out that Coxsackie viruses are partly to blame for type 1 diabetes, efforts at preventing diabetes might involve treating or preventing the virus, says Lernmark.

"So far, all we can do is look for GAD, IA-2, and insulin antibodies and tell people they're going to develop diabetes, and we can say that the earlier you're diagnosed, the better off you will be. But we have nothing to offer that will prevent diabetes," says Lernmark. "If we can understand how the disease starts, we'll be in a much better position to treat it.

"We may be able to treat mothers or children when the virus is present and suppress the virus. We may be able to treat them with anti-viral drugs. Or, perhaps we could try and develop a vaccine that would cover many of the viruses, and then treat women before they get pregnant," he adds. "But we have to work our way backwards to the event that starts diabetes before we can try to find a way to stop it."

Section 51.6

Does Hepatitis C Infection Increase Risks for Diabetes?

By David A. Cooke, MD, © 2008 Omnigraphics, Inc.

An infectious disease like hepatitis C wouldn't come to mind for most doctors if asked what causes diabetes. Indeed, for many years no one knew that the two diseases had any relationship at all. However, studies over the past decade have uncovered a strong link, and this has drawn the interest of liver specialists and endocrinologists alike.

Hepatitis C is a moderately common viral infection that affects about 3% of the world's population. The disease is seen in virtually all parts of the world, and it is estimated that about 1.8% of Americans have hepatitis C. The virus is spread through blood and body fluids, and infection may occur via blood transfusions, IV drug use, sexual contact, and mother-to-child transmission. Still, contaminated needles are the most common source of infection. In the United States, hepatitis C is very common in jails; about 20% of prisoners are infected.

In addition, health care workers, the poor, and racial minority populations tend to be at increased risk. However, in some patients it is unclear how infection was acquired.

Once a person is exposed to hepatitis C, the virus mainly infects the liver, although other organs can be affected. While some people are able to rid themselves of the infection, most develop long-term infections that last for decades. Frequently, people do not know they are infected, as there may be few or no symptoms. However, over many years the virus can cause severe liver damage, and lead to cirrhosis and liver failure.

Most diabetics do not have hepatitis C infection, but people with hepatitis C are unusually prone to developing diabetes. Having hepatitis C more than triples the risk of diabetes, and about one quarter of people with hepatitis C are diabetic. People with hepatitis C are mainly type 2 diabetics; hepatitis C and type 1 diabetes have not been convincingly linked.

How could hepatitis C infection cause diabetes?

Hepatitis C targets the liver, and the liver plays a key role in digestion and metabolism. It would make sense that liver disease might increase the risk of diabetes. In fact, patients with hepatitis C and advanced liver disease are significantly more likely to develop diabetes. However, there is more to hepatitis C and diabetes than just liver disease. People with hepatitis C are far more likely to become diabetic, compared to people with other kinds of liver disease.

A number of theories have been developed to explain the hepatitis C–diabetes connection. In addition to liver damage, researchers have looked at pancreatic damage, autoimmunity, and generalized inflammation as possible causes. At this point, no single theory has provided a complete answer. However, the best available evidence suggests that hepatitis C infection triggers increased insulin resistance.

Insulin resistance is the fundamental problem underlying all forms of type 2 diabetes. Insulin is a hormone produced in the pancreas, a large gland in the abdomen, in response to eating a meal. Insulin directs cells throughout the body to take glucose (sugar) out of the blood stream and use it for nourishment. However, in some people, cells do not respond appropriately to normal levels of insulin. Instead, significantly higher insulin levels are needed to get the expected result. This is known as insulin resistance. Type 2 diabetes occurs when insulin resistance becomes so high that the pancreas can't make enough insulin to keep blood sugars in a normal range.

There are many causes of insulin resistance, including obesity, inactivity, and genetics. Infection can also cause insulin resistance, because hormones released when the body is fighting infection tend to counter the effects of insulin. Hepatitis C tends to cause a chronic, persistent infection lasting years or decades, and high levels of the virus may circulate in the blood. It may be that the body's unsuccessful attempts to clear this infection cause insulin resistance and ultimately lead to type 2 diabetes. Still, there are probably more pieces to this puzzle. Hepatitis B can also cause persistent infection like hepatitis C, yet the diabetes risk is much higher with hepatitis C.

What does all this mean for people with diabetes or hepatitis C?

First, hepatitis C should always be considered in patients with type 2 diabetes, especially if they have risk factors for the infection. While only a minority of type 2 diabetics have hepatitis C, it is still a higher rate of infection than would be expected by chance. In particular, mild liver test abnormalities, which are commonly seen in diabetic patients, should not automatically be assumed to be due to the diabetes itself.

Second, patients who are known to have hepatitis C should be closely monitored for the development of diabetes. This risk appears to be highest amongst people who are more than 40 years old, as well as those with more severe liver damage. Early recognition of diabetes, if it develops, may help prevent complications from the disease later on.

There is a great deal that is still not understood about either hepatitis C infection or type 2 diabetes. Study of this unexpected interaction between the two conditions may eventually yield important insights into treatment for both diseases.

Section 51.7

Greater Diabetes Risk in Patients Taking High Blood Pressure Medications

"NHLBI Media Availability: Greater Diabetes Risk in Patients Taking High Blood Pressure Medications," a press release issued by the National Heart, Lung, and Blood Institute, November 13, 2006.

In a long-term study of older adults with high blood pressure from the National Heart, Lung, and Blood Institute of the National Institutes of Health, participants without diabetes who were taking high blood pressure medications experienced increased average fasting glucose levels. This was true regardless of which class of medication was used: diuretic, ACE inhibitor (angiotensin-converting enzyme inhibitor), or calcium channel blocker. During a four year period, the glucose changes led to new diagnoses of diabetes in approximately one in ten participants (diuretic 11.0 percent, ACE inhibitor 7.8 percent, and calcium channel blocker 9.3 percent.) However, the results of this Antihypertensive and Lipid-Lowering Treatment to Prevent Heart Attack Trial (ALLHAT) analysis showed no significant evidence that the new onset diabetes increased the risk of stroke, heart failure, or death from any cause, but it did increase the risk of heart attack. In those taking a diuretic, the relationship between new diabetes and coronary disease was actually less than in those taking the other drugs and not significant for the diuretic. According to the authors, this suggests that the glucose changes induced by diuretics do not lead to heart disease in the same way as diabetes caused by overweight, inactivity, and genetic predisposition. This finding is strongly supported by previous findings in a 14-year follow-up of the Systolic Hypertension in the Elderly Program (SHEP).

Chapter 52

Stress and Diabetes: A Review of the Links

Evidence suggests that stressful experiences might affect diabetes, in terms of both its onset and its exacerbation. In this article, the authors review some of this evidence and consider ways in which stress might affect diabetes, both through physiological mechanisms and via behavior. They also discuss the implications of this for clinical practice and care.

In recent years, the complexities of the relationship between stress and diabetes have become well known but have been less well researched. Some studies have suggested that stressful experiences might affect the onset and/or the metabolic control of diabetes, but findings have often been inconclusive. In this article, we review some of this research before going on to consider how stress might affect diabetes control and the physiological mechanisms through which this may occur. Finally, we discuss the implications for clinical practice and care. Before going any further, however, the meaning of the term stress must be clarified because it can be used in different ways. Stress may be thought of as *a)* a physiological response to an external stimulus, or *b)* a psychological response to external stimuli, or *c)* stressful events themselves, which can be negative or positive or both. In this article, we address all three aspects of stress: stressful events or experiences (sometimes referred to as stressors) and the physiological and psychological/behavioral responses to these.

Role of Stress in the Onset of Diabetes

Stressful experiences have been implicated in the onset of diabetes in individuals already predisposed to developing the disease. As early as the beginning of the 17th century, the onset of diabetes was linked to "prolonged sorrow" by an English physician.[1]

Since then, a number of research studies have identified stressors such as family losses and workplace stress as factors triggering the onset of diabetes, both type 1 and type 2. For example, Thernlund et al.[2] suggested that negative stressful experiences in the first two years of life may increase the risk of developing type 1 diabetes in children. Other factors, such as high family chaos and behavioral problems, were also implicated. Other research has also supported the hypothesis that stressful experiences can lead to increased risk for developing type 1 or type 2 diabetes.[3–5]

In a large population-based survey of glucose intolerance, Mooy et al.[6] demonstrated an association between stressful experiences and the diagnosis of type 2 diabetes. Although this was a cross-sectional study, the authors investigated stress levels in people with previously undetected diabetes in order to rule out the possibility that the disease itself influenced reports of stressful experiences. They also took other factors into account, such as alcohol consumption, physical activity level, and education.

Bjorntop[7] has attempted to explain the physiological links between stressful experiences and the onset of diabetes. He argues that the psychological reaction to stressors of defeatism or helplessness leads to the activation of the hypothalamo-pituitary-adrenal (HPA) axis, leading in turn to various endocrine abnormalities, such as high cortisol and low sex steroid levels, that antagonize the actions of insulin. At the same time, an increase in visceral adiposity (increased girth) is seen, which plays an important role in diabetes by contributing to insulin resistance.[8] Increased visceral adiposity can be measured by waist-to-hip ratio. In the Mooy et al. study of type 2 diabetes,[6] there was only a weak association between stressful experiences and waist-to-hip ratio, suggesting that other factors, so far unidentified, may play a mediating role.

Where stressful experiences have been implicated in the onset of type 1 diabetes, researchers have often attempted to explain this in terms of the effects of stress on the autoimmune system.[2] Bottazo et al.[9] hypothesized that environmental factors (e.g., viruses or toxic agents) trigger the autoimmune destruction of the ß-cells in genetically predisposed individuals.

However, not all studies have demonstrated a link between stressful experiences and the development of diabetes. In a recent review, Cosgrove [10] argued that many of the studies that have demonstrated a link between stressful events and type 1 diabetes have been of small size and lacked appropriate control groups. Cosgrove cited one large Swedish study[11] indicating that there was no association between stressful events and the onset of type 1 diabetes. However, this study included a wide age range (15–34 years) of newly diagnosed people. Often quite vast differences in the type and intensity of life changes are found at the different ages within this range, and changes in social supports (known to be a buffer to stress) are frequent during these years, especially in the teenage years. This may have masked any association between stressful experiences and the development of diabetes.

Given the numerous measurement strategies and different study populations that have been investigated through the years, definite conclusions are difficult to reach. Smaller in-depth studies have usually demonstrated a link between stress and diabetes, whereas larger studies using self-report checklists to measure the occurrence of stressful experiences have sometimes failed to support this link. Much more conclusive is the evidence regarding the relationship between stressful experiences and metabolic control in those already diagnosed with diabetes, and it is to this research that we now turn.

Stress and Diabetes Control

In recent years, some researchers have turned their attention to the possibilities of stressful experiences influencing diabetes control.[12–15] This potential influence is important, not only for the often debilitating effects poor blood glucose control can have on daily life, but also because of the known association between chronically high blood glucose levels and the development of diabetes complications.[16]

It is a complex area of research, much of it having been conducted in children and adolescents, with fewer studies in adults or in those with type 2 diabetes, and using a number of different measurement tools. Stressful experiences have been recorded using anything from simple checklists to longer self-report questionnaires, to in-depth interviewing techniques. Most studies in this area have not determined the type or severity of stress that may influence changes in glycemic control, nor have they been able to fully address the role of other factors in mediating the impact of stress on glycemic control. Moreover, it is difficult to determine the temporal relationship between stress and health, not least because poor health often leads to adverse experiences.

A number of laboratory studies have been conducted to demonstrate the effects of specific stressful situations (for example, arithmetic problem solving, unpleasant interviews) on blood glucose levels. Many of these studies have demonstrated that these types of stressors can destabilize blood glucose levels, at least for hours at a time.[17] However, a major criticism of this approach is that it does not mirror the real world in which individuals with diabetes live.

Other studies have focused on that real world and have attempted to measure naturally occurring stress.[18–21] These later studies are not without problems however, such as, the myriad possibilities for measurement and/or observation, which makes cross-study comparisons difficult. Stress may take the form of day-today hassles, and it may be that major life events (death of a close relative, losing a job) are an added layer of complexity, along with long-term chronic difficulties (e.g., providing long-term care for a relative or long-term unemployment).

In an attempt to overcome some of the previous methodological limitations, a prospective in-depth investigation into the relationship between stressful experiences and changes in glycemic control over time was designed.[21] Individuals with type 1 diabetes were interviewed using an in-depth interview schedule and then followed up quarterly for a year with measures of diabetes control (hemoglobin A1c [A1C]). Unlike previous studies, the participants were asked about both negative and positive stressors in their lives. The results showed that those whose glycemic control deteriorated over time were more likely to report negative stress, whereas those whose control improved over the follow-up period reported positive stress. Negative stressors included interpersonal conflicts, death of a close tie, and disturbed behavior of someone close, whereas positive stressors were events such as engagement to be married, birth of a child, or a desired change in employment (Figure 52.1).

Studies such as the one reported above have their limitations. For example, not all individuals perceive stressors in the same way; what is a negative stressor in one person's life might actually be a positive one in another's, so the context in which stress occurs is also important. Some people react to stressful events in a way that makes them psychologically vulnerable, for example, they may experience feelings of hopelessness or anxiety, particularly in the context of social isolation or poverty. Others may respond to stress in positive terms or as a "challenge," or they may feel better able to cope with the stress because they have several social supports or the support of a loving family. It is easier to categorize major stressors into those that are positive and those that are negative; it is more difficult for more minor stress or "hassles." Long-term chronic difficulties are also important, but may change in perceived level of severity or negativity over time.

Findings from Smith's study[22] of women's experiences of diabetes-related stress indicated that a wide variety of factors were important, including relationships with other people (including health care professionals), the interaction between diabetes and daily life and work, and fear of the future. Minor stressors and hassles were seen as an integral part of living with diabetes in this study and were related to both work and family life, which often took priority over the management of diabetes.

The impact of stressful experiences on diabetes is clearly varied and may depend on other psychosocial factors. One of these is social support, and research has shown this may provide a buffering effect in times of stress.[13] Psychological support is also important. In a recent meta-analysis of randomized controlled trials, Ismail et al.[23] concluded that people with type 2 diabetes who received behavioral-based diabetes education or psychological interventions were likely to show improvements in both glycemic control and psychological distress.

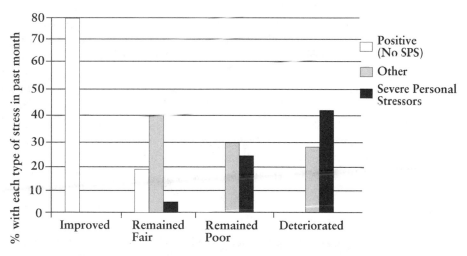

Differences between the groups significantly different $P = 0.000$.

Figure 52.1. Relationship between stress and glycemic control. From Ref. 21.

The relationship between stressful experiences and metabolic control is thought to differ greatly among individuals in terms of both the strength and the direction of the relationship,[24] and these differences have serious implications for the design of effective interventions to reduce the impact of stressors. Precisely how stressors affect glycemic control remains controversial, and there may be both physiological and behavioral pathways between stressors and health status. The mechanisms through which this may take place may be direct (through physiological effects on the neuroendocrine system)[25] or indirect (through alterations in health care practices in times of stress).[18, 26] It is to these pathways that we now turn.

Behavior

The behavioral mechanisms through which stressful experiences might affect diabetes control are varied and often complex. There are, of course, many different types of stress, there are shorter- and longer-term stressors, and people may respond to these very differently. Difficulties in measurement such as those mentioned above also apply to measuring behavior. At the same time, differences in resources such as social supports, ability to cope, and other psychosocial variables will all affect both the response to and the behavior resulting from stressful experiences.

Reactions to external stressors, for example, feelings of anxiety or depression, may lead to difficulties with self-care manifested through less physical activity, poorer diet, or difficulties with medication taking.[27, 28] Experiences of stress may lead to other unhealthy behaviors, such as smoking, which in turn are linked to poor blood glucose control but also to a greater risk of developing diabetes complications.[29] Data from Smith's study[22] indicated a range of behavior described as occurring in response to stress. These behaviors ranged from unhealthy lifestyle patterns associated with alcohol and tobacco consumption to increased physical activity and relaxation, such as walking, yoga, swimming, meditation, and hypnotherapy.

One particular type of stress was investigated in a Swedish study. Agardh et al.[30] demonstrated that work stress, as indicated by low decision latitude (or fewer opportunities for decision making), along with a low sense of coherence, significantly increased risk for type 2 diabetes. Low sense of coherence is thought to negatively affect people's ability to cope with stressors[31] and also to be linked to unhealthy lifestyle patterns that could lead to poor health.

Research also supports the behavioral link. Peyrot et al.[32] found that stress and coping affected glycemic control by interfering with self-care practices. Coping behavior was also shown to affect glycemic control in a study of type 1 and type 2 diabetes that used sophisticated statistical techniques to demonstrate a "network" of interlinked variables in relation to the achievement of treatment goals.[33] For example, active coping behavior was associated with higher self-efficacy and greater satisfaction with doctor-patient relationships. The researchers suggested that their findings have clinical implications for diabetes care because coping behavior (a key factor in their analysis) was linked to self-care but could also be influenced by the health care professionals involved in that care. However, little work has been carried out to try to implement the findings of coping research into clinical practice.[34] Changes in clinical practice have usually involved behavioral interventions (task-oriented) rather than cognitive ones or have only included coping implicitly rather than explicitly.[34]

Diabetes-related distress may also affect self-care behavior,[35, 36] as demonstrated when the Problem Areas in Diabetes (PAID) scale was developed.[35] The scale covers negative emotions related to living with diabetes, for example, "feeling alone with diabetes" and "worrying about the future and the possibility of serious complications." Although often associated with depression,[36, 37] diabetes-related distress has been found to be predictive of diabetes self-care behavior as well as blood glucose control.[36, 38]

Depression and diabetes-related distress can occur together and can have serious implications for the management of diabetes, because those affected may feel unable or unmotivated to carry out self-care behaviors such as blood glucose testing or healthy eating. A different group of researchers in the United States has identified both diabetes-related stress and other stressors as important in predicting self-care behavior.[27] If study participants reported, "My life is out of control because of my diabetes" or "I have other problems more serious than diabetes," they were less likely to report attention to diet or exercise as part of their diabetes self-care.

In summary, studies strongly suggest that stressful experiences have an impact on diabetes self-care behavior; however, there are many different factors that may mediate this relationship. Before turning to the implications for clinical practice, we consider the physiological mechanisms behind stress and its impact on diabetes.

Physiological Mechanisms behind Stressful Experiences

Any stressful event might be judged by people in different ways, based on factors such as previous experience, psychological factors, and social influences. An event that is seen by one individual as particularly threatening might be seen as totally harmless by another individual. However, when a situation is regarded as threatening, that is, seen as having the potential to cause harm to the individual, a specific pattern of physiological responses is elicited, known as the stress response or "fight/flight" response. This pattern of responses has developed as a result of human evolution and is aimed at priming the individual for action, so that the situation can be dealt with by either fighting or fleeing the threat. The actions initiated by the central nervous system in response to a threat affect the entire body and are associated with three different bodily systems: the autonomic nervous system, the neuroendocrine system, and the immune system.[39, 40]

The autonomic nervous system is concerned with the regulation of smooth muscle, cardiac muscle, and glands and regulates the functions over which there is no conscious control, such as cardiovascular function, digestion, and metabolism. It consists of two distinct branches: the parasympathetic and the sympathetic nervous system, the latter being the most dominant in times of stress. The sympathetic system is involved with the preparation of the body for action. It increases oxygen and nutrient supplies to the muscles by increasing the blood flow to the skeletal muscles and freeing glucose and lipids from its stores. It also prepares the immune system to deal with possible injury.

With regard to the effects of stress on the neuroendocrine system, the HPA axis is of considerable importance.[39] Upon encountering a threat or a stressor, the hypothalamus secretes corticotropin-releasing factor, which causes the release of adrenocorticotropin. This in turn travels to the adrenal cortex, where it leads to the secretion of glucocorticoid hormones, in particular cortisol.

Cortisol exerts considerable influence over bodily functions, both when the body is at rest and during stress. In normal circumstances, it is secreted according to a circadian (daily) rhythm, with cortisol levels highest in the morning and lowest in the evening. However, exposures to stress stimulate the HPA axis to release additional amounts of cortisol to maintain homeostasis and reduce the effects of stress. Cortisol influences a wide range of processes, including the breakdown of carbohydrates, lipids, and proteins to provide the body with energy. It also has an effect on bone and cell growth and may modulate salt and water balance. Cortisol has an immunosuppressive effect and therefore plays a role in the regulation of immune and inflammatory processes.

That the central nervous system communicates with and exerts an influence on the immune system is now well established; brain lesions can alter a variety of immune measures, and both the autonomic and the neuroendocrine system have been shown to influence the state of the immune system.[41] Because both the neuroendocrine and the autonomic system are influenced by psychosocial factors, it follows that the immune system is also affected by such factors, although the precise nature of these complex interactions remains to be determined.

Although there is still much unknown about the effects of acute stress on the immune system and studies have been limited in the number of immune parameters studied, one review[42] revealed that stress influences both circulating cell numbers and the function of immune cells. The cells generating the immune defense are generally known as white blood cells and consist of several subgroups including the lymphocytes (ß-cells, T-cells, and natural killer cells), which have received much attention in stress research.[41]

Although research into the effects of stress continues, it seems clear that there is a range of responses to stressful experiences, both physiological and behavioral/emotional. The final section of this article focuses on the implications of stress research for practice in the care of individuals with diabetes.

Implications for Practice: Stress Management

In addition to the physiological impact that stress has on glycemia, research has shown that stress interferes with the ability to self-manage diabetes. Doing everyday self-care tasks, such as monitoring glucose frequently, following a meal plan, and correctly preparing or remembering to take insulin or oral medications at the right time, is difficult during times of stress. Moreover, diabetes self-management tasks themselves may become a source of stress. Learning to prevent and control the negative responses to stress is helpful, particularly if the causes are relatively permanent. For example, if cooking dinner, bathing children, and doing laundry constitute a typical stressful evening, that stress is a relatively permanent part of life for several years and must be dealt with accordingly.

Assessment of stress levels in practice is a relatively underdeveloped area. One approach is to identify those life events during the previous year that typically act as stressors. Using a scale such as the Recent Life Changes Questionnaire[43] or the Revised Social Readjustment Rating Scale,[44] individuals identify events that have occurred in their life from a list that includes births, deaths, marriage, retirement, social issues, financial worries, work-related stress, and so forth. The weighted ratings provide the basis for an overall score that can be compared to norms. However, these scales are rather long and take some time to complete, which may not always be appropriate in a practice setting.

Polonsky[45] describes a diabetes-specific exercise to help people with diabetes develop an understanding of the relationship between stress and blood glucose levels. In this exercise, individuals rate their perceived stress each evening on a 0–10 Likert scale and record their glucose levels before breakfast and dinner and at bedtime. The individual then looks for blood glucose level patterns for days when perceived stress is high, medium, and low. The premise behind this exercise is that those individuals whose blood glucose levels are sensitive to stress may be more sensitive to stress management strategies. Although validation data are not available, individuals may find this approach helpful in understanding and managing stress-related aberrant glucose readings. Finally, surveys tools, such as the individual items on the PAID scale that measure diabetes-related distress, may also reflect accumulated stress resulting from living with diabetes. PAID scores are associated with A1C levels.[35, 36, 38]

Clinicians must take care to differentiate stress response from depression and anxiety. Depression is more common in diabetes than in the general population.[46,47] Although both under-diagnosed and under-treated,[48, 49] depression is responsive to both medication and psychotherapy. Tools such as the Beck Depression Inventory[50] or the Hospital Anxiety and Depression Scale[51] are useful in screening for depression. Asking simple questions such as, "During the past month, have you been bothered by feeling down, depressed, or hopeless?" and "During the past month, have you been bothered by little interest or pleasure in doing things?" can be as successful as surveys when screening for depression.[52]

Three approaches to stress management go hand in hand, albeit with some overlap: 1) when possible, removing or minimizing the source of stress, 2) changing the response to the stressful situation, and 3) modifying the longer-term effects of stress. Some interventions directly target people with diabetes in order to prevent diabetes-related stress and improve quality of life or glycemia.

1. Remove or minimize the source of stress.

Time management and organizational techniques may reduce small stressors that often compound until a crescendo is reached. Self-help books[53, 54] may be useful for patients to find successful ways to put structure in their lives and manage their time and life stressors. Minimizing the source of stress is helpful. For example, if repetitive noise at work is causing stress, one solution could be substituting white noise for the repetitive noise by softly playing relaxing classical music. Setting up a meeting with the employer or coworkers to get help with one's workload may also alleviate stress. Often, the most difficult challenge is actually identifying the source of stress and separating that source from the responses to stress. Effective problem-solving strategies are important for minimizing the source of stress.

Diabetes-specific approaches that may help individuals cope better with diabetes include setting specific, realistic self-management goals. Many individuals set global vague goals that may serve to exacerbate stress. "Lose weight," "Take better care of my diabetes," and "Improve my glycemic control" are examples of vague unhelpful goals. Realistic, measurable, and achievable goals specifically stating the measurement criteria that indicate success are more helpful as motivators. Examples of realistic, measurable goals are, "I will walk 20 minutes each day on Monday, Wednesday, Friday, and Saturday at 5:00 p.m.;" "I will drink diet cola instead of cola with sugar;" and "I will lose six pounds over the next nine weeks by following my meal plan and increasing my walking to 30 minutes, five days per week." Evaluation does not necessarily have to focus on whether a goal is met, but rather on how successful one's effort has been in trying to achieve it. Thus, instead of "No, I did not reach my target A1C," evaluation would be "My A1C has improved by 0.5 percentage points, thus, I am about half way to my first goal of a 1–percentage point improvement."

2. *Change the response to stress.*

Most stress management techniques emphasize changing the response to stress. When the response to chronic or acute stress results in rage and reactive behavior, a thought-stopping and reflective technique can be helpful in preventing negative consequences of the impulsive behaviors associated with anxiety and rage (Table 52.1). Other approaches involve learning how to induce a more relaxed feeling.

Benson's relaxation response,[55] first reported as a means to lower blood pressure, can be useful in inducing relaxation quickly in times of stress, for example, while driving in traffic, or before taking an exam. Practicing the relaxation response is extremely important because the technique is difficult to learn. However, once learned, the relaxation response quickly brings about the physiological responses associated with relaxation.

515

Table 52.1. A Thought-Stopping Strategy for Acute Rage

Stop	To interrupt a negative spiral of anger, say "stop" out loud or to yourself.
Breathe	Take several deep breaths, exhaling slowly.
Reflect	Think about the situation and what could happen if...If you choose to act in anger, what could happen? What are all the negative things that may happen? What would you accomplish? Be thorough and reflect on the consequences of your actions, how your actions will affect others, how they will affect you in the long term.
Choose	Based on your reflection above, decide how you will act.
Then Act	Your actions are then based on rational thought rather than on anger. The actions may not change, but what is different is that you are in control and have thought about the consequences of your actions.

3. Modifying the longer-term effects of stress.

Other approaches to stress that may be useful for individuals with diabetes include using distraction and involvement in pleasurable activities that help to minimize the influence of stress-producing activities. (For other examples, see Table 52.2.) For example, active participation in a hobby (even a sedentary one) or exercise program can help combat stress. Typically passive activities, such as watching television, may not help alleviate stress, although attending a concert, theater performance, or movie with friends can have beneficial effects as a distraction. If one is not able to put aside worries from work, then distraction may be effective.

If a person with diabetes is experiencing severe stress, referral to a mental health professional may be the most effective approach.

Reports from research investigating the effect of stress management on glycemic control have been inconsistent.[56–60] Several of these studies were underpowered, and others had design problems. However, recent reports have shown that stress management may affect diabetes and its treatment. In a small study with a pre-/post-design and no control group,[61] 20 study participants demonstrated improved glycemic control and state and trait anxiety scores after 12 weeks of treatment

Table 52.2. Useful Interventions for Managing Stress

Changing stress-producing situations
- Time management
- Improved organization skills
- Learning problem-solving skills

Changing the physiological response to stress
- Stop, Breathe, Reflect, and Choose (Table 52.1)
- Relaxation with or without tapes
- Deep muscle relaxation
- Head-to-toe relaxation
- Pleasant scenes
- Breath-focused relaxation
- Yoga, Tai Chi, meditation
- Hot baths, scented candles

De-emphasizing stress with distractions
- Hobbies
- Attending pleasant activities, such as theater, movies, concerts

with an anti-anxiety medication (fludiazepam). Surwit et al.[14] used a randomized, controlled design to investigate the use of stress management techniques for groups of type 2 diabetes patients. They found that those using stress management had a small improvement in A1C (0.5 percentage points) at the 1-year follow-up compared to those who were not. Although Boardway et al.[62] found that adolescents receiving stress management improved stress levels but not glycemic control or adherence, evidence now exists that stress management training may potentiate intensive treatment. For adolescents enrolled in an intensive diabetes management clinic, Grey et al.[63, 64] demonstrated that preventive strategies such as teaching coping skills to adolescents with type 1 diabetes in order to better prepare them for stressful life events can lead to improvements in both glycemic control and quality of life and that the improvement was maintained over time.

In summary, research has indicated that stressful experiences have an impact on diabetes. Stress may play a role in the onset of diabetes, it can have a deleterious effect on glycemic control and can affect lifestyle. Emerging evidence strongly suggests, however, that interventions that help individuals prevent or cope with stress can have an important positive effect on quality of life and glycemic control.

The clinical implications of this research illustrate the need for greater understanding of the effects of stress, as well as a serious acceptance of the need for psychosocial support for people in this predicament.

References

1.   Willis T: Pharmaceutice rationalis or an exercitation of the operations of medicines in human bodies. In *The Works of Thomas Willis*. London, Dring, Harper, Leigh, 1679

2.   Thernlund GM, Dahlquist G, Hansson K, Ivarsson SA, Kudvigsson, Sjoblad S, Hagglof B: Psychological stress and the onset of IDDM in children. *Diabetes Care* 18:1323–1329, 1995

3.   Kisch ES: Stressful events and the onset of diabetes mellitus. *Isr J Med Sci* 21:356–358, 1985

4.   Vialettes B, Ozanon JP, Kaplansky S, Farnarier C, Sauvaget E, Lassman-Vague V, Vague P: Stress antecedents and immune status in recently diagnosed type 1 (insulin-dependent) diabetes mellitus. *Diabetes Metab* 15:45–50, 1989

5.   Kawakami N, Araki S, Takatsuka N, Shimizu H, Ishibashi H: Overtime, psychosocial working conditions, and occurrence of non-insulin dependent diabetes mellitus in Japanese men. *J Epidemiol Community Health* 53:359–363, 1999

6·   Mooy JM, De Vries H, Grootenhuis PA, Bouter LM, Heine RJ: Major stressful life events in relation to prevalence of undetected type 2 diabetes. *Diabetes Care* 23:197–201, 2000

7.   Bjorntop P: Body fat distribution, insulin resistance, and metabolic diseases. *Nutrition* 13:795–803, 1997

8.   Bjorntop P: Visceral fat accumulation: the missing link between psychological factors and cardiovascular disease? *J Intern Med* 230:195–201, 1991

9.   Bottazo GF, Pujol-Borrell R, Gale E: Etiology of diabetes: the role of autoimmune mechanisms. In *The Diabetes Annual*. Alberti KG, Krall LP, Eds. Amsterdam, Elsevier/North Holland, 1985, p. 16–52

10.   Cosgrove M: Do stressful life events cause type 1 diabetes? *Occup Med* 54:250–254, 2004

11. Littorin B, Sundkvist G, Nystrom L, Carlson A, Landin-Olsson M, Ostman J, Arnqvist HJ, Bjork E, Blohme G, Bolinder J, Eriksson JW, Schiersten B, Wibell L: Family characteristics and life events before the onset of autoimmune type 1 diabetes in young adults. *Diabetes Care* 24:1033–1037, 2001

12. Delamater AM, Cox DJ: Psychological stress, coping, and diabetes. *Diabetes Spectrum* 7:18–49, 1994

13. Viner R, McGrath M, Trudinger P: Family stress and metabolic control in diabetes. *Arch Dis Child* 74:418–421, 1996

14. Surwit RS, van Tilburg MA, Zucker N, McCaskill CC, Parekh P, Feinglos MN, Edwards CL, Williams P, Lane JD: Stress management improves long-term glycemic control in type 2 diabetes. *Diabetes Care* 25:30–34, 2002

15. DeVries JH, Snoek FJ, Heine RJ: Persistent poor glycaemic control in adult Type 1 diabetes: a closer look at the problem. *Diabet Med* 21:1263–1268, 2004

16. The DCCT Research Group: The effect of intensive treatment of diabetes on the development and progression of long-term complications in insulin-dependent diabetes mellitus. *N Engl J Med* 329:977–986, 1993

17. Goetsch VL, VanDorsten B, Pbert LA, Ullrich IH, Yeater RA: Acute effects of laboratory stress on blood glucose in non-insulin-dependent diabetes. *Psychosom Med* 55:492–496, 1993

18. Hanson CL, Henggeler SW, Burghen GA: Model of associations between psychosocial variables and health-outcome measures of adolescents with IDDM. *Diabetes Care* 10:752–758, 1987

19. Delamater A, Kurtz SM, Bubb J, White NH, Santiago JV: Stress and coping in relation to metabolic control of adolescents with type 1 diabetes. *J Dev Behav Pediatr* 8:136–140, 1987

20. Lloyd CE, Robinson N, Stevens LK, Fuller JH: The relationship between stress and the development of diabetic complications. *Diabet Med* 8:146–150, 1990

21. Lloyd CE, Dyer PH, Lancashire RJ, Harris T, Daniels JE, Barnett AH: Association between stress and glycaemic control

in adults with type 1 (insulin dependent) diabetes. *Diabetes Care* 22:1278–1283, 1999

22. Smith J: The enemy within: stress in the lives of women with diabetes. *Diabet Med 19* (Suppl. 2):98–99, 2002

23. Ismail K, Winkley K, Rabe-Hesketh S: Systematic review and meta-analysis of randomized controlled trials of psychological interventions to improve glycaemic control in patients with type 2 diabetes. *Lancet* 363:1589–1597, 2004

24. Kramer JR, Ledolter J, Manos GN, Bayless ML: Stress and metabolic control in diabetes mellitus: methodological issues and an illustrative analysis. *Ann Behav Med* 22:17–28, 2000

25. Konen JC, Summerson JH, Dignan MB: Family function, stress and locus of control: relationships to glycaemia in adults with diabetes mellitus. *Arch Fam Med* 2:393–402, 1993

26. Lloyd CE, Wing RR, Orchard TJ, Becker DJ: Psychosocial correlates of glycemic control: the Pittsburgh Epidemiology of Diabetes Complications (EDC) Study. *Diabetes Res Clin Pract* 21:187–195, 1993

27. Albright TL, Parchman M, Burge SK, the RRNeST Investigators: Predictors of self-care behavior in adults with type 2 diabetes: an RRNeST Study. *Fam Med* 33:354–360, 2001

28. Lin EHB, Katon W, Von Korff M, Rutter C, Simon GE, Oliver M, Ciechanowski P, Ludman EJ, Bush T, Young B: Relationship of depression and diabetes self-care, medication adherence, and preventive care. *Diabetes Care* 27:2154–2160, 2004

29. Spangler JG, Summerson JH, Bell RA, Konen JC: Smoking status and psychosocial variables in type 1 diabetes mellitus. *Addict Behav* 26:21–29, 2001

30. Agardh EE, Ahlbom A, Andersson T, Efendic S, Grill V, Hallqvist J, Norman A, Ostenson CG: Work stress and low sense of coherence is associated with type 2 diabetes in middle-aged Swedish women. *Diabetes Care* 26:719–724, 2003

31. Antonovsky A: Unraveling the Mystery of Health: How People Manage Stress and Stay Well. San Francisco, Calif. *Jossey-Bass*, 1987

32. Peyrot M, McMurry JF, Kruger DF: A biopsychosocial model of glycemic control in diabetes: stress, coping and regimen adherence. *J Health Soc Behav* 40:141–158, 1999

33. Rose M, Fliege H, Hildebrandy M, Schirop T, Klapp BF: The network of psychological variables in patients with diabetes and their importance for quality of life and metabolic control. *Diabetes Care* 25:35–42, 2002

34. De Ridder D, Schreurs K: Developing interventions for chronically ill patients: is coping a helpful concept? *Clin Psychol Rev* 21:205–240, 2001

35. Polonksy WH, Anderson BJ, Lohrer PA, Welch G, Jacobson AM, Aponte JE, Schwartz CE: Assessment of diabetes-related distress. *Diabetes Care* 18:754–760, 1995

36. Welch GW, Jacobson AM, Polonsky WH: The Problem Areas In Diabetes scale: an evaluation of its clinical utility. *Diabetes Care* 20:760–766, 1997

37. Skinner TC, Cradock S, Meekin D, Cansfield J: Routine screening for depression and diabetes emotional distress: a pilot study. *Diabet Med 19* (Suppl.):A345, 2002

38. Weinger K, Jacobson AM: Psychosocial and quality of life correlates of glycemic control during intensive treatment of type 1 diabetes. *Patient Educ Couns* 42:123–131, 2001

39. Willemsen G, Lloyd C: The physiology of stressful life experiences. In *Working for Health.* Heller T, Muston R, Sidell M, Lloyd C, Eds. London, Open University/Sage, 2001

40. Kiecolt-Glaser JK, McGuire L, Robles TF, Glaser R: Psychoneuroimmunology: psychological influences on immune function and health. *J Consult Clin Psychol* 70:537–547, 2002

41. Staines N, Brostoff J, James K: *Introducing Immunology.* 2nd ed. St Louis, Mo., Mosby, 1994

42. Herbert TB, Cohen S: Stress and immunity in humans: a meta-analytic review. *Psychosom Med* 55:364–379, 1993

43. Miller MA, Rahe RH: Life changes scaling for the 1990s. *J Psychosom Res* 43:279–292, 1997

44. Hobson CJ, Delunas L: National norms and life-event frequencies for the Revised Social Readjustment Rating Scale. *Int J Stress Manag* 8:299–314, 2001

45. Polonksy WH: *Diabetes Burnout.* Alexandria, Va., American Diabetes Association, 1999

46. Lloyd CE, Dyer PH, Barnett AH: Prevalence of symptoms of depression and anxiety in a diabetes clinic population. *Diabet Med* 17:198–202, 2000

47. Anderson RJ, Freedland KE, Clouse RE, Lustman PJ: The prevalence of comorbid depression in adults with diabetes: a meta-analysis. *Diabetes Care* 24:1069–1078, 2001

48. Perez-Stable EJ, Miranda J, Munoz RF, Ying YW: Depression in medical outpatients: underrecognition and misdiagnosis. *Arch Intern Med* 150:1083–1088, 1990

49. Kovacs M, Obrosky DS, Goldston D, Drash A: Major depressive disorder in youths with IDDM: a controlled prospective study of course and outcome. *Diabetes Care* 20:45–51, 1997

50. Beck AT, Steer RA: Internal consistencies of the original and revised Beck Depression Inventory. *J Clin Psychol* 40:1365–1367, 1984

51. Zigmond AS, Snaith RP: The Hospital Anxiety and Depression Scale. *Acta Psychiatr Scand* 67:361–370, 1983

52. Whooley MA, Avins AL, Miranda J, Browner WS: Case-finding instruments for depression: two questions are as good as many. *J Gen Intern Med* 12:439–445, 1997

53. Morganstern J: *Organizing From the Inside Out.* New York, Henry Holt, 1998

54. Morganstern J: *Time Management From the Inside Out.* New York, Henry Holt, 2000

55. Benson H, Stuart EM: *The Wellness Book: The Comprehensive Guide to Maintaining Health and Treating Stress Related Illness.* New York, Simon & Schuster, 1992

56. Stenstrom U, Goth A, Carlsson C, Andersson PO: Stress management training as related to glycemic control and mood in

adults with type 1 diabetes mellitus. *Diabetes Res Clin Pract* 60:147–152, 2003

57. Bradley C: Contributions of psychology to diabetes management. *Br J Clin Psychol* 33:11–21, 1994

58. Aikens J, Kiolbasa TA, Sobel R: Psychological predictors of glycemic change with relaxation training in non-insulin-dependent diabetes mellitus. *Psychother Psychosom* 66:302–306, 1997

59. Lane JD, McCaskill CC, Ross SL, Feinglos MN, Surwit RS: Relaxation training for NIDDM: predicting who may benefit. *Diabetes Care* 16:1087–1094, 1993

60. Mendez FJ, Belendez M: Effects of a behavioral intervention on treatment adherence and stress management in adolescents with IDDM. *Diabetes Care* 20:1370–1375, 1997

61. Okada S, Ichiki K, Tanokuchi S, Ishii K, Hamada H, Ota Z: Improvement of stress reduces glycosylated haemoglobin levels in patients with type 2 diabetes. *J Int Med Res* 23:119–122, 1995

62. Boardway RH, Delamater AM, Tomaskowsky J, Gutai JP: Stress management training for adolescents with diabetes. *J Pediatr Psychol* 18:29–45, 1993

63. Grey M, Boland EA, Davidson M, Yu C, Tamborlane WV: Coping skills training for youths with diabetes on intensive therapy. *Appl Nurs Res* 12:3–12, 1999

64. Grey M, Boland EA, Davidson M, Li J, Tamborlane WV: Coping skills training for youth with diabetes mellitus has long-lasting effects on metabolic control and quality of life. *J Pediatr* 137:107–113, 2000

Chapter 53

Diabetes Prevention Program

The Diabetes Prevention Program (DPP) was a major clinical trial, or research study, aimed at discovering whether either diet and exercise or the oral diabetes drug metformin (Glucophage) could prevent or delay the onset of type 2 diabetes in people with impaired glucose tolerance (IGT).

The answer is yes. In fact, the DPP found that over the three years of the study, diet and exercise sharply reduced the chances that a person with IGT would develop diabetes. Metformin also reduced risk, although less dramatically. The DPP resolved these questions so quickly that, on the advice of an external monitoring board, the program was halted a year early. The researchers published their findings in the February 7, 2002, issue of the *New England Journal of Medicine*.

DPP Study Design and Goals

In the DPP, participants from 27 clinical centers around the country were randomly split into different treatment groups. The first group, called the lifestyle intervention group, received intensive training in diet, exercise, and behavior modification. By eating less fat and fewer calories and exercising for a total of 150 minutes a week, they aimed to lose seven percent of their body weight and maintain that loss.

"Diabetes Prevention Program," National Diabetes Information Clearinghouse (NDIC), National Institute of Diabetes and Digestive and Kidney Diseases, NIH Pub. No. 06-5099, August 2006.

The second group took 850 mg of metformin twice a day. The third group received placebo pills instead of metformin. The metformin and placebo groups also received information on diet and exercise, but no intensive counseling efforts. A fourth group was treated with the drug troglitazone (Rezulin), but this part of the study was discontinued after researchers discovered that troglitazone can cause serious liver damage.

All 3,234 study participants were overweight and had IGT, which are well recognized risk factors for the development of type 2 diabetes. In addition, 45 percent of the participants were from minority groups—African American, Hispanic American/Latino, Asian American or Pacific Islander, or American Indian—that are at increased risk of developing diabetes.

Type 2 Diabetes and Pre-Diabetes

Diabetes is a disorder that affects the way your body uses digested food for growth and energy. Normally, the food you eat is broken down into glucose. The glucose then passes into your bloodstream, where it is used by your cells for growth and energy. For glucose to reach your cells, however, insulin must be present. Insulin is a hormone produced by your pancreas, a hand-sized gland behind your stomach.

Most people with type 2 diabetes have two problems: the pancreas may not produce enough insulin, and fat, muscle, and liver cells cannot use it effectively. This means that glucose builds up in the blood, overflows into the urine, and passes out of the body—without fulfilling its role as the body's main source of fuel.

About 20.8 million people in the United States have diabetes. Of those, 14.6 million are diagnosed and 6.2 million are undiagnosed. Ninety to 95 percent of people with diabetes have type 2 diabetes. Diabetes is the main cause of kidney failure, limb amputation, and new-onset blindness in American adults. People with diabetes are also two to four times more likely than people without diabetes to develop heart disease.

Pre-diabetes, also called impaired glucose tolerance (IGT) or impaired fasting glucose (IFG), is a condition in which your blood glucose (blood sugar) levels are higher than normal but not high enough for a diagnosis of diabetes. Having pre-diabetes puts you at higher risk for developing type 2 diabetes. If you have pre-diabetes, you are also at increased risk for developing heart disease.

You are more likely to develop type 2 diabetes if any of these risk factors apply to you:

- you are overweight

- you are 45 years old or older

- you have a parent, brother, or sister with diabetes

- your family background is African American, American Indian, Asian American, Hispanic American/Latino, or Pacific Islander

- you have had gestational diabetes or gave birth to at least one baby weighing more than 9 pounds

- your blood pressure is 140/90 or higher, or you have been told that you have high blood pressure

- your HDL cholesterol is 35 or lower, or your triglyceride level is 250 or higher

- you are fairly inactive, or you exercise fewer than three times a week

Pre-diabetes is becoming more common in the United States, according to new estimates provided by the U.S. Department of Health and Human Services. About 40 percent of U.S. adults ages 40 to 74—or 41 million people—had pre-diabetes in 2000. New data suggest that at least 54 million U.S. adults had pre-diabetes in 2002. Those with pre-diabetes are likely to develop type 2 diabetes within 10 years, unless they take steps to prevent or delay diabetes. The results of the Diabetes Prevention Program showed that modest weight loss and regular exercise can prevent or delay type 2 diabetes.

DPP Results

The DPP's striking results tell us that millions of high-risk people can use diet, exercise, and behavior modification to avoid developing type 2 diabetes. The DPP also suggests that metformin is effective in delaying the onset of diabetes.

Participants in the lifestyle intervention group—those receiving intensive counseling on effective diet, exercise, and behavior modification—reduced their risk of developing diabetes by 58 percent. This finding was true across all participating ethnic groups and for both men and women. Lifestyle changes worked particularly well for participants aged 60 and older, reducing their risk by 71 percent. About five percent of the lifestyle intervention group developed diabetes each year during the study period, compared with 11 percent in those who did not get the intervention. Researchers think that weight loss—achieved through better eating habits and exercise—reduces the risk

527

of diabetes by improving the ability of the body to use insulin and process glucose.

Participants taking metformin reduced their risk of developing diabetes by 31 percent. Metformin was effective for both men and women, but it was least effective in people aged 45 and older. Metformin was most effective in people 25 to 44 years old and in those with a body mass index of 35 or higher (at least 60 pounds overweight). About 7.8 percent of the metformin group developed diabetes each year during the study, compared with 11 percent of the group receiving the placebo.

Future Research

Researchers will perform other analyses to try to determine the relative contribution of diet and exercise to the reduction in diabetes. The DPP was not designed to examine diet versus exercise, however, so the analyses may not provide a definitive answer. Researchers will also analyze the information from the study to try to determine how lifestyle intervention and metformin affect the development of heart and blood vessel diseases, which are more common in people with pre-diabetes and type 2 diabetes.

The DPP did not examine whether combining lifestyle changes and metformin would further reduce the risk of developing diabetes.

DPP researchers plan to continue examining the roles of lifestyle and metformin in preventing type 2 diabetes. They will also continue to monitor participants to learn more about the study's long-term effects. The National Institute of Diabetes and Digestive and Kidney Diseases (NIDDK) is encouraging new research to look at cost-effective methods of delivering lifestyle modifications in group settings and over the internet, as well as methods to sustain behavior change and weight loss. The National Diabetes Education Program (NDEP)—a joint project of the National Institutes of Health (NIH), the Centers for Disease Control and Prevention (CDC), and more than 200 public and private organizations—will disseminate the findings and protocols stemming from the DPP.

The U.S. Government does not endorse or favor any specific commercial product or company. Trade, proprietary, or company names appearing in this document are used only because they are considered necessary in the context of the information provided. If a product is not mentioned, this does not mean or imply that the product is unsatisfactory.

Additional Information on the DPP

- NIDDK's Questions & Answers About the DPP available online at http://www.niddk.nih.gov/patient/dpp/dpp-q&a.htm

- NDEP available online at http://www.ndep.nih.gov/diabetes/ prev/prevention.htm

If you wish to perform your own search of the database, you may access and search the NIDDK Reference Collection database online, available at http://catalog.niddk.nih.gov/resources.

Part Seven

Additional Help and Information

Chapter 54

Diabetes Dictionary

acanthosis nigricans: A skin condition characterized by darkened skin patches; common in people whose body is not responding correctly to the insulin that they make in their pancreas (insulin resistance). This skin condition is also seen in people who have pre-diabetes or type 2 diabetes.

acarbose: An oral medicine used to treat type 2 diabetes. It blocks the enzymes that digest starches in food. The result is a slower and lower rise in blood glucose throughout the day, especially right after meals. Belongs to the class of medicines called alpha-glucosidase inhibitors. (Brand name: Precose.)

ACE inhibitor: An oral medicine that lowers blood pressure; ACE stands for angiotensin converting enzyme. For people with diabetes, especially those who have protein (albumin) in the urine, it also helps slow down kidney damage.

acetohexamide: An oral medicine used to treat type 2 diabetes. It lowers blood glucose by helping the pancreas make more insulin and by helping the body better use the insulin it makes. Belongs to the class of medicines called sulfonylureas. (Brand name: Dymelor.)

adult-onset diabetes: Former term for type 2 diabetes.

Excerpted from "Diabetes Dictionary," National Diabetes Information Clearinghouse, National Institute of Diabetes and Digestive and Kidney Diseases, NIH. Pub. No. 07-3016, October 2006.

AGEs: Pronounced A-G-EEZ. Stands for advanced glycosylation endproducts. AGEs are produced in the body when glucose links with protein. They play a role in damaging blood vessels, which can lead to diabetes complications.

albuminuria: A condition in which the urine has more than normal amounts of a protein called albumin. Albuminuria may be a sign of nephropathy (kidney disease).

alpha cell: A type of cell in the pancreas. Alpha cells make and release a hormone called glucagon. The body sends a signal to the alpha cells to make glucagon when blood glucose falls too low. Then glucagon reaches the liver where it tells it to release glucose into the blood for energy.

alpha-glucosidase inhibitor: A class of oral medicine for type 2 diabetes that blocks enzymes that digest starches in food. The result is a slower and lower rise in blood glucose throughout the day, especially right after meals. (Generic names: acarbose and miglitol.)

amylin: A hormone formed by beta cells in the pancreas. Amylin regulates the timing of glucose release into the bloodstream after eating by slowing the emptying of the stomach.

amyotrophy: A type of neuropathy resulting in pain, weakness, and/ or wasting in the muscles.

antibodies: Proteins made by the body to protect itself from "foreign" substances such as bacteria or viruses. People get type 1 diabetes when their bodies make antibodies that destroy the body's own insulin-making beta cells.

A1C: A test that measures a person's average blood glucose level over the past two to three months. Hemoglobin is the part of a red blood cell that carries oxygen to the cells and sometimes joins with the glucose in the bloodstream. Also called hemoglobin A1C or glycosylated hemoglobin, the test shows the amount of glucose that sticks to the red blood cell, which is proportional to the amount of glucose in the blood.

ARB: An oral medicine that lowers blood pressure; ARB stands for angiotensin receptor blocker.

aspart insulin: A rapid-acting insulin. On average, aspart insulin starts to lower blood glucose within 10 to 20 minutes after injection. It has its strongest effect one to three hours after injection but keeps working for three to five hours after injection.

atherosclerosis: Clogging, narrowing, and hardening of the body's large arteries and medium-sized blood vessels. Atherosclerosis can lead to stroke, heart attack, eye problems, and kidney problems.

autonomic neuropathy: A type of neuropathy affecting the lungs, heart, stomach, intestines, bladder, or genitals.

background retinopathy: A type of damage to the retina of the eye marked by bleeding, fluid accumulation, and abnormal dilation of the blood vessels. Background retinopathy is an early stage of diabetic retinopathy. Also called simple or nonproliferative retinopathy.

basal rate: A steady trickle of low levels of longer-acting insulin, such as that used in insulin pumps.

beta cell: A cell that makes insulin. Beta cells are located in the islets of the pancreas.

biguanide: A class of oral medicine used to treat type 2 diabetes that lowers blood glucose by reducing the amount of glucose produced by the liver and by helping the body respond better to insulin. (Generic name: metformin.)

blood glucose: The main sugar found in the blood and the body's main source of energy. Also called blood sugar.

blood glucose level: The amount of glucose in a given amount of blood. It is noted in milligrams in a deciliter, or mg/dL.

blood glucose meter: A small, portable machine used by people with diabetes to check their blood glucose levels. After pricking the skin with a lancet, one places a drop of blood on a test strip in the machine. The meter (or monitor) soon displays the blood glucose level as a number on the meter's digital display.

blood glucose monitoring: Checking blood glucose level on a regular basis in order to manage diabetes. A blood glucose meter (or blood glucose test strips that change color when touched by a blood sample) is needed for frequent blood glucose monitoring.

blood pressure: The force of blood exerted on the inside walls of blood vessels. Blood pressure is expressed as a ratio (example: 120/80, read as "120 over 80"). The first number is the systolic pressure, or the pressure when the heart pushes blood out into the arteries. The second number is the diastolic pressure, or the pressure when the heart rests.

blood urea nitrogen (BUN): A waste product in the blood from the breakdown of protein. The kidneys filter blood to remove urea. As kidney function decreases, the BUN levels increase.

body mass index (BMI): A measure used to evaluate body weight relative to a person's height. BMI is used to find out if a person is underweight, normal weight, overweight, or obese. To find BMI: Multiply body weight in pounds by 703. Divide that number by height in inches. Divide that number by height in inches again. Below 18.5 is underweight; 18.5–24.9 is normal; 25.0–29.9 is overweight; 30.0 and above is obese.

bolus: An extra amount of insulin taken to cover an expected rise in blood glucose, often related to a meal or snack.

borderline diabetes: A former term for type 2 diabetes or impaired glucose tolerance.

brittle diabetes: A term used when a person's blood glucose level moves often from low to high and from high to low.

capsaicin: An ingredient in hot peppers that can be found in ointment form for use on the skin to relieve pain from diabetic neuropathy.

carbohydrate: One of the three main nutrients in food. Foods that provide carbohydrate are starches, vegetables, fruits, dairy products, and sugars.

carbohydrate counting: A method of meal planning for people with diabetes based on counting the number of grams of carbohydrate in food.

cardiovascular disease: Disease of the heart and blood vessels (arteries, veins, and capillaries).

cataract: Clouding of the lens of the eye.

cerebrovascular disease: Damage to blood vessels in the brain. Vessels can burst and bleed or become clogged with fatty deposits. When blood flow is interrupted, brain cells die or are damaged, resulting in a stroke.

certified diabetes educator (CDE): A health care professional with expertise in diabetes education who has met eligibility requirements and successfully completed a certification exam.

Charcot foot: A condition in which the joints and soft tissue in the foot are destroyed; it results from damage to the nerves.

chlorpropamide: An oral medicine used to treat type 2 diabetes. It lowers blood glucose levels by helping the pancreas make more insulin and by helping the body better use the insulin it makes. Belongs to the class of medicines called sulfonylureas. (Brand name: Diabinese.)

cholesterol: A type of fat produced by the liver and found in the blood; it is also found in some foods. Cholesterol is used by the body to make hormones and build cell walls.

coma: A sleep-like state in which a person is not conscious. May be caused by hyperglycemia (high blood glucose) or hypoglycemia (low blood glucose) in people with diabetes.

combination oral medicines: A pill that includes two or more different medicines.

combination therapy: The use of different medicines together (oral hypoglycemic agents or an oral hypoglycemic agent and insulin) to manage the blood glucose levels of people with type 2 diabetes.

congestive heart failure: Loss of the heart's pumping power, which causes fluids to collect in the body, especially in the feet and lungs.

conventional therapy: A term used in clinical trials where one group receives treatment for diabetes in which A1C and blood glucose levels are kept at levels based on current practice guidelines. However, the goal is not to keep blood glucose levels as close to normal as possible, as is done in intensive therapy. Conventional therapy includes use of medication, meal planning, and exercise, along with regular visits to health care providers.

coronary heart disease: Heart disease caused by narrowing of the arteries that supply blood to the heart. If the blood supply is cut off the result is a heart attack.

C-peptide: "Connecting peptide," a substance the pancreas releases into the bloodstream in equal amounts to insulin. A test of C-peptide levels shows how much insulin the body is making.

creatinine: A waste product from protein in the diet and from the muscles of the body. Creatinine is removed from the body by the kidneys; as kidney disease progresses, the level of creatinine in the blood increases.

dawn phenomenon: The early-morning (4 A.M. to 8 A.M.) rise in blood glucose level.

Diabetes Control and Complications Trial (DCCT): A study by the National Institute of Diabetes and Digestive and Kidney Diseases, conducted from 1983 to 1993 in people with type 1 diabetes. The study showed that intensive therapy compared to conventional therapy significantly helped prevent or delay diabetes complications. Intensive therapy included multiple daily insulin injections or the use of an insulin pump with multiple blood glucose readings each day. Complications followed in the study included diabetic retinopathy, neuropathy, and nephropathy.

diabetes educator: A health care professional who teaches people who have diabetes how to manage their diabetes. Some diabetes educators are certified diabetes educators (CDEs). Diabetes educators are found in hospitals, physician offices, managed care organizations, home health care, and other settings.

diabetes insipidus: A condition characterized by frequent and heavy urination, excessive thirst, and an overall feeling of weakness. This condition may be caused by a defect in the pituitary gland or in the kidney. In diabetes insipidus, blood glucose levels are normal.

diabetes mellitus: A condition characterized by hyperglycemia resulting from the body's inability to use blood glucose for energy. In type 1 diabetes, the pancreas no longer makes insulin and therefore blood glucose cannot enter the cells to be used for energy. In type 2 diabetes, either the pancreas does not make enough insulin or the body is unable to use insulin correctly.

Diabetes Prevention Program (DPP): A study by the National Institute of Diabetes and Digestive and Kidney Diseases conducted from 1998 to 2001 in people at high risk for type 2 diabetes. All study participants had impaired glucose tolerance, also called pre-diabetes, and were overweight. The study showed that people who lost 5 to 7 percent of their body weight through a low-fat, low-calorie diet and moderate exercise (usually walking for 30 minutes five days a week) reduced their risk of getting type 2 diabetes by 58 percent. Participants who received treatment with the oral diabetes drug metformin reduced their risk of getting type 2 diabetes by 31 percent.

diabetic diarrhea: Loose stools, fecal incontinence, or both that result from an overgrowth of bacteria in the small intestine and diabetic neuropathy in the intestines. This nerve damage can also result in constipation.

diabetic ketoacidosis (DKA): An emergency condition in which extremely high blood glucose levels, along with a severe lack of insulin, result in the breakdown of body fat for energy and an accumulation of ketones in the blood and urine. Signs of DKA are nausea and vomiting, stomach pain, fruity breath odor, and rapid breathing. Untreated DKA can lead to coma and death.

diabetic myelopathy: Damage to the spinal cord found in some people with diabetes.

diabetic retinopathy: Diabetic eye disease; damage to the small blood vessels in the retina. Loss of vision may result.

diabetogenic: Causing diabetes. For example, some drugs cause blood glucose levels to rise, resulting in diabetes.

diabetologist: A doctor who specializes in treating people who have diabetes.

dialysis: The process of cleaning wastes from the blood artificially. This job is normally done by the kidneys. If the kidneys fail, the blood must be cleaned artificially with special equipment. The two major forms of dialysis are hemodialysis and peritoneal dialysis.

dietitian: A health care professional who advises people about meal planning, weight control, and diabetes management. A registered dietitian (RD) has more training.

D-phenylalanine derivative: A class of oral medicine for type 2 diabetes that lowers blood glucose levels by helping the pancreas make more insulin right after meals. (Generic name: nateglinide.)

Dupuytren contracture: A condition associated with diabetes in which the fingers and the palm of the hand thicken and shorten, causing the fingers to curve inward.

edema: Swelling caused by excess fluid in the body.

electromyography (EMG): A test used to detect nerve function. It measures the electrical activity generated by muscles.

endocrine gland: A group of specialized cells that release hormones into the blood. For example, the islets in the pancreas, which secrete insulin, are endocrine glands.

539

end-stage renal disease (ESRD): See kidney failure.

euglycemia: A normal level of glucose in the blood.

exchange lists: One of several approaches for diabetes meal planning. Foods are categorized into three groups based on their nutritional content. Lists provide the serving sizes for carbohydrates, meat and meat alternatives, and fats. These lists allow for substitution for different groups to keep the nutritional content fixed.

fasting blood glucose test: A check of a person's blood glucose level after the person has not eaten for 8 to 12 hours (usually overnight). This test is used to diagnose pre-diabetes and diabetes. It is also used to monitor people with diabetes.

fat: 1) One of the three main nutrients in food. Foods that provide fat are butter, margarine, salad dressing, oil, nuts, meat, poultry, fish, and some dairy products. 2) Excess calories are stored as body fat, providing the body with a reserve supply of energy and other functions.

50/50 insulin: Premixed insulin that is 50 percent intermediate-acting (NPH) insulin and 50 percent short-acting (regular) insulin.

fructosamine test: Measures the number of blood glucose molecules linked to protein molecules in the blood. The test provides information on the average blood glucose level for the past three weeks.

fructose: A sugar that occurs naturally in fruits and honey. Fructose has four calories per gram.

gangrene: The death of body tissue, most often caused by a lack of blood flow and infection. It can lead to amputation.

gastroparesis: A form of neuropathy that affects the stomach. Digestion of food may be incomplete or delayed, resulting in nausea, vomiting, or bloating, making blood glucose control difficult.

gestational diabetes mellitus (GDM): A type of diabetes mellitus that develops only during pregnancy and usually disappears upon delivery, but increases the risk that the mother will develop diabetes later. GDM is managed with meal planning, activity, and, in some cases, insulin.

glargine insulin: Very-long-acting insulin. On average, glargine insulin starts to lower blood glucose levels within one hour after injection and keeps working evenly for 24 hours after injection.

glimepiride: An oral medicine used to treat type 2 diabetes. It lowers blood glucose by helping the pancreas make more insulin and by helping the body better use the insulin it makes. Belongs to the class of medicines called sulfonylureas. (Brand name: Amaryl.)

glipizide: An oral medicine used to treat type 2 diabetes. It lowers blood glucose by helping the pancreas make more insulin and by helping the body better use the insulin it makes. Belongs to the class of medicines called sulfonylureas. (Brand names: Glucotrol, Glucotrol XL.)

glomerular filtration rate: Measure of the kidney's ability to filter and remove waste products.

glomerulus: A tiny set of looping blood vessels in the kidney where the blood is filtered and waste products are removed. (Plural: glomeruli.)

glucagon: A hormone produced by the alpha cells in the pancreas. It raises blood glucose. An injectable form of glucagon, available by prescription, may be used to treat severe hypoglycemia.

glucose: One of the simplest forms of sugar.

glucose tablets: Chewable tablets made of pure glucose used for treating hypoglycemia.

glyburide: An oral medicine used to treat type 2 diabetes. It lowers blood glucose by helping the pancreas make more insulin and by helping the body better use the insulin it makes. Belongs to the class of medicines called sulfonylureas. (Brand names: DiaBeta, Glynase PresTab, Micronase; ingredient in Glucovance.)

glycemic index: A ranking of carbohydrate-containing foods, based on the food's effect on blood glucose compared with a standard reference food.

glycogen: The form of glucose found in the liver and muscles.

glycosuria: The presence of glucose in the urine.

hemodialysis: The use of a machine to clean wastes from the blood after the kidneys have failed. The blood travels through tubes to a dialyzer, a machine that removes wastes and extra fluid. The cleaned blood then goes back into the body.

honeymoon phase: Temporary remission of hyperglycemia that occurs in some people newly diagnosed with type 1 diabetes, when some

541

insulin secretion resumes for a short time, usually a few months, before stopping again.

hormone: A chemical produced in one part of the body and released into the blood to trigger or regulate particular functions of the body. For example, insulin is a hormone made in the pancreas that tells other cells when to use glucose for energy. Synthetic hormones, made for use as medicines, can be the same or different from those made in the body.

human leukocyte antigens (HLA): Proteins located on the surface of the cell that help the immune system identify the cell either as one belonging to the body or as one from outside the body. Some patterns of these proteins may mean increased risk of developing type 1 diabetes.

hyperglycemia: Excessive blood glucose. Fasting hyperglycemia is blood glucose above a desirable level after a person has fasted for at least eight hours. Postprandial hyperglycemia is blood glucose above a desirable level one to two hours after a person has eaten.

hyperinsulinemia: A condition in which the level of insulin in the blood is higher than normal. Caused by overproduction of insulin by the body. Related to insulin resistance.

hyperlipidemia: Higher than normal fat and cholesterol levels in the blood.

hyperosmolar hyperglycemic nonketotic syndrome (HHNS): An emergency condition in which one's blood glucose level is very high and ketones are not present in the blood or urine. If HHNS is not treated, it can lead to coma or death.

hypertension: A condition present when blood flows through the blood vessels with a force greater than normal. Also called high blood pressure. Hypertension can strain the heart, damage blood vessels, and increase the risk of heart attack, stroke, kidney problems, and death.

hypoglycemia: A condition that occurs when one's blood glucose is lower than normal, usually less than 70 mg/dL. Signs include hunger, nervousness, shakiness, perspiration, dizziness or light-headedness, sleepiness, and confusion. If left untreated, hypoglycemia may lead to unconsciousness. Hypoglycemia is treated by consuming a carbohydrate-rich food such as a glucose tablet or juice. It may also be treated with an injection of glucagon if the person is unconscious or unable to swallow. Also called an insulin reaction.

hypoglycemia unawareness: A state in which a person does not feel or recognize the symptoms of hypoglycemia. People who have frequent episodes of hypoglycemia may no longer experience the warning signs of it.

IDDM (insulin-dependent diabetes mellitus): Former term for type 1 diabetes.

impaired fasting glucose (IFG): A condition in which a blood glucose test, taken after an 8- to 12-hour fast, shows a level of glucose higher than normal but not high enough for a diagnosis of diabetes. IFG, also called pre-diabetes, is a level of 100 mg/dL to 125 mg/dL. Most people with pre-diabetes are at increased risk for developing type 2 diabetes.

impaired glucose tolerance (IGT): A condition in which blood glucose levels are higher than normal but are not high enough for a diagnosis of diabetes. IGT, also called pre-diabetes, is a level of 140 mg/dL to 199 mg/dL two hours after the start of an oral glucose tolerance test. Most people with pre-diabetes are at increased risk for developing type 2 diabetes. Other names for IGT that are no longer used are "borderline," "subclinical," "chemical," or "latent" diabetes.

implantable insulin pump: A small pump placed inside the body to deliver insulin in response to remote-control commands from the user.

inhaled insulin: An experimental treatment for taking insulin using a portable device that allows a person to breathe in insulin.

injection site rotation: Changing the places on the body where insulin is injected. Rotation prevents the formation of lipodystrophies.

insulin: A hormone that helps the body use glucose for energy. The beta cells of the pancreas make insulin. When the body cannot make enough insulin, insulin is taken by injection or through use of an insulin pump.

insulin adjustment: A change in the amount of insulin a person with diabetes takes based on factors such as meal planning, activity, and blood glucose levels.

insulin-dependent diabetes mellitus (IDDM): Former term for type 1 diabetes.

insulin pen: A device for injecting insulin that looks like a fountain pen and holds replaceable cartridges of insulin. Also available in disposable form.

insulin pump: An insulin-delivering device about the size of a deck of cards that can be worn on a belt or kept in a pocket. An insulin pump connects to narrow, flexible plastic tubing that ends with a needle inserted just under the skin. Users set the pump to give a steady trickle or basal amount of insulin continuously throughout the day. Pumps release bolus doses of insulin (several units at a time) at meals and at times when blood glucose is too high, based on programming done by the user.

insulin reaction: When the level of glucose in the blood is too low (at or below 70 mg/dL). Also known as hypoglycemia.

insulin receptors: Areas on the outer part of a cell that allow the cell to bind with insulin in the blood. When the cell and insulin bind, the cell can take glucose from the blood and use it for energy.

insulin resistance: The body's inability to respond to and use the insulin it produces. Insulin resistance may be linked to obesity, hypertension, and high levels of fat in the blood.

intensive therapy: A treatment for diabetes in which blood glucose is kept as close to normal as possible through frequent injections or use of an insulin pump; meal planning; adjustment of medicines; and exercise based on blood glucose test results and frequent contact with a person's health care team.

intermediate-acting insulin: A type of insulin that starts to lower blood glucose within one to two hours after injection and has its strongest effect 6 to 12 hours after injection, depending on the type used.

intermittent claudication: Pain that comes and goes in the muscles of the leg. This pain results from a lack of blood supply to the legs and usually happens when walking or exercising.

intramuscular injection: Inserting liquid medication into a muscle with a syringe. Glucagon may be given by subcutaneous or intramuscular injection for hypoglycemia.

islet cell autoantibodies (ICA): Proteins found in the blood of people newly diagnosed with type 1 diabetes. They are also found in people who may be developing type 1 diabetes. The presence of ICA indicates that the body's immune system has been damaging beta cells in the pancreas.

islet transplantation: Moving the islets from a donor pancreas into a person whose pancreas has stopped producing insulin. Beta cells in the islets make the insulin that the body needs for using blood glucose.

islets: Groups of cells located in the pancreas that make hormones that help the body break down and use food. For example, alpha cells make glucagon and beta cells make insulin. Also called islets of Langerhans.

jet injector: A device that uses high pressure instead of a needle to propel insulin through the skin and into the body.

juvenile diabetes: Former term for insulin-dependent diabetes mellitus (IDDM), or type 1 diabetes.

ketone: A chemical produced when there is a shortage of insulin in the blood and the body breaks down body fat for energy. High levels of ketones can lead to diabetic ketoacidosis and coma. Sometimes referred to as ketone bodies.

ketonuria: A condition occurring when ketones are present in the urine, a warning sign of diabetic ketoacidosis.

ketosis: A ketone buildup in the body that may lead to diabetic ketoacidosis. Signs of ketosis are nausea, vomiting, and stomach pain.

kidney failure: A chronic condition in which the body retains fluid and harmful wastes build up because the kidneys no longer work properly. A person with kidney failure needs dialysis or a kidney transplant. Also called end-stage renal disease, or ESRD.

kidneys: The two bean-shaped organs that filter wastes from the blood and form urine. The kidneys are located near the middle of the back. They send urine to the bladder.

Kussmaul breathing: The rapid, deep, and labored breathing of people who have diabetic ketoacidosis.

lancet: A spring-loaded device used to prick the skin with a small needle to obtain a drop of blood for blood glucose monitoring.

latent autoimmune diabetes in adults (LADA): A condition in which type 1 diabetes develops in adults.

lente insulin: An intermediate-acting insulin. On average, lente insulin starts to lower blood glucose levels within one to two hours after injection. It has its strongest effect 8 to 12 hours after injection but keeps working for 18 to 24 hours after injection. Also called L insulin.

lipid profile: A blood test that measures total cholesterol, triglycerides, and HDL cholesterol. LDL cholesterol is then calculated from the results. A lipid profile is one measure of a person's risk of cardiovascular disease.

lipoatrophy: Loss of fat under the skin resulting in small dents. Lipoatrophy may be caused by repeated injections of insulin in the same spot.

lipodystrophy: Defect in the breaking down or building up of fat below the surface of the skin, resulting in lumps or small dents in the skin surface. (See lipohypertrophy or lipoatrophy.) Lipodystrophy may be caused by repeated injections of insulin in the same spot.

lipohypertrophy: Buildup of fat below the surface of the skin, causing lumps. Lipohypertrophy may be caused by repeated injections of insulin in the same spot.

lispro insulin: A rapid-acting insulin. On average, lispro insulin starts to lower blood glucose within five minutes after injection. It has its strongest effect 30 minutes to one hour after injection but keeps working for three hours after injection.

long-acting insulin: A type of insulin that starts to lower blood glucose within four to six hours after injection and has its strongest effect 10 to 18 hours after injection. See ultralente insulin.

macrosomia: Abnormally large; in diabetes, refers to abnormally large babies that may be born to women with diabetes.

maturity-onset diabetes of the young (MODY): A kind of type 2 diabetes that accounts for 1 to 5 percent of people with diabetes. Of the six forms identified, each is caused by a defect in a single gene.

meglitinide: A class of oral medicine for type 2 diabetes that lowers blood glucose by helping the pancreas make more insulin right after meals. (Generic name: repaglinide.)

metabolic syndrome: The tendency of several conditions to occur together, including obesity, insulin resistance, diabetes or pre-diabetes, hypertension, and high lipids.

metabolism: The term for the way cells chemically change food so that it can be used to store or use energy and make the proteins, fats, and sugars needed by the body.

metformin: An oral medicine used to treat type 2 diabetes. It lowers blood glucose by reducing the amount of glucose produced by the liver and helping the body respond better to the insulin made in the pancreas. Belongs to the class of medicines called biguanides. (Brand names: Glucophage, Glucophage XR; an ingredient in Glucovance.)

mg/dL: milligrams per deciliter, a unit of measure that shows the concentration of a substance in a specific amount of fluid. In the United States, blood glucose test results are reported as mg/dL. Medical journals and other countries use millimoles per liter (mmol/L). To convert to mg/dL from mmol/L, multiply mmol/L by 18. Example: 10 mmol/L × 18 = 180 mg/dL.

microalbumin: Small amounts of the protein called albumin in the urine detectable with a special lab test.

miglitol: An oral medicine used to treat type 2 diabetes. It blocks the enzymes that digest starches in food. The result is a slower and lower rise in blood glucose throughout the day, especially right after meals. Belongs to the class of medicines called alpha-glucosidase inhibitors. (Brand name: Glyset.)

mixed dose: A combination of two types of insulin in one injection. Usually a rapid- or short-acting insulin is combined with a longer acting insulin (such as NPH insulin) to provide both short-term and long-term control of blood glucose levels.

mmol/L: Millimoles per liter, a unit of measure that shows the concentration of a substance in a specific amount of fluid. In most of the world, except for the United States, blood glucose test results are reported as mmol/L. In the United States, milligrams per deciliter (mg/dL) is used. To convert to mmol/L from mg/dL, divide mg/dL by 18. Example: 180 mg/dL ÷ 18 = 10 mmol/L.

monofilament: A short piece of nylon, like a hairbrush bristle, mounted on a wand. To check sensitivity of the nerves in the foot, the doctor touches the filament to the bottom of the foot.

mononeuropathy: Neuropathy affecting a single nerve.

nateglinide: An oral medicine used to treat type 2 diabetes. It lowers blood glucose levels by helping the pancreas make more insulin right after meals. Belongs to the class of medicines called D-phenylalanine derivatives. (Brand name: Starlix.)

necrobiosis lipoidica diabeticorum: A skin condition usually on the lower part of the legs. Lesions can be small or extend over a large area. They are usually raised, yellow, and waxy in appearance and often have a purple border.

nephrologist: A doctor who treats people who have kidney problems.

nephropathy: Disease of the kidneys. Hyperglycemia and hypertension can damage the kidneys' glomeruli. When the kidneys are damaged, protein leaks out of the kidneys into the urine. Damaged kidneys can no longer remove waste and extra fluids from the bloodstream.

nerve conduction studies: Tests used to measure for nerve damage; one way to diagnose neuropathy.

neurologist: A doctor who specializes in problems of the nervous system, such as neuropathy.

neuropathy: Disease of the nervous system. The three major forms in people with diabetes are peripheral neuropathy, autonomic neuropathy, and mononeuropathy. The most common form is peripheral neuropathy, which affects mainly the legs and feet.

noninsulin-dependent diabetes mellitus (NIDDM): Former term for type 2 diabetes.

noninvasive blood glucose monitoring: Measuring blood glucose without pricking the finger to obtain a blood sample.

NPH insulin: An intermediate-acting insulin; NPH stands for neutral protamine Hagedorn. On average, NPH insulin starts to lower blood glucose within one to two hours after injection. It has its strongest effect 6 to 10 hours after injection but keeps working about 10 hours after injection. Also called N insulin.

obesity: A condition in which a greater than normal amount of fat is in the body; more severe than overweight; having a body mass index of 30 or more.

oral glucose tolerance test (OGTT): A test to diagnose pre-diabetes and diabetes. The oral glucose tolerance test is given by a health care professional after an overnight fast. A blood sample is taken, then the patient drinks a high-glucose beverage. Blood samples are taken at intervals for two to three hours. Test results are compared with a standard and show how the body uses glucose over time.

oral hypoglycemic agents: Medicines taken by mouth by people with type 2 diabetes to keep blood glucose levels as close to normal as possible. Classes of oral hypoglycemic agents are alpha-glucosidase inhibitors, biguanides, D-phenylalanine derivatives, meglitinides, sulfonylureas, and thiazolidinediones.

overweight: An above-normal body weight; having a body mass index of 25 to 29.9.

pancreas: An organ that makes insulin and enzymes for digestion. The pancreas is located behind the lower part of the stomach and is about the size of a hand.

peripheral neuropathy: Nerve damage that affects the feet, legs, or hands. Peripheral neuropathy causes pain, numbness, or a tingling feeling.

peripheral vascular disease (PVD): A disease of the large blood vessels of the arms, legs, and feet. PVD may occur when major blood vessels in these areas are blocked and do not receive enough blood. The signs of PVD are aching pains and slow-healing foot sores.

peritoneal dialysis: Cleaning the blood by using the lining of the abdomen as a filter. A cleansing solution called dialysate is infused from a bag into the abdomen. Fluids and wastes flow through the lining of the belly and remain "trapped" in the dialysate. The dialysate is then drained from the belly, removing the extra fluids and wastes from the body.

pioglitazone: An oral medicine used to treat type 2 diabetes. It helps insulin take glucose from the blood into the cells for energy by making cells more sensitive to insulin. Belongs to the class of medicines called thiazolidinediones. (Brand name: Actos.)

podiatrist: A doctor who treats people who have foot problems. Podiatrists also help people keep their feet healthy by providing regular foot examinations and treatment.

point system: A meal planning system that uses points to rate the caloric content of foods.

polydipsia: Excessive thirst; may be a sign of diabetes.

polyphagia: Excessive hunger; may be a sign of diabetes.

polyuria: Excessive urination; may be a sign of diabetes.

postprandial blood glucose: The blood glucose level taken one to two hours after eating.

pre-diabetes: A condition in which blood glucose levels are higher than normal but are not high enough for a diagnosis of diabetes. People with pre-diabetes are at increased risk for developing type 2 diabetes and for heart disease and stroke. Other names for pre-diabetes are impaired glucose tolerance and impaired fasting glucose.

premixed insulin: A commercially produced combination of two different types of insulin. See 50/50 insulin and 70/30 insulin.

preprandial blood glucose: The blood glucose level taken before eating.

proinsulin: The substance made first in the pancreas and then broken into several pieces to become insulin.

proliferative retinopathy: A condition in which fragile new blood vessels grow along the retina and in the vitreous humor of the eye.

protein: 1) One of the three main nutrients in food. Foods that provide protein include meat, poultry, fish, cheese, milk, dairy products, eggs, and dried beans. 2) Proteins are also used in the body for cell structure, hormones such as insulin, and other functions.

proteinuria: The presence of protein in the urine, indicating that the kidneys are not working properly.

rapid-acting insulin: A type of insulin that starts to lower blood glucose within 5 to 10 minutes after injection and has its strongest effect 30 minutes to three hours after injection, depending on the type used. See aspart insulin and lispro insulin.

rebound hyperglycemia: A swing to a high level of glucose in the blood after a low level. See Somogyi effect.

Recognized Diabetes Education Programs: Diabetes self-management education programs that are approved by the American Diabetes Association.

regular insulin: Short-acting insulin. On average, regular insulin starts to lower blood glucose within 30 minutes after injection. It has its strongest effect two to five hours after injection but keeps working five to eight hours after injection. Also called R insulin.

renal: Having to do with the kidneys. A renal disease is a disease of the kidneys. Renal failure means the kidneys have stopped working.

renal threshold of glucose: The blood glucose concentration at which the kidneys start to excrete glucose into the urine.

repaglinide: An oral medicine used to treat type 2 diabetes. It lowers blood glucose by helping the pancreas make more insulin right after meals. Belongs to the class of medicines called meglitinides. (Brand name: Prandin.)

retina: The light-sensitive layer of tissue that lines the back of the eye.

rosiglitazone: An oral medicine used to treat type 2 diabetes. It helps insulin take glucose from the blood into the cells for energy by making cells more sensitive to insulin. Belongs to the class of medicines called thiazolidinediones. (Brand name: Avandia.)

secondary diabetes: A type of diabetes caused by another disease or certain drugs or chemicals.

self-management: In diabetes, the ongoing process of managing diabetes. Includes meal planning, planned physical activity, blood glucose monitoring, taking diabetes medicines, handling episodes of illness and of low and high blood glucose, managing diabetes when traveling, and more. The person with diabetes designs his or her own self-management treatment plan in consultation with a variety of health care professionals such as doctors, nurses, dietitians, pharmacists, and others.

70/30 insulin: Premixed insulin that is 70 percent intermediate-acting (NPH) insulin and 30 percent short-acting (regular) insulin.

sharps container: A container for disposal of used needles and syringes; often made of hard plastic so that needles cannot poke through.

short-acting insulin: A type of insulin that starts to lower blood glucose within 30 minutes after injection and has its strongest effect two to five hours after injection. See regular insulin.

sliding scale: A set of instructions for adjusting insulin on the basis of blood glucose test results, meals, or activity levels.

Somogyi effect: When the blood glucose level swings high following hypoglycemia. The Somogyi effect may follow an untreated hypoglycemic episode during the night and is caused by the release of stress hormones. (Also called rebound hyperglycemia.)

551

sorbitol: 1) A sugar alcohol (sweetener) with four calories per gram. 2) A substance produced by the body in people with diabetes that can cause damage to the eyes and nerves.

split mixed dose: Division of a prescribed daily dose of insulin into two or more injections given over the course of the day.

subcutaneous injection: Putting a fluid into the tissue under the skin with a needle and syringe.

sucrose: A two-part sugar made of glucose and fructose. Known as table sugar or white sugar, it is found naturally in sugar cane and in beets.

sugar diabetes: Former term for diabetes mellitus.

sulfonylurea: A class of oral medicine for type 2 diabetes that lowers blood glucose by helping the pancreas make more insulin and by helping the body better use the insulin it makes. (Generic names: acetohexamide, chlorpropamide, glimepiride, glipizide, glyburide, tolazamide, tolbutamide.)

syringe: A device used to inject medications or other liquids into body tissues. The syringe for insulin has a hollow plastic tube with a plunger inside and a needle on the end.

team management: A diabetes treatment approach in which medical care is provided by a team of health care professionals including a doctor, a dietitian, a nurse, a diabetes educator, and others. The team act as advisers to the person with diabetes.

thiazolidinediones: A class of oral medicine for type 2 diabetes that helps insulin take glucose from the blood into the cells for energy by making cells more sensitive to insulin. (Generic names: pioglitazone and rosiglitazone.)

tolazamide: An oral medicine used to treat type 2 diabetes. It lowers blood glucose by helping the pancreas make more insulin and by helping the body better use the insulin it makes. Belongs to the class of medicines called sulfonylureas. (Brand name: Tolinase.)

tolbutamide: An oral medicine used to treat type 2 diabetes. It lowers blood glucose by helping the pancreas make more insulin and by helping the body better use the insulin it makes. Belongs to the class of medicines called sulfonylureas. (Brand name: Orinase.)

triglyceride: The storage form of fat in the body. High triglyceride levels may occur when diabetes is out of control.

type 1 diabetes: A condition characterized by high blood glucose levels caused by a total lack of insulin. Occurs when the body's immune system attacks the insulin-producing beta cells in the pancreas and destroys them. The pancreas then produces little or no insulin. Type 1 diabetes develops most often in young people but can appear in adults.

type 2 diabetes: A condition characterized by high blood glucose levels caused by either a lack of insulin or the body's inability to use insulin efficiently. Type 2 diabetes develops most often in middle-aged and older adults but can appear in young people.

ultralente insulin: Long-acting insulin. On average, ultralente insulin starts to lower blood glucose within four to six hours after injection. It has its strongest effect 10 to 18 hours after injection but keeps working 24 to 28 hours after injection. Also called U insulin.

unit of insulin: The basic measure of insulin. U-100 insulin means 100 units of insulin per milliliter (mL) or cubic centimeter (cc) of solution. Most insulin made today in the United States is U-100.

United Kingdom Prospective Diabetes Study (UKPDS): A study in England, conducted from 1977 to 1997 in people with type 2 diabetes. The study showed that if people lowered their blood glucose, they lowered their risk of eye disease and kidney damage. In addition, those with type 2 diabetes and hypertension who lowered their blood pressure also reduced their risk of stroke, eye damage, and death from long-term complications.

urea: A waste product found in the blood that results from the normal breakdown of protein in the liver. Urea is normally removed from the blood by the kidneys and then excreted in the urine.

uremia: The illness associated with the buildup of urea in the blood because the kidneys are not working effectively. Symptoms include nausea, vomiting, loss of appetite, weakness, and mental confusion.

urine testing: Also called urinalysis; a test of a urine sample to diagnose diseases of the urinary system and other body systems. In people with diabetes, a doctor may check for glucose, a sign of diabetes or other diseases; protein, a sign of kidney damage, or nephropathy; white blood cells, a sign of urinary tract infection; or ketones, a sign of diabetic ketoacidosis or other conditions. Urine may also be checked for signs of bleeding. Some tests use a single urine sample. For others, 24-hour collection may be needed. And sometimes a sample is "cultured" to see exactly what type of bacteria grows.

very-long-acting insulin: A type of insulin that starts to lower blood glucose within one hour after injection and keeps working evenly for 24 hours after injection. See glargine insulin.

wound care: Steps taken to ensure that a wound such as a foot ulcer heals correctly. People with diabetes need to take special precautions so wounds do not become infected.

Chapter 55

Cookbooks for People with Diabetes or Kidney Failure

The All-Natural Diabetes Cookbook: 150 High-Flavor Recipes Made with Real Foods
By Jackie Newgent. (2007). American Diabetes Association: Alexandria, VA. 224 pp.

The Art of Cooking for the Diabetic (3rd edition)
By Mary Abbott Hess, R.D. (1996). Contemporary Books: Chicago, IL, or New York, NY. 528 pp.

Cleveland Clinic Foundation Creative Cooking For Renal Diabetic Diets
By Pat Ellis. (1985). Senay Publishing Incorporated: Willoughby, OH. 184 pp.

Cocinando para Latinos con Diabetes / Diabetic Cooking for Latinos
By Olga Fuste. (2002). American Diabetes Association: Alexandria, VA. 450 pp.

The list of books included in this chapter was compiled from resources at the National Institute of Diabetes and Digestive and Kidney Diseases and other sources deemed accurate; inclusion does not constitute endorsement and there is no implication associated with omission.

The Complete Quick and Hearty Diabetic Cookbook (Second Edition)
By American Diabetes Association. (2007). American Diabetes Association: Alexandria, VA. 268 pp.

The Complete Step-by-Step Diabetic Cookbook (3rd edition)
By registered Dietitians from the University of Alabama at Birmingham. (1995). Oxmoor House: Birmingham, AL. 368 pp.

Cooking for David: A Culinary Dialysis Cookbook
By Sara Colman and Dorothy Gordon. (2000). Culinary Kidney Cooks: Huntington Beach, CA. 272 pp.

Cooking with the Diabetic Chef: Expert Chef Chris Smith Shares His Secrets to Creating More than 150 Simply Delicious Meals for People with Diabetes
By Chris Smith and the American Diabetes Association Staff. (2000). American Diabetes Association: Alexandria, VA. 169 pp.

The Diabetes Carbohydrate and Fat Gram Guide
By Lea Ann Holzmeister and American Diabetes Association Staff. (2006) The McGraw-Hill Companies: Columbus, OH. 603 pp.

Diabetes Cookbook
By American Diabetes Association, DK Publishing, and Simon Smith. (2000). DK Publishing, Inc.: New York, NY. 128 pp.

Diabetes and Heart Healthy Cookbook
By American Diabetes Association and American Hearth Association. (2004). The McGraw-Hill Companies: Columbus, OH. 300 pp.

The Diabetes Menu Cookbook: Delicious Special-Occasion Recipes for Family and Friends
By Barbara Scott-Goodman. (2006). Wiley, John, and Sons, Incorporated: Hoboken, NJ. 256 pp.

The Diabetic Gourmet Cookbook: More Than 200 Healthy Recipes from Homestyle Favorites to Restaurant Classics
By Diabetic Gourmet Magazine. (2004) Wiley, John, and Sons, Incorporated: Hoboken, NJ. 232 pp.

The Diabetic's Innovative Cookbook: A Positive Approach to Living with Diabetes
By Joseph Juliano, M.D., and Dianne Young. (1994). Henry Holt and Company: New York, NY. 416 pp.

Diabetic Meals In 30 Minutes—or Less!
Robyn Webb, M.S. (2006). American Diabetes Association: Alexandria, VA. 180 pp.

Fix-It and Forget-It Diabetic Cookbook
By Phyllis Pellman Good and American Diabetes Association. (2005). Good Books: Intercourse, PA. 284 pp.

Healthy and Hearty Diabetic Cooking
The Canadian Diabetes Association Publisher. (1993). Diabetes Self-Management Books, R.A. Rappaport Publishing, Inc.: New York, NY. 337 pp.

Italian Diabetic Meals in 30 Minutes or Less
By Robyn Webb. (2005). The McGraw-Hill Companies: Columbus, OH. 160 pp.

The Joslin Diabetes Great Chefs Cook Health Cookbook
By Frances Towner Giedt, Bonnie Sanders Polin, and Alan C. Moses. (2003). Simon and Schuster Adult Publishing Group: New York, NY. 320 pp.

The Joy of Snacks (2nd edition)
By Nancy Cooper, R.D. (1991). Chronimed Publishing Company: Minneapolis, MN. 295 pp.

Kidney Friendly Comfort Foods: A Collection of Recipes for Eating Well with Chronic Kidney Disease (1st Edition)
By Isaac Hayes. (2005). Shire: Oxford, UK.

MicroWave Diabetes Cookbook
By Betty Marks. (1993). Surrey Books: Chicago, IL. 200 pp.

Month of Meals (five books are available)
American Diabetes Association. (1990-1994). American Diabetes Association: Alexandria, VA. 70 pp.

Mr. Food Every Day's a Holiday Diabetic Cookbook
By Art Ginsburg and Nicole Johnson. (2002). American Diabetes Association: Alexandria, VA. 192 pp.

The New Family Cookbook for People with Diabetes
By American Dietetic Association and American Diabetic Association. (2007). Simon and Schuster Adult Publishing Group: New York, NY. 539 pp.

The Official Pocket Guide to Diabetic Exchanges
By American Diabetes Association. (2003). American Diabetes Association: Alexandria, VA. 64 pp.

The UCSD Healthy Diet for Diabetes: A Comprehensive Nutritional Guide and Cookbook
By Susan Algert, R.D., Barbara Grasse, R.D., and Annie Durning, R.D. (1990). Houghton Mifflin Company: Boston, MA. 373 pp.

What to Eat when You Get Diabetes: Easy and Appetizing Ways to Make Healthful Changes in Your Diet
By Carolyn Leontos. (2000). Wiley, John, and Sons, Incorporated: Hoboken, NJ. 256 pp.

Magazines with Frequent Recipes

Diabetes Forecast
American Diabetes Association. (Monthly periodical). American Diabetes Association: Alexandria, VA. For more information, call 800-DIABETES or 800-342-2383.

Diabetes Self-Management (Bimonthly)
R.A. Rappaport Publishing, Inc.: New York, NY. For more information, call 800-234-0923.

Chapter 56

Directory of Diabetes Organizations

Agency for Healthcare Research and Quality
U.S. Department of Health and Human Services
540 Gaither Road,
Suite 2000
Rockville, MD 20850
Phone: 301-427-1364
Website: http://www.ahrq.gov

American Association for Clinical Chemistry
1850 K St., NW,
Suite 625
Washington, DC 20006
Website: http://
www.labtestsonline.org
E-mail:
2labtestsonline@aacc.org

American Association of Clinical Endocrinologists
254 Riverside Avenue, Suite 200
Jacksonville, FL 32202
Phone: 904-353-7878
Fax: 904-353-8185
Website: http://www.aace.com

American Association of Diabetes Educators
200 West Madison, Suite 800
Chicago, IL 60606
Phone: 800-338-3633 or
312-424-2426
Diabetes Educator Access Line:
800-TEAMUP4 (800-832-6874)
Fax: 312-424-2427
Website: http://
www.diabeteseducator.org or
http://www.aadenet.org
E-mail: aade@aadenet.org

This chapter includes a list of organizations that offer information about diabetes, its management, and complications. It was compiled from many sources deemed authoritative. Inclusion does not constitute endorsement and there is no implication associated with omission. All contact information was updated and verified in December 2007.

American College of Physicians

190 N Independence Mall West
Philadelphia, PA 19106-1572
Toll-Free: 800-523-1546
Phone: 215-351-2600
Website: http://www.acponline.org

American Diabetes Association

1701 North Beauregard Street,
Suite 100
Alexandria, VA 22311
Phone: 800-DIABETES
(800-342-2383) (National Call
Center); 703-549-1500 (National
Service Center)
Fax: 703-549-6995
Website: http://www.diabetes.org
E-mail: askada@diabetes.org

American Dietetic Association

120 South Riverside Plaza,
Suite 2000
Chicago, IL 60606-6995
Phone: 800-877-1600 or
800-877-0877; 800-877-1600, ext.
5000 (referral to registered dietitians)
Fax: 312-899-4899
Website: http://www.eatright.org
E-mail: knowledge@eatright.org

American Podiatric Medical Association

9312 Old Georgetown Road
Bethesda, MD 20814-1621
APMA Foot Care Information
Center: 800-FOOT-CARE
Phone: 301-571-9200
Fax: 301-530-2752
Website: http://www.apma.org

Centers for Disease Control and Prevention

National Center for Chronic
Disease Prevention and Health
Promotion
Division of Diabetes Translation
Mail Stop K-10
4770 Buford Highway, NE
Atlanta, GA 30341-3717
Toll-Free: 800-CDC-INFO
(800-232-4636)
Phone: 770-448-5000
Fax: 770-488-5966
TTY: 888-232-6348
Website: http://www.cdc.gov/
diabetes
E-mail: diabetes@cdc.gov

Department of Veterans Affairs

Veterans Health Administration
(VHA)
Program Chief, Diabetes
Veterans Health Administration
810 Vermont Avenue, NW
Washington, DC 20420
Phone: 202-273-5400
Fax: 202-273-9142
Website: http://www1.va.gov/
diabetes

Diabetes Action Research and Education Foundation

426 C Street, NE
Washington, DC 20002
Phone: 202-333-4520
Fax: 202-558-5240
Website: http://
www.diabetesaction.org
E-mail: info@diabetesaction.org

Diabetes Exercise and Sports Association
8001 Montcastle Drive
Nashville, TN 37221
Phone: 800-898-4322
Fax: 615-673-2077
Website: http://www.
diabetes-exercise.org
E-mail:
desa@diabetes-exercise.org

Endocrine Society
8401 Connecticut Avenue,
Suite 900
Chevy Chase, MD 20815-5817
Phone: 301-941-0200 or
888-363-6274
Fax: 301-941-0259
Website: http://www.
endo-society.org
E-mail:
pcorrea@endo-society.org

Indian Health Service
Indian Health Service National
Diabetes Program
5300 Homestead Road, NE
Albuquerque, NM 87110
Phone: 505-248-4182 or
505-248-4236
Fax: 505-248-4188
Website: http://www.ihs.gov/
medicalprograms/diabetes/
index.asp
E-mail:
diabetesprogram@mail.ihs.gov

International Diabetes Federation
Avenue Emile De Mot 19
B-1000 Brussels, Belgium

Phone: 132 2-5385511
Fax: +32-2-5385114
Website: http://www.idf.org
E-mail: info@idf.org

Juvenile Diabetes Research Foundation International
120 Wall Street, Floor 19
New York, NY 10005-4001
Phone: 800-533-CURE (2873)
Fax: 212-785-9595
Website: http://www.jdrf.org
E-mail: info@jdrf.org

Life Options
c/o Medical Education Institute,
Inc.
414 D'Onofrio Drive, Suite 200
Madison, WI 53719
Phone: 800-468-7777
Fax: 608-833-8366
Website: http://
www.lifeoptions.org

LifeMed Media
101 Franklin Street
Westport, CT 06880
Toll-Free: 866-dLifeNow
(866-354-3366)
Phone: 203-454-6985
Fax: 203-454-6986
Website: http://www.dlife.com
E-mail: info@dlife.com

National Certification Board for Diabetes Educators
330 East Algonquin Road, Suite 4
Arlington Heights, IL 60005
Phone: 847-228-9795
Phone requests for exam
applications: 913-541-0400
Fax: 847-228-8469

Website: http://www.ncbde.org
E-mail: info@ncbde.org

*National Diabetes
Education Program*
1 Diabetes Way
Bethesda, MD 20892-3560
Phone: 800-438-5383
Fax: 703-738-4929
Website: http://www.ndep.nih.gov
E-mail: ndep@mail.nih.gov

*National Diabetes
Information Clearinghouse*
1 Information Way
Bethesda, MD 20892-3560
Phone: 800-860-8747
Fax: 703-738-4929
Website: http://
diabetes.niddk.nih.gov/
index.htm
E-mail: ndic@info.niddk.nih.gov

*National Digestive Diseases
Information Clearinghouse*
2 Information Way
Bethesda, MD 20892-3570
Phone: 800-891-5389
Fax: 703-738-4929
Website: http://
digestive.niddk.nih.gov
E-mail:
nddic@info.niddk.nih.gov

National Eye Institute
31 Center Drive
MSC 2510
Bethesda, MD 20892-2510
Phone: 301-496-5248
Website: www.nei.nih.gov
E-mail: 2020@nei.nih.gov

*National Heart, Lung, and
Blood Institute Information
Center*
P.O. Box 30105
Bethesda, MD 20824-0105
Phone: 301-592-8573
Fax: 240-629-3246
TTY: 240-629-3255
Website: http://
www.nhlbi.nih.gov
E-mail: nhlbiinfo@
nhlbi.nih.gov

*National Institute of Child
Health and Human
Development*
P.O. Box 3006
Rockville, MD 20847
Phone: 800-370-2943
TTY: 888-320-6942
Fax: 301-984-1473
Website: http://
www.nichd.nih.gov
E-mail:
NICHDInformationResource
Center@mail.nih.gov

*National Institute of
Diabetes and Digestive and
Kidney Diseases*
National Institutes of Health
Building 31,
Room 9A06
31 Center Drive,
MSC 2560
Bethesda, MD 20892-2560
Phone: 301-496-3583
Website: http://
www.niddk.nih.gov
E-mail:
dkwebmaster@extra.niddk.nih.gov

National Kidney and Urologic Diseases Information Clearinghouse
3 Information Way
Bethesda, MD 20892-3580
Phone: 800-891-5390
Fax: 703-738-4929
Website: http://www.kidney.niddk.nih.gov
E-mail: nkudic@info.niddk.nih.gov

National Kidney Disease Education Program
3 Kidney Information Way
Bethesda, MD 20892
Phone: 866-4-KIDNEY or 866-454-3639
Fax: 301-402-8182
Website: http://www.nkdep.nih.gov
E-mail: nkdep@info.niddk.nih.gov

National Kidney Foundation, Inc.
30 East 33rd Street
New York, NY 10016
Phone: 800-622-9010 or 212-889-2210
Fax: 212-689-9261
Website: http://www.kidney.org
E-mail: info@kidney.org

Office of Minority Health Resource Center
P.O. Box 37337
Washington, DC 20013-7337
Phone: 800-444-6472
Fax: 301-251-2160
Website: http://www.omhrc.gov
E-mail: info@omhrc.gov

Pedorthic Footwear Association
2025 M Street, NW, Suite 800
Washington, DC 20036
Phone: 202-367-1145 or 800-673-8447
Fax: 202-367-2145
Website: http://www.pedorthics.org
E-mail: info@pedorthics.org

Weight-control Information Network
1 WIN Way
Bethesda, MD 20892-3665
Phone: 877-946-4627 or 202-828-1025
Fax: 202-828-1028
Website: win.niddk.nih.gov
E-mail: win@info.niddk.nih.gov

Chapter 57

Diabetes Research and Training Centers' Prevention and Control Divisions

The Diabetes Research and Training Center (DRTC) program was established in 1977 by the Diabetes Research and Education Act (Public Law 91-354) in response to a recommendation by the National Commission on Diabetes. Currently, five DRTCs are supported by the National Institute of Diabetes and Digestive and Kidney Diseases (NIDDK). The DRTCs, which carry out basic and clinical research, are located at major academic institutions.

Each DRTC includes a Prevention and Control Division that focuses on issues related to diabetes translation, including diabetes education, professional training, and community outreach. (The Prevention and Control Divisions were formerly called Demonstration and Education Divisions.) The researchers in the Prevention and Control Divisions develop and demonstrate innovative approaches to providing quality diabetes care. Several of the centers carry out their programs onsite in model demonstration units, while other centers conduct their programs in community settings. The Prevention and Control Divisions have developed links with major diabetes professional and voluntary organizations as well as with groups in the communities served by the centers.

The Prevention and Control Divisions offer continuing education seminars, workshops in state-of-the-art diabetes management for

From "Diabetes Research and Training Centers' Prevention and Control Divisions," National Diabetes Information Clearinghouse, National Institute of Diabetes and Digestive and Kidney Diseases, NIH Pub. 04-3267, October 2003. Contact information was updated and verified in December 2007.

professionals, an array of tested evaluation and assessment instruments, and professional expertise in developing and implementing diabetes programs in a variety of settings.

Each center offers a range of educational materials, including videotapes, curricula, and program guides for health professionals. The following briefly describes the current activities at each DRTC Prevention and Control Division.

The Albert Einstein College of Medicine DRTC Prevention and Control Component

Dr. Elizabeth A. Walker directs the Prevention and Control (P&C) component of the Albert Einstein College of Medicine in the Bronx. The multidisciplinary clinical and behavioral research team develops and evaluates interventions for preventive diabetes care and self-management, focusing on the health disparities of underserved and high-risk populations.

The P&C cores provide services to investigators with peer-reviewed National Institute of Health (NIH) support or other funding to address diabetes-related issues in translation of research, in facilitation of clinical research, and in evaluation of health promotion interventions.

Einstein P&C research has lead to the development and evaluation of:

- Interventions to promote ophthalmic screening in diabetes: This funded research has demonstrated that a multicomponent health education intervention, including print, video, and tailored telephone counseling, can be highly effective in improving the ophthalmic screening rates among African Americans with diabetes. A more broad-based telephone intervention for both Spanish- and English-speaking populations in the Bronx is under evaluation for cost-effectiveness.

- Interactive multimodal weight-control intervention: This research addresses techniques to optimize staff time in providing a weight control intervention. The American Diabetes Association has published the patient workbook and the staff curriculum from this research under the titles *The Complete Weight Loss Workbook: Proven Techniques for Controlling Weight-Related Health Problems* and *The Leaders Guide for the Complete Weight Loss Workbook*. The interactive computer system that helps patients individually tailor the weight loss approach has been converted to HTML code to make it usable via the internet. Related collaborative investigations have lead to the development of materials to facilitate addressing Weight, Activity, Variety, and Excess (WAVE) as nutritional issues in primary care.

- Risk perceptions for developing diabetes: This survey research explores perception of risk for developing diabetes relative to environmental risks, and other disease risks in lay, expert and at risk for diabetes populations. Under evaluation is a survey for perception of risk for diabetes complications, a similar assessment for individuals with diagnosed diabetes.

- Medication adherence has been studied in the Diabetes Prevention Program in individuals at high risk for developing type 2 diabetes. The intervention includes a structured interview for assessment of barriers to adherence, strategies to improve adherence to medication, and the use of a toolbox approach and motivational interviewing to tailor the plan for the individual.

Health professional education programs include:

- A diabetes management preceptorship offered in conjunction with graduate or postgraduate training programs for physicians, advanced-practice nurses, dietitians, and clinical health psychology trainees.

- A weekly basic science and clinical research conference, including topics in the multidisciplinary management of diabetes, new findings on diabetes clinical research, and basic research.

University of Chicago's DRTC Prevention and Control Division

Dr. Donald Steiner directs the Prevention and Control Division of the University of Chicago DRTC. Many of the programs focus on improving the quality of care and outcomes of vulnerable patients with diabetes, including indigent and minority persons. University of Chicago faculty from the medical and social sciences collaborate to design and implement diabetes programs that can work in diverse settings. Current projects include:

- Improving Diabetes Care in Midwest Community Health Centers: The Chicago DRTC is collaborating with the Midwest Clinicians' Network, a consortium of 70 community health centers in 10 Midwestern states that serve the indigent. We are improving diabetes care in the health centers with rapid quality improvement methods, chronic care models, training to enhance communication between providers and patients, and programs to empower patients to take a more active role in their care.

- Chicago Department of Public Health Neighborhood Clinics: Within Chicago neighborhood clinics that care for the poor, American Diabetes Association practice guidelines are being disseminated, as well as introducing patient flow sheets, providing continuing medical education to providers, and performing audits of charts for key processes of diabetes care and feeding results back to the clinics. Programs to improve providers' skills at communicating with patients and facilitating behavioral change are also being implemented.

- Pathways Lifestyle Modification Program for African American Women: Pathways is a successful weight loss program tested in a clinical setting as part of a church-based lay educator program in inner city African American churches. The study demonstrated that a culturally relevant lifestyle program can provide significant weight loss in African American women who typically do not benefit from such efforts. It also provided evidence that lay women can be trained to conduct successful lifestyle modification programs in their own neighborhoods. We are currently testing whether a similar program promoting lifestyle changes in diet and physical activity are sufficient to cause weight loss in subjects with early diabetes.

Other programs developed by the Chicago DRTC include:

- From Basics Forward, a comprehensive continuing education program for diabetes educators conducted nationally by the American Association of Diabetes Educators.

- In Control, a clinical patient education program for 9- to 12-year-old children with diabetes and their parents.

- Choices, a problem-solving curriculum to meet the special needs of adolescents with diabetes management problems.

- Get Going, an exercise program for inner-city minority women with diabetes.

- Por Su Salud (For Your Health), a community-based lifestyle intervention that focuses on assisting inner city Hispanic women overcome some of the risk factors for diabetes through healthy eating and physical activity.

University of Michigan's DRTC Prevention and Control Division

Dr. William Herman directs the Prevention and Control Division of the DRTC at the University of Michigan in Ann Arbor. This division has developed model clinical and educational programs, as well as educational programs and materials for health-care professionals and people with diabetes. Many of the center's programs for diabetes education and empowerment focus on communities and community organizations.

Along with clinical and educational programs, the University of Michigan DRTC also facilitates disease, cost-of-disease, and quality-of-life modeling to assess the relative effectiveness, cost-effectiveness, and cost utility of alternative strategies for the prevention, detection, and management of type 2 diabetes. In addition, this DRTC supports and coordinates studies that evaluate interventions directed at improving health outcomes of people with diabetes and studies that evaluate barriers that prevent adoption and dissemination of state-of-the-art diabetes care. Specific projects have been developed to evaluate culture-specific diabetes education programs, diabetes care for the underinsured, and people with diabetes in managed care systems.

The University of Michigan DRTC Prevention and Control Division also develops instructional materials and standardized instruments to measure knowledge (Diabetes Knowledge Test), patient self-care skills and practices (Diabetes Care Profile), attitudes of patients and health professionals (Diabetes Attitude Scale), and patient empowerment (Diabetes Empowerment Scale). The center offers an undergraduate course for students at the University of Michigan, other training opportunities for health professionals, and patient education materials. These materials and instruments are available from the center at http://www.med.umich.edu/mdrtc on the internet.

Vanderbilt University's DRTC Prevention and Control Division

The Prevention and Control Division at Vanderbilt University in Nashville, TN, works closely with Meharry Medical College, Fisk University, Tennessee State University, the county hospital, the local and state health departments, the NAACP, local churches, and concerned citizens to reduce and in time eliminate local racial disparities in cardiovascular disease and diabetes. The work is funded through a CDC REACH 2010 project grant plus other federal and foundation grants. Collaborations designed to reduce disparities involve assessments of community eating behaviors, lifestyles, attitudes toward disease and the health care system, and standards of care. A variety of questionnaires, videos, training materials, and slide presentations related to these efforts are available.

The Vanderbilt University DRTC has a long history of research on improving the teaching skills of health professionals involved in diabetes education and management. The center's widely attended Effective Patient Teaching (EPT) course emphasizes teaching, promoting adherence, and imparting problem-solving skills. By special arrangement with the Vanderbilt University DRTC, professionals can be trained to present the EPT program to colleagues in their own institutions.

The center also offers the program Sugar Is Not a Poison: The Dietitian's New Role in Diabetes Management to prepare dietitians for their expanded role in diabetes management. The program has been presented throughout the United States. The curriculum emphasizes skills needed for modern diabetes management, therefore the course is useful for all dietitians who work with people with diabetes.

Other training materials available from the Vanderbilt University DRTC include manuals on interviewing, teaching, and problem-solving and brief videotapes for problem-based patient learning.

The DRTC staff have also developed:

- Questionnaires for evaluating the reactions of adults and adolescents with diabetes in situations that challenge adherence to their meal plans and coping strategies.

- The Personal Diabetes Questionnaire (PDQ), a web-based assessment of situations that make patient adherence to self-management recommendations difficult.

- The Self-Monitoring Analysis System (SMAS), a software package for microanalysis of eating behavior.

- Psychological Assessment Applications Generator (PAAG), a software package for developing, administering, scoring, and interpreting psychological tests.

- Assessment tools and teaching aids for promoting diabetes detection, treatment, and prevention in African-American communities.

- Primary Care Management of Diabetes Mellitus, a set of 178 PowerPoint slides for use in teaching health professionals about diabetes. A comprehensive content outline on diabetes, the slide series may be downloaded from the VDRTC's internet site.

Contact Steve Davis, M.D. (Director, Prevention/Control and Clinical Research Component), David Schlundt, Ph.D. (Behavioral Health Disparities Core), or James Pichert, Ph.D. (Clinical Outcomes and Behavioral Sciences Core) for information about programs and materials available from the Prevention and Control component of the Vanderbilt University DRTC.

Washington University's DRTC Prevention and Control Division

Dr. Edwin B. Fisher directs the Prevention and Control Division of the Washington University DRTC in St. Louis. The Washington University DRTC division is currently involved in many projects designed to improve prevention of and care for people with diabetes. Current projects at the Washington University DRTC include:

- Evaluation and enhancement of care for type 2 diabetes among low-income, minority patients of neighborhood health centers.

- Translation to a Native American community of peer- and community-based approaches to promoting a reduced-fat diet.

- Promotion of exercise among participants in an activity and health program for older adults.

- Study of social support provided by staff in diabetes care and especially in the Diabetes Prevention Program.

Independently funded research projects affiliated with the DRTC also address:

- child and family factors in Type 1 diabetes.

- depression and diabetes.

- use of a peer "coach" to enhance diabetes management in low-income, minority patients with type 2 diabetes.

- over 70 active protocols in patient oriented research in diabetes and endocrinology implemented through the Clinical Research Center closely linked with the DRTC.

A master's program in health care services is affiliated with this DRTC. This program for nurses, dietitians, physical and occupational therapists, and other professionals offers interdisciplinary training in health promotion, disease prevention, chronic disease care, patient education and counseling, and program development and evaluation. The curriculum covers programs serving diverse audiences in a variety of settings.

Diabetes Research and Training Centers Prevention and Control Divisions

Albert Einstein College of Medicine DRTC
Director, Prevention and Control Division
The Diabetes Research and Training Center
701 Belfer Building
Albert Einstein College of Medicine
1300 Morris Park Avenue
Bronx, NY 10461
Phone: 718-430-2908
Fax: 718-430-8557

University of Chicago DRTC
Howard Hughes Medical Institute
University of Chicago
5841 South Maryland Avenue, MC 1027
Room N-216
Chicago, IL 60637
Phone: 773-702-1334
Fax: 773-702-4292

University of Michigan DRTC
Michigan Diabetes Research and Training Center
400 N. Ingalls, Room G148
Ann Arbor, MI 48109-5482
Phone: 734-763-5730
Fax: 734-647-2307
Website: www.med.umich.edu/mdrtc

Vanderbilt University DRTC
Division of Diabetes, Endocrinology, and Metabolism
707 Light Hall
Nashville, TN 37232-0615
Phone: 615-322-7004
Fax: 615-936-1250

Vanderbilt Diabetes Center
315 Medical Arts Building
1211 21st Avenue South
Nashville, TN 37212
Phone: 615-936-1149
Fax: 615-936-1152

Washington University DRTC
Division of Health Behavior Research
Washington University
4444 Forest Park Avenue, Campus Box 8504
St. Louis, MO 63108
Phone: 314-286-1900
Fax: 314-286-1919

Diabetes Endocrinology Research Centers (DERCs)

The NIDDK supports two types of centers to foster diabetes research: Diabetes Research and Training Centers and Diabetes Endocrinology Research Centers. These centers facilitate progress in research by providing shared resources to enhance the efficiency of biomedical research and foster collaborations within and among institutions with established, comprehensive bases of research relevant to diabetes mellitus. They focus on basic and clinical research.

Individual centers produce a variety of diabetes education materials. For information about publications and programs, contact the individual centers listed.

Joslin Diabetes Center DERC
Harvard Medical School
One Joslin Place, Room 620
Boston, MA 02215
Phone: 617-732-2635
Fax: 617-732-2487
Website: http://www.joslin.harvard.edu

Massachusetts General Hospital DERC
Diabetes Unit Medical Service
Department of Molecular Biology
Simches Research Building
Wellman 8
55 Fruit Street
Boston, MA 02114

Phone: 617-726-6909
Fax: 617-726-6909

University of Colorado DERC
Barbara Davis Center for Childhood Diabetes
1775 North Ursula Street
P.O. Box 6511, Mail Stop Box B-140
Aurora, CO 80045
Phone: 303-724-6837
Fax: 303-724-6838
Website: www.uchsc.edu/misc/diabetes/derc/index.htm

University of Iowa DERC
Iowa Diabetes-Endocrinology Research Center
VA/JDF Diabetes Research Center
3E19 VA Medical Center
Iowa City, IA 52246
Phone: 319-338-0581, ext. 7625
Fax: 319-339-7025
Website: www.int-med.uiowa.edu/faculty.htm

University of Massachusetts Medical School DERC
373 Plantation Street, Suite 218
Worcester, MA 01605
Phone: 508-856-3800
Fax: 508-856-4093
Website: http://www.umassmed.edu/diabetes

University of Pennsylvania DERC
Division of Endocrinology, Diabetes and Metabolism
700 Clinical Research Building
415 Curie Boulevard
Philadelphia, PA 19104-6149
Phone: 215-898-0198
Fax: 215-898-5408
Website: www.uphs.upenn.edu/endocrin/faculty/lazar.html

University of Washington DERC
P.O. Box 358285
DVA Puget Sound Health Care System
1660 S. Columbian Way
Seattle, WA 98108
Phone: 206-764-2688
Fax: 206-764-2693
Website: depts.washington.edu/diabetes/index.html

574

Yale University School of Medicine DERC
Department of Internal Medicine
P.O. Box 208020
333 Cedar Street
Section of Endocrinology
New Haven, CT 06520-8020
Phone: 203-785-4183
Fax: 203-737-5558
Website: info.med.yale.edu/intmed/endocrin/faculty/sherwin.html

Chapter 58

Getting High Quality Medical Care in a Changing Healthcare Landscape

When searching for good medical care, it used to be that the hunt focused on whether the physician was the best in his or her profession, had a good bedside manner, was conveniently located, and referred patients to the hospital with the most up-to-date equipment.

But nowadays, rules imposed by insurers for scheduling and receiving care can sometimes place roadblocks between you and the physicians and hospitals you prefer.

For people with diabetes, this new healthcare environment can be especially disconcerting. In an effort to save money on the spiraling cost of medical treatment, employers can decide to switch healthcare insurance options they offer employees—and all of a sudden you may discover that visits to your family doctor or diabetes doctor are no longer covered, and you need to seek out a new physician or physicians to provide your medical care. For people with diabetes, this can mean learning new philosophies and methods of care which may differ from lifelong established systems that the patient has successfully used to manage the disease.

So, What Do You Do in This New Healthcare World?

Here's some general guidelines to follow:

- Understand what's going on in healthcare these days, so you can better understand and work with the changing roles of healthcare providers, and the different pressures they are facing.

- Be knowledgeable about your own diabetes so you can ask questions and pinpoint areas where you and your primary care physician need to focus extra attention—and perhaps get additional help from a specialist—to keep your diabetes on track.

- Be your own advocate. Know what preventive care and screening the American Diabetes Association recommends, and ask your physician when it is time to have these various aspects of your care provided. Try to find an insurer that supports (i.e., pays for) getting these preventive measures done. Don't hesitate to call or write your health insurer and provide them with a clear and compelling argument as to why you need them to pay for some aspect of your healthcare that they don't cover—a referral, or an educational program for example. Include in your arguments any research that supports your need for the referral, and be sure to note that the insurance company will benefit if a needed referral will decrease your risks of developing more costly medical problems down the road.

- Choose your primary care physician wisely. Look for someone who is both knowledgeable about diabetes and who seems interested in working cooperatively with you.

- Make sure your primary care physician will, and more importantly can refer you periodically to a quality diabetes or other specialist, or to education programs for help with hard to manage problems.

- If possible, be prepared to pay for some things out of pocket, particularly diabetes education, and an occasional second opinion from a physician who may not be covered by your insurance.

- When possible, choose the health plan that enables you the greatest freedom to see different physicians and pays for the care you need.

- Don't hesitate to express concern if you have questions about the quality of your care.

The Changing Roles of Physicians

Today's world of medicine is very specialized, yet efforts to contain costs are placing increasing burdens on primary care physicians—the traditional family physician—to provide as much medical care to patients as possible, because their care is the least costly. Yet, in caring for your diabetes, it is likely that your medical needs will require both a primary care physician and a team of healthcare professionals who can back your primary care physician up when needed. "If at all possible, you should find a medical setting where your diabetes is cared for by a team of professionals, each an expert in a particular aspect of your total care," notes Dr. Richard S. Beaser of Joslin Diabetes Center. This team should include the primary care physician, a diabetes expert who is usually an endocrinologist, a dietitian, nurse educator, exercise physiologist, and someone who will provide psychological counseling and support when needed. Other team members may be added as needed to treat or prevent complications.

Your desire to have your diabetes treated by a team of specialists—and your insurer's desire, in many cases, to have as much care as possible provided by a primary care physician—may seem to be at odds. "Some believe that those two needs are in conflict," notes Kenneth E. Quickel Jr., M.D., president emeritus of Joslin in Boston. "But in fact, the best, most cost-effective care in the long run will occur for people with diabetes when the primary care physician and the specialty care team work in collaboration with each other."

Physician as Traffic Cop

Your primary care physician is trained to care for you as a total person and treat a wide range of medical problems, from colds and the flu, to checking your cholesterol levels and checking your diabetes care. This person serves as a traffic cop, in many ways, coordinating your overall medical treatment.

But in addition to acting like a traffic cop, this physician also serves in many health insurance settings as a gatekeeper, managing day-to-day health needs and regulating the flow of patients to more costly forms of care. In essence your primary care physician works on your behalf and the insurer's behalf to be sure that you are receiving care for your medical needs in the most cost-effective way possible. Frequently, payments to primary care physicians from insurers are tied to how effectively they can reduce the use of expensive tests and services—and the physician may be penalized for a perceived overuse of specialists and expensive tests.

"Back in 1916 Elliott P. Joslin wrote that 'the number of cases of diabetes is so great that it at once becomes evident that their care must rest in the hands of the general practitioner. It is ridiculous to expect that the treatment of diabetics should all be under the supervision of a specialist,'" notes Dr. Quickel. "So, while this role of 'gatekeeper' is just a fact of life today, in fact it has always been important for the primary care physician to work with the diabetes specialist. Picking an excellent primary care physician is as important for people with diabetes these days as it is to pick an excellent diabetologist or endocrinologist, and being certain that they can work together is essential.

Diabetes Specialists as Primary Care Physicians

In some health insurance programs diabetes specialists are registering as primary care physicians, as well as diabetes specialists, to enable patients to pick a diabetes expert to serve as their primary care physician. This is due, in part, to the fact that most diabetologists are first trained in general internal medicine or pediatrics before they receive additional training in diabetes and endocrinology. But they are also doing this because the line where primary care ends and diabetes care begins can be very blurred. In the Boston market, some of Joslin's diabetologists are enrolled as primary care physicians in some health plans for this very reason. "Joslin physicians have frequently served as primary care physicians for patients over the past 50 years or more, because diabetes is a lifelong disease that affects so many aspects of a person's health," notes Dr. Quickel.

Other insurers don't allow diabetes specialists—even though they are certified to practice general internal medicine—to enroll as primary care physicians. In some cases, they may even insist that specialists associated with a medical school be classified as 'tertiary care physicians,' which severely limits your ability to be referred to them. The insurers do this because the insurance company perceives these specialists and the institutions they hospitalize patients in as exceptionally high priced. So the same Joslin physician may be enrolled as a primary care physician in one health plan, and a tertiary care specialist in another.

"In the perfect world, our preferred role is to serve as the diabetes expert, and to leave the primary care to the primary care physicians," notes Dr. Richard Jackson, a senior physician at Joslin. "But because patients sometimes want and need more from us than insurers will allow them to get if we enroll in these health plans as specialists only, we do in some cases enroll as primary care physicians."

The Ideal

The ideal scenario is that you identify a primary care physician who is knowledgeable about diabetes, has an interest in the disease—and knows his or her limitations and will refer you for additional care when needed, irrespective of any disincentives insurers may place on making the referral. "Most physicians aren't going to let the insurers get in the way of making a referral for a patient who really needs it simply because of some small financial incentive," notes Dr. Quickel. "But a primary care physician has to know a lot about a mind-boggling number of different diseases and conditions. He or she may not be as immediately up-to-date on new thoughts in diabetes care as a diabetes specialist, whose role is to know a lot about one disease or group of diseases and their complications. What this means is that the primary care physician can manage most of your medical issues—including many of those surrounding your diabetes. But at a certain point, the primary care physician may need to seek a specialist's advice if things aren't going as well as they need to."

"What we're really advocating is a holistic approach, focused on preventing problems," notes Dr. Jackson. "By focusing on preventing problems rather than acting upon them when they occur, we can actually lower the cost of healthcare by limiting the amount of money patients need to spend on specialists to treat costly complications like artery disease, a heart attack, stroke, or other problems."

Be Knowledgeable about Your Disease

How can you as the patient know if the diabetes portion of your medical care is going as it should? "By being a knowledgeable patient," says Joan Hill, RD, CDE, former director of educational services at Joslin.

Following are some key questions you should know the answer to in assessing both how your diabetes is going and how your primary care physician and diabetes healthcare team's combined management of your disease is fairing. "If you don't know the answers to these questions, ask the person who provides the bulk of your diabetes care (whether that is a primary care physician, a Joslin specialist, a nurse practitioner, or a diabetes specialist elsewhere) the answers to these questions at your next visit," Hill says.

These are also good questions to discuss with a new primary care physician or diabetes specialist that you may be switching to as a result of a change in health plans, notes Jackson.

Be Your Own Advocate

If you don't know the answers to all of these questions, discuss them with the clinician most involved in your diabetes care over the next couple of visits. Then ask yourself how you felt while you were asking your physician some or all of these questions. If you felt increasingly comfortable as the conversation continued, this may suggest that the physician was a good listener, and didn't send out "bad vibes" suggesting that he/she didn't like being questioned about his medical practices. If, on the other hand, you felt that you needed to stop asking questions fairly quickly, was that because the physician—either overtly or covertly—was sending you signals that he/she didn't like being questioned about his knowledge of your disease? Or was it just your own discomfort with questioning a traditional authority figure?

"You're paying for your health insurance—get what you need and are paying for," says Dr. Jackson.

What to Do If You Are Uncomfortable

Many people will find it difficult to discuss these questions with their physician. "Many of us have been raised to believe that we can't question the parish priest or the doctor, that they will take care of us and it's just as well not to ask too much," says Hill. "But as research like the Diabetes Control and Complications Trial (DCCT) increasingly shows us, the results of careful blood sugar control will reduce complications risk. It becomes increasingly important to make sure that all the members of your healthcare team know what they are doing—and that includes you. You, the patient, are the most important member of the team managing your disease. You have every right, as a result, to know that the other members of the team are working with you, and have the skills to make your life with diabetes as manageable and risk-free as possible."

What do you do if you are genuinely uncomfortable with your healthcare provider, and your choices are limited to the physicians enrolled as provider for your insurance company?

"Ask around," recommends Hill. "Go to meetings of the local diabetes association, and try to find other people with diabetes who have found good primary care physicians and/or good diabetes specialists-primary care physicians who may be covered under your insurance. Check out the primary care physicians of friends who don't have diabetes, but who say their physician is approachable and seems knowledgeable about whatever medical conditions they have. Perhaps such a physician will also be knowledgeable about diabetes—or perhaps if he/she isn't, at least he/she will be willing to refer you to someone who is for your diabetes care, and continue to provide your overall non-diabetes medical care."

Can your employer help?

You may also want to consider letting your employer's human resources or benefits department know if you are uncomfortable with the quality of the care you are receiving under your health plan, particularly if the health coverage has been recently changed and you feel your healthcare is suffering because of it. While insurance companies, on average, will have an individual as a subscriber for three years or so before the subscriber either switches insurers or switches jobs, statistics show that your employer will, in all likelihood, have you as an employee for much longer. Poor healthcare can result in poorer performance on the job, lost work days and lost productivity, not to mention higher insurance costs in the long run if you develop complications. Your employer is likely to be very interested in knowing if you are concerned about the quality of your medical care as a result of a change in health coverage. And the insurance carrier may be more likely to listen to the voice of an employer who is paying for insurance for hundreds or thousands of workers, rather than listening to you, who is the voice of only one.

Perhaps even more importantly, your employer may be interested in knowing of ways that they can continue to offer a lower cost health plan that meets the needs of most of their employees, while offering some additional work-site programs to help meet the needs of their workers with diabetes, or others with problems such as obesity, high blood pressure, high blood fat levels, etc. Perhaps you can talk with your employee benefits department about providing on-site nutrition counseling free of charge to people with these kinds of problems; or perhaps offering a fitness benefit or weight loss program in addition to the basic health plan, which might enable you to develop an exercise or weight loss program at lower cost to help manage your diabetes; or perhaps a stress management program free at work to help lower blood pressure.

Be Prepared to Pay Out-of-Pocket

People need to recognize that increasingly, having health insurance does not automatically entitle you to have all your medical care for free. People with diabetes have long had to pay for diabetes education out-of-pocket—and in some cases have balked at doing so. "Part of being an educated consumer is having a good diabetes education," notes Hill. "While insurers are increasingly covering some diabetes education, you may still have to pay something for that."

In addition, a change in health insurance coverage and a resulting change in healthcare providers may leave you longing for your former diabetes healthcare team. You may find that advocating for yourself to get the referral you want to see your former team just isn't working. Or the effort of managing your diabetes and all the other things going on in your life may leave you without the emotional energy you may need to do all the spade work required to get that referral. Or, admit it, some people just feel too uncomfortable to complain on their own behalf. Or the environment at your workplace may make you feel uncomfortable about calling attention to your medical issues with your employer's benefits department.

If any of these situations is the case for you, then perhaps, if possible, you should simply plan to spend out of pocket once a year for a good diabetes-specific medical evaluation (doctor visit, lab tests, diabetes education, eye exam) with your former diabetes specialists, even if they aren't covered under your health plan. See it as augmenting the care you are receiving and getting covered by your insurer. "After all, to make sure your car is running smoothly you would spend $500–$1000 a year on tune-ups, oil changes, and other things which are over and above your warranty," says Dr. Jackson. "Why not do the same thing for your body?"

This can serve two useful purposes—first, it can help reassure you that your diabetes care is on track, and provide you information about how you can improve your overall diabetes care. Second, if problems with your existing medical care are uncovered, you can use this information to go back to your own physician and health plan and seek improvements. Or perhaps you can parlay the information into an out-of-plan referral to the physician team you wanted to see in the first place, or some additional action (i.e. specialty referrals) within the plan to physicians who may be categorized as super specialists, only to be referred to in the most dire of circumstances.

How Do You Choose Your Insurance Wisely?

Despite changes in the market place most people covered by insurance at work still find that they have some choice in health coverage. What should you look for when the annual opportunity to make your health plan selection comes along? What should you look for in health insurance coverage if you are going to change jobs and someone in your family has diabetes? How do you minimize upheaval in your healthcare team coverage? Here's some questions to make sure you know the answer to when considering health plans:

- Are the physicians I currently see covered under the insurance plan?

- If they are, how easy or difficult is it to gain access to these specialists I am seeing? How easy, in general, is it to get a referral?

Just seeing the name of your physicians on a list of providers may suggest that you'll be able to see them whenever you wanted, just as in the past. This may not be the case, however. Some plans, for example, list certain physicians as part of their health network. But they are as tertiary care providers, which means that you can only be seen by one of these physicians if your primary care physician recommends it and the medical director of the health plan OKs it. "Getting this approval is a long process and your request will often be rejected. Instead, the plan will offer to cover you seeing a specialist in the local area—an endocrinologist in the community not associated with the physician you want to see, even though the physician you want to see may be in your local community."

So, before signing up with a new health plan, don't just check with the health plan's provider book to see if your specialists are covered under the plan. Also check with your specialists themselves to see how difficult it is to get a referral under the health plan you are considering.

Other questions to know the answers to include:

- What co-pays and deductibles are required in the health plan I am considering? How do these differ with physicians I may see who are "out-of-network?"

- Does the insurance plan cover such things as diabetes education? Weight loss programs? Fitness programs? One-on-one counseling with dietitians, certified diabetes educators, etc.? Can the costs of these services be included in your deductible? Does the insurance plan cover costs associated with these programs at any institution, or only at certain places?

- What coverage is provided for medical supplies such as blood sugar monitoring equipment and supplies? What does the drug benefit include? Are insulin and syringes covered?

- What is the mental health benefit? Will it cover such things as a diabetes-related support group or one-on-one counseling? How difficult or easy is it to get a referral to such a program through your health plan?

- If the person with diabetes to be covered under the health plan has a diabetes complication, what rules governing preexisting conditions may limit how much money your insurance will cover to pay for those complications? Or for diabetes care itself?

- Is the person to be covered under the plan who has diabetes planning on becoming pregnant? If so, will the health plan cover the more frequent testing and doctor visits required? Who are the specialists in diabetes and pregnancy covered under the plan? Where will the baby be delivered and what are the neonatology services available?

Keep in mind that each insurance plan has numerous different sub-plans that it sells to employer groups. The only way you will know for sure if your care at Joslin is covered, for example, is to check with your insurance carrier.

"Getting healthcare just isn't what it used to be," notes Hill. "People just have to be prepared to be more aggressive consumers to get the care they used to simply get by paying their health insurance premiums and their doctor bills. It takes a lot of work. But now, more than ever, an informed, intelligent consumer who is willing to be a little aggressive will get the best healthcare."

Chapter 59

Financial Help for Diabetes Care or Kidney Failure

Financial Help for Diabetes Care

Diabetes treatment is expensive. According to the American Diabetes Association, people who have this disease spend an average of $13,243 a year on health care expenses.

Many people who have diabetes need help paying some of the bills. It's a good idea to start by looking for an insurance plan that covers as many diabetes-related expenses as possible. A variety of governmental and nongovernmental programs exist to help, depending on whether you qualify.

Medicare

Medicare is a Government program providing health care services for people who are 65 years and older. People who are disabled or have become disabled also can apply for Medicare, and limited coverage is available for people of all ages with kidney failure. To learn if you're eligible, check with your local Social Security office or call the Medicare Hotline. Medicare now includes coverage for glucose monitors, test strips, and lancets as well as medical nutrition therapy services for people with diabetes or kidney disease when referred by a doctor.

This chapter contains information from two documents produced by the National Institute of Diabetes and Digestive and Kidney Diseases: "Financial Help for Diabetes Care," August 2004; and "Financial Help for Treatment of Kidney Failure," August 2007. Contact information was updated in December 2007.

Diabetes self-management training, therapeutic shoes, glaucoma screening, and flu and pneumonia shots are also covered.

For more information about Medicare benefits, call the National Diabetes Education Program at 800-438-5383 and request copies of *The Power to Control Diabetes Is in Your Hands* and *Expanded Medicare Coverage of Diabetes Services*, or read them online at http://www.ndep.nih.gov (click on "Control" under "About Diabetes and Pre-Diabetes"). You can also read the booklet Medicare Coverage of Diabetes Supplies & Services (PDF) online or request a copy from:

Centers for Medicare & Medicaid Services
7500 Security Boulevard
Baltimore, MD 21244-1850
Phone: 800-MEDICARE (633-4227)
Website: http://www.medicare.gov

Medicaid

Medicaid is a state health assistance program for people based on financial need. Your income must be below a certain level to qualify for Medicaid funds. To apply, talk with a social worker or contact your local department of human services. Check the government pages of your phone book.

State Children's Health Insurance Program

The U.S. Department of Health and Human Services has established the State Children's Health Insurance Program (SCHIP) to help children without health insurance. SCHIP provides health coverage for children whose families earn too much to qualify for Medicaid but too little to afford private health insurance. Consumers can obtain information about the program by calling toll-free 877-KIDS-NOW (543-7669), or by checking http://www.insurekidsnow.gov.

Health Insurance

Because health insurance is meant to cover unexpected future illnesses, diabetes that has already been diagnosed presents a problem. It is considered a preexisting condition so finding coverage may be difficult. Many insurance companies have a specific waiting period during which they do not cover diabetes-related expenses for new enrollees, although they will cover other medical expenses that arise during this time.

Recent state and Federal laws, however, may help. Many states now require insurance companies to cover diabetes supplies and education. The Health Insurance Portability Act, passed by Congress in 1996, limits insurance companies from denying coverage because of a preexisting condition. To find out more about these laws, contact your state insurance regulatory office. This office can also help you find an insurance company that offers individual coverage.

Managed Care

Most HMOs keep costs down by limiting the choice of doctors to those who belong to the network, restricting access to specialists, reducing hospital stays, and emphasizing preventive care. In most managed care plans, especially Medicare HMOs, you select a primary care physician who will be responsible for directing your care and referring you to specialists when he or she feels it's necessary. Some plans also cover extra benefits like prescription drugs.

For more information on managed care organizations, particularly the quality of care offered to patients, you may want to contact the National Committee for Quality Assurance (NCQA) at 888-275-7585 or see http://www.ncqa.org on the internet.

Medicare also has many publications to help you learn more about managed care. Go to http://www.medicare.gov on the internet or call 800-MEDICARE (633-4227) for more information.

Health Insurance after Leaving a Job

If you lose your health coverage when you leave your job, you may be able to buy group coverage for up to 18 months under a Federal law called the Consolidated Omnibus Budget Reconciliation Act or COBRA. Buying group coverage is cheaper than going out alone to buy individual coverage. If you have a disability, you can extend COBRA coverage for up to 29 months. COBRA may also cover young people who were insured under a parent's policy but have reached the age limit and are trying to obtain their own insurance.

For more information, call the Department of Labor at 866-487-2365 or see http://www.dol.gov/dol/topic/health-plans/cobra.htm on the internet.

If you don't qualify for coverage or if your COBRA coverage has expired, you can still seek other options:

- Some states require employers to offer conversion policies, in which you stay with your insurance company but buy individual coverage.

589

- Some professional or alumni organizations offer group coverage for members.

- Your state may be one of 29 with a high-risk pool for people unable to get coverage.

- Some insurance companies also offer stopgap policies designed for people who are between jobs.

Contact your state insurance regulatory office for more information on these and other options. Information on consumer health plans is also available at the U.S. Department of Labor's website at http://www.dol.gov/dol/topic/health-plans/consumerinfhealth.htm.

Health Care Services

The Bureau of Primary Health Care, a service of the Health Resources and Services Administration, offers health care for people regardless of their insurance status or ability to pay. To find local health centers, call 800-400-2742 and ask for a directory, or visit the bureau's website at http://www.bphc.hrsa.gov on the internet.

The Department of Veterans Affairs (VA) runs hospitals and clinics that serve veterans who have service-related health problems or who simply need financial aid. If you're a veteran and would like to find out more about VA health care, call 800-827-1000 or visit their website at http://www.va.gov.

Many local governments have public health departments that can help people who need medical care. Your local county or city government's health and human services office can provide further information.

Hospital Care

If you're uninsured and need hospital care, you may be able to get help. In 1946, Congress passed the Hospital Survey and Construction Act, which was sponsored by Senators Lister Hill and Harold Burton and is now known as the Hill-Burton Act. Although the program originally provided hospitals with Federal grants for modernization, today it provides free or reduced-charge medical services to low-income people. The program is administered by the Department of Health and Human Services. For more information, call 800-638-0742 or visit http://www.hrsa.gov/hillburton/default.htm on the internet.

Prosthetic Care

If you've had an amputation, paying for your rehabilitation expenses may be a concern. The following organizations provide financial assistance or information about locating financial resources for people who need prosthetic care:

Amputee Coalition of America
900 East Hill Avenue, Suite 205
Knoxville, TN 37915-2568
Phone: 888-AMP-KNOW (267-5669)
Fax: 865-525-7917
TTY: 865-525-4512
Website: http://www.amputee-coalition.org

Easter Seals
230 West Monroe Street, Suite 1800
Chicago, IL 60606
Toll-Free: 800-221-6827
Phone: 312-726-6200
Fax: 312-726-1494
TTY: 312-726-1494
Website: http://www.easterseals.com

Prescription Assistance

If you can't pay for your medicines and supplies without help, you should tell your health care provider. Your doctor may be able to direct you to local programs or even provide free samples.

You or your doctor can order a free filament to check feet for nerve damage. The filament (with instructions for use) is available by calling the Bureau of Primary Health Care's (BPHC's) Lower Extremity Amputation Prevention Program (LEAP) at 888-ASK-HRSA (275-4772) or by accessing http://www.bphc.hrsa.gov/leap on the internet.

The Medicare program offers a searchable database of prescription drug assistance programs at http://www.medicare.gov/Choices/Overview.asp. This website gives information on public and private programs offering discounted or free medication. You can also learn about Medicare health plans with prescription coverage.

In addition, drug companies that sell insulin or diabetes medications usually have patient assistance programs. Such programs are available only through a physician. The Pharmaceutical Research and Manufacturers of America and its member companies

591

sponsor an interactive website with information on drug assistance programs at https://www.pparx.org.

Also, since programs targeted at the homeless sometimes provide aid, try contacting a local shelter for more information on how to obtain free medications and medical supplies. Check your phone book under Human Service Organizations or Social Service Organizations for the number of the nearest shelter.

Food and Nutrition

Food, nutrition education, and access to health care services are also available through the U.S. Department of Agriculture's Women, Infants, and Children (WIC) program. Pregnant women who meet residential, financial need, and nutrition risk criteria are eligible for assistance. Gestational diabetes is considered a medically based nutrition risk and would qualify a woman for assistance through the WIC program if she meets the financial need requirements and has lived in a particular state the required amount of time. The WIC website provides a page of contact information for each state and Indian tribe, or you can contact the national headquarters at the following address:

WIC at FNS Headquarters
Supplemental Food Programs Division
Food and Nutrition Service—USDA
3101 Park Center Drive
Alexandria, VA 22302
Phone: 703-305-2746
Website: http://www.fns.usda.gov/wic

Local Resources

Finally, for help in financing some of the many expenses related to diabetes, you may also want to seek out available local resources, such as the following charitable groups:

- Lions Clubs International, which can help with vision care

- Rotary Clubs, which provide humanitarian and educational assistance

- Elks Clubs, which provide charitable activities that benefit youth and veterans

- Shriners, which offer need-based treatment for children at Shriners hospitals throughout the country

- Kiwanis Clubs, which conduct fund-raising events and projects to help the community and especially children

- Religious organizations

In many areas, nonprofit or special interest groups such as those listed previously can sometimes provide financial assistance or help with fund-raising. In addition, some local governments may have special trusts set up to help people in need. You can find out more about such groups at your local library or your local city or county government's health and human services office.

Financial Help for Treatment of Kidney Failure

If you have permanent kidney failure, you may be worried about paying for the expensive treatments you need.

In 1972, Congress passed legislation making people of any age with permanent kidney failure eligible for Medicare, a program that helps people over 65 and people with disabilities pay for medical care, usually up to 80 percent. Other public and private resources can help with the remaining 20 percent. Your dialysis or transplant center has a social worker who can help you locate and apply for financial assistance.

Medicare

Medicare is a federally administered health insurance program for people 65 and older and people of any age with permanent kidney failure. To qualify for Medicare on the basis of kidney failure, you must:

- checkmark need regular dialysis, or

- checkmark have had a kidney transplant.

You must also:

- checkmark have paid into Social Security through your employer,

- checkmark worked under the Railroad Retirement Board, or as a government employee (or be the child or spouse of someone who has), or

- checkmark you must already be receiving Social Security, Railroad Retirement, or Office of Personnel Management benefits.

593

You can enroll for Medicare at your local Social Security office (check the blue pages in your phone directory to locate the office).

Medicare has two parts: Part A (hospital insurance) and Part B (medical insurance). Part B covers doctors' services, outpatient hospital services, and many other health services and supplies. While Medicare Part A has no premiums, Part B requires you to pay premiums, deductibles, and coinsurance. Part B is voluntary. Most of the services and supplies needed by people with permanent kidney failure are covered by Medicare Part B.

You will apply for Medicare when you start dialysis treatments. Your Medicare benefits then begin the third month after the month your course of regular dialysis treatments begins. For example, if you begin receiving regular dialysis treatments in July, your Medicare coverage would start on October 1. Coverage can begin earlier if you take self-care dialysis training (for home hemodialysis or peritoneal dialysis) before the third month or have a transplant within the first three months.

If you're covered by a group health plan, Medicare is a secondary payer during a 30-month coordination period. Your group health plan pays at its regular level for this period. Since you usually can't get Medicare in the first three months, your group health plan is the only payer for health services. In the third month, Medicare begins to cover only that portion of your health services that isn't covered by your group health plan. Medicare then becomes the primary payer for your health insurance claims at the end of the 30-month period.

You may wish to wait to enroll in Medicare Part A and Part B until the end of the 30-month coordination period if your group health plan will pay for all of your health care expenses. In doing so, you'll avoid paying the Medicare Part B premium.

Enrolling in Medicare Parts A and B could help pay a yearly deductible or coinsurance payment required by some group health plans.

Contact your local Social Security office or call the nationwide toll-free number at 800-772-1213 if you want to apply for Medicare. Often, the social worker at your hospital or dialysis center will help you apply.

Private Insurance

Private insurance frequently pays for the entire cost of treatment. Or it may pay for the 20 percent that Medicare doesn't cover. Private insurance may also pay for your prescription drugs. Read your private health insurance policy carefully to make sure it covers kidney failure. Talk with your insurance agent or company benefits counselor if you have any questions about your benefits.

Medicaid

Medicaid is a state program. Your income must be below a certain level to receive Medicaid funds. If you aren't eligible for Medicare, Medicaid may pay for your treatments. In some states, it pays the 20 percent that Medicare doesn't cover. It may also pay for some of your medicines. To apply for Medicaid, talk with your social worker or contact your local department of human services or social services.

State Children's Health Insurance Program

The U.S. Department of Health and Human Services has established the State Children's Health Insurance Program (SCHIP) to help children without health insurance. SCHIP provides health coverage for children whose families earn too much to qualify for Medicaid but too little to afford private health insurance. Consumers can obtain information about the program by calling toll-free 877-KIDS-NOW (543-7669), or by checking http://www.insurekidsnow.gov.

Department of Veterans Affairs (VA) Benefits

If you're a veteran, the VA can help pay for treatment or provide other benefits. Contact your local VA office for more information, or call 800-827-1000 to reach the national office. If you're retired from the military, you may also call the Department of Defense at 800-538-9552.

Social Security Disability Insurance (SSDI) and Supplemental Security Income (SSI)

These benefits from the Social Security Administration help you with the costs of daily living. To receive Social Security Disability Insurance (SSDI), you must be unable to work and have earned the required number of work credits.

You can receive Supplemental Security Income (SSI) if you don't own much and have a low income. People who get SSI usually get food stamps and Medicaid, too. To find out if you qualify for SSDI and SSI, talk to your social worker or call your local Social Security office or the nationwide number, 800-772-1213.

Patient Assistance Programs From Prescription Drug Companies

Medicare pays for erythropoietin to treat anemia in kidney failure and for immunosuppressants to prevent rejection of a transplanted kidney. But other self-administered drugs that you need may not be covered by Medicare. If you have trouble paying for all the medications your doctor prescribes, you may qualify for assistance from private programs. Most drug manufacturers have patient assistance programs giving discounts to patients who can show that they can't afford the cost of their prescribed medications.

The Partnership for Prescription Assistance provides a website that directs patients, caregivers, and doctors to more than 275 public and private patient assistance programs, including more than 150 programs offered by pharmaceutical companies. The website features an application wizard that helps you determine which programs might be available to you. The web address is http://www.pparx.org.

Additional Patient Assistance Programs

The United Network for Organ Sharing (UNOS) offers a website called Transplant Living, which includes a section on financing a transplant. The web address is http://www.transplantliving.org/beforethetransplant/finance/finance.aspx. For more information about UNOS, contact them at:

United Network for Organ Sharing (UNOS)
700 North 4th Street
Richmond, VA 23219
Toll-Free: 804-782-4800
Fax: 804-782-4817
Website: http://www.unos.org

Additional Organizations That Can Help

Several groups offer information and services to patients with kidney disease. You may wish to contact one of the following:

American Association of Kidney Patients
3505 East Frontage Road, Suite 315
Tampa, FL 33607
Phone: 800-749-2257
Fax: 813-636-8122
Website: http://www.aakp.org
E-mail: info@aakp.org

American Kidney Fund
6110 Executive Boulevard, Suite 1010
Rockville, MD 20852
Toll-Free: 800-638-8299
Phone: 301-881-3052
Fax: 301-881-0898
Website: http://www.kidneyfund.org
E-mail: helpline@akfinc.org

Life Options Rehabilitation Program
c/o Medical Education Institute, Inc.
414 D'Onofrio Drive, Suite 200
Madison, WI 53719
Phone: 800-468-7777 or 608-232-2333
Website: http://www.lifeoptions.org; http://www.kidneyschool.org
E-mail: lifeoptions@MEIresearch.org

National Kidney Foundation
30 East 33rd Street
New York, NY 10016
Toll-Free: 800-622-9010
Phone: 212-889-2210
Fax: 212-689-9261
Website: http://www.kidney.org
E-mail: info@kidney.org

Additional Reading

If you would like to learn more about financial assistance for kidney failure treatments, you may be interested in reading these publication:

Medicare Coverage of Kidney Dialysis and
Kidney Transplant Services
Publication Number CMS-10128
U.S. Department of Health and Human Services
Centers for Medicare and Medicaid Services
7500 Security Boulevard
Baltimore, MD 21244-1850
Phone: 800-MEDICARE (800-633-4227)
Website: http://www.medicare.gov

Index

Index

Page numbers followed by 'n' indicate a footnote. Page numbers in *italics* indicate a table or illustration.

A

A1C test
  blood glucose levels *173*, 180
  defined 534
  described 80
  overview 191–94
  recommended frequency 80, 176,
    181
  wintertime 534
AAKP *see* American Association of
  Kidney Patients
"The ABCs of A1C Testing ...
  The Best Test of Blood Sugar
  Control for People with Diabetes"
  (VA) 191n
acanthosis nigricans
  defined 533
  type 2 diabetes mellitus 42
acarbose 36, 257, 262, 533
ACCORD (Action to Control
  Cardiovascular Risk in Diabetes)
  study 481–82
ACE inhibitors *see* angiotensin
  converting enzyme inhibitors

acetohexamide 259, 533
Action for Health in Diabetes
  (Look AHEAD) 482
Actoplus Met (metformin,
  pioglitazone) 261
Actos (pioglitazone) 260, 262, 267
acupuncture
  diabetes 273–74
  neuropathies 356
ADA *see* Americans with
  Disabilities Act
Addison disease, described 63
adolescents
  diabetes statistics 11
  maturity-onset diabetes of the
    young 56
  type 1 diabetes mellitus 26
adult-onset diabetes *see* type 2
  diabetes mellitus
advanced glycosylation
  endproducts (AGE), defined 534
aerobic exercise, suggestions 129
African Americans
  diabetes statistics 8–9, 12
  foot ulcers 309
  gestational diabetes 48
  insulin resistance 32
  kidney disorders 318
  type 2 diabetes 41

AGE *see* advanced glycosylation endproducts

age factor
blood urea nitrogen 198
creatinine 202
diabetes, healthy living 165–68
diabetes statistics 8, 11–13, 17

Agency for Healthcare Research and Quality (AHRQ)
contact information 559
diabetes medications publication 262n

AHRQ *see* Agency for Healthcare Research and Quality

Alaska Natives
diabetes statistics 13
type 2 diabetes 41

albumin
kidney disease 319, 391–92
proteinuria 322

albuminuria, defined 534

alcohol use
blood glucose levels 99
diabetes 119–21
food pyramid 105, 106, *107*
neuropathy 314

alendronate 380

ALLHAT *see* Antihypertensive and Lipid-Lowering Treatment to Prevent Heart Attack Trial

alpha cells, defined 534

alpha-glucosidase inhibitors 36, 257, 534, 549

alpha-lipoic acid 277

alprostadil 358

alternative site testing, described 215

Amaryl (glimepiride) 259

American Association for Clinical Chemistry
contact information 559
publications
blood urea nitrogen test 196n
creatinine tests 199n, 203n
glucose tolerance tests 184n
microalbumin tests 203n

American Association of Clinical Endocrinologists, contact information 559

American Association of Diabetes Educators, contact information 559

American Association of Kidney Patients (AAKP)
contact information 596
home hemodialysis publication 426n

American College of Physicians
contact information 560
selenium supplements publication 496n

American Diabetes Association
contact information 560
insulin delivery methods publication 226n

American Dietetic Association, contact information 560

American Indians
diabetes statistics 13
gestational diabetes 48
insulin resistance 32
type 2 diabetes 41

American Kidney Fund, contact information 597

American Podiatric Medical Association (APMA)
contact information 560
foot ulcers publication 309n

Americans with Disabilities Act (ADA; 1990) 162–65

"Am I at Risk for Type 2 Diabetes" (NIDDK) 39n

amitriptyline 356

amputations
diabetes statistics 19
nerve damage 87
neuropathies 355
peripheral neuropathy 350

Amputee Coalition of America, contact information 591

amylin, defined 534

amyloidosis
nephrotic syndrome 327
overview 324–26

"Amyloidosis and Kidney Disease" (NIDDK) 324n

amyotrophy, defined 534

androgen deprivation therapy, research 492–93

"Androgen Deprivation Therapy
May Increase Risk of Diabetes
and Cardiovascular Disease"
(CancerConsultants.com) 492n
anemia
overview 333–35
treatment 396
"Anemia and Diabetes" (NAAC) 333n
angiotensin converting enzyme
inhibitors (ACE inhibitors)
defined 533
hypertension 320, 324, 328, 504
kidney disease 395
angiotensin receptor blockers (ARB)
defined 534
hypertension 320, 324, 328
kidney disease 395
antibodies
defined 534
diabetes research 498–501
Antihypertensive and Lipid-Lowering
Treatment to Prevent Heart Attack
Trial (ALLHAT) 504
APMA *see* American Podiatric
Medical Association
ARB *see* angiotensin receptor
blockers
arteriovenous fistula
depicted *419*
described 419
arteriovenous graft
depicted *420*
described 419–20
artificial pancreas, described 27
Asian Americans
diabetes statistics 13
gestational diabetes 48
insulin resistance 32
type 2 diabetes 41
aspart insulin
defined 534–35
described 217–19, *222*, 222–23
aspirin therapy, heart disease 301
asthma 64
atherosclerosis, defined 535
athlete's foot, described 138–39
automobile driving
diabetes 156–58
hypoglycemia prevention 288

autonomic nerves, described 337
autonomic neuropathy
affected nerves 349, *351*
defined 535
described 349, 350–52
Avandamet (metformin,
rosiglitazone) 261, 267
Avandaryl (glimepiride,
rosiglitazone) 261, 267
Avandia (rosiglitazone) 260, 262,
267, 268, 551

B

background neuropathy,
defined 535
Baker, Lois 490n
BARI-2D *see* Bypass Angioplasty
Revascularization Investigation
2 Diabetes
barium beefsteak meal,
gastroparesis 360
barium x-ray, gastroparesis 360
basal rate, defined 535
basic metabolic panel (BMP),
described 196–97, 200
BCBC *see* Beta Cell Biology
Consortium
Beaser, Richard S. 579
Bell's palsy 353
Beta Cell Biology Consortium
(BCBC) 482
bezoars
gastroparesis 360
treatment 362
biguanides 36, 258, 535, 549
biofeedback
diabetes 274
neuropathies 356
Blagg, Christopher 426n
blindness
daily guidelines 85–86
diabetes statistics 19
see also diabetic retinopathy
blisters, described 138
blood glucose
defined 535
gestational diabetes 52

blood glucose levels
  defined 535
  diabetes control 177
  dry skin 139
  fiber 108–9
  mouth problems *142*
  targets 5–6, 91–92
  see also hyperglycemia;
    hypoglycemia
blood glucose meter
  defined 535
  overview 209–16
blood glucose monitoring
  daily guidelines 79
  defined 535
blood glucose test
  diabetes control 172–73,
    175
  insulin resistance 32–33
blood lipids control, statistics 21
blood pressure
  autonomic neuropathy 350
  daily guidelines 85
  defined 535–36
  diabetes control 173–74, 176
  insulin resistance 34
  kidney disease 391, 395
  measurement 315–16
  recommendations 178, 180
  type 2 diabetes mellitus 42
  see also hypertension
blood pressure control,
  statistics 20–21
blood sugar *see* blood glucose
blood tests *see* blood glucose test;
  hemoglobin A1C test
blood urea nitrogen (BUN)
  defined 536
  kidney disease 393
  overview 196–99
BMI *see* body mass index
BMP *see* basic metabolic panel
body mass index (BMI)
  chart *35*
  defined 536
  diabetes 294
  insulin resistance 34
  type 2 diabetes mellitus 43
bolus, defined 536

bone density test, osteoporosis 379
bone problems, diabetes 375–80
borderline diabetes *see* impaired
  glucose tolerance; type 2 diabetes
  mellitus
botulinum toxin, gastroparesis 364
brittle diabetes, defined 536
BUN *see* blood urea nitrogen
BUN/creatinine ratio 199, 202–3
bunions, described 138
"BUN: The Test Sample, The Test,
  Common Questions" (American
  Association for Clinical Chemistry)
  196n
Burton, Harold 590
Byetta (exenatide) 223–24
Bypass Angioplasty
  Revascularization Investigation 2
  Diabetes (BARI-2D) 483

C

CAD *see* coronary artery disease
calcitonin 380
calcitriol 376, 389
calcium, renal osteodystrophy
  376–77
calcium acetate 377
calcium carbonate 377
calorie counting
  versus exchange diet 109–10
  hemodialysis 433
CAM therapy *see* complementary
  and alternative medicine
CancerConsultants.com, androgen
  deprivation therapy publication
  492n
"Can I Reuse My Insulin Syringe?"
  (Michigan Diabetes Research and
  Training Center) 250n
CAPD *see* continuous ambulatory
  peritoneal dialysis
capsaicin, defined 536
captopril 320
carbohydrate counting
  chart *113*
  defined 536
  described 109–19

"Carbohydrate Counting:
As Easy As 1-2-3" (Joslin
Diabetes Center) 111n
carbohydrates
defined 536
described 285
glucose 184
cardiovascular disease,
defined 536
see also heart disease
carpal tunnel syndrome,
amyloidosis 326
Carver, Catherine 154
cataracts
defined 536
described 365
CCPD see continuous cycler-assisted
peritoneal dialysis
CDE see certified diabetes educator
Center for Inherited Disease
Research (CIDR) 483
Centers for Disease Control and
Prevention (CDC)
contact information 560
publications
diabetes maintenance 177n
exercise 127n
flu shots 269n
groups affected 15n
Centers for Medicare and
Medicaid Services, contact
information 588
central diabetes insipidus,
described 68
central obesity, described 298
cerebrovascular disease
defined 536
described 302–3
certified diabetes educator
(CDE), defined 536, 538
Charcot foot, defined 537
chemical diabetes see impaired
glucose tolerance
children
diabetes statistics 11
hypoglycemia 291
renal osteodystrophy 375–77
type 1 diabetes mellitus 23–27
chlorpropamide 259, 537

cholesterol
defined 537
kidney disease 395
cholesterol levels
daily guidelines 85
diabetes control 174
heart disease 298–99
insulin resistance 30–31, 34–36
recommendations 178–79, 181
chromium 278
chronic kidney disease (CKD),
stages 393–94
Cialis (tadalafil) 358
CIDR see Center for Inherited
Disease Research
cilostazol 308
cinacalcet hydrochloride 377
CITR see Collaborative Islet
Transplant Registry
CKD see chronic kidney disease
Clancy, Carolyn 262
"Class Action" (McCarren) 256n
Cleveland Clinic, kidney pancreas
transplantation publication 457n
clinical trials
diabetes research 33, 479–87, 538
hypertension medications 504
CMP see comprehensive
metabolic panel
COBRA see Consolidated Omnibus
Budget Reconciliation Act
codeine 356
coenzyme Q10 278–79
Collaborative Islet Transplant
Registry (CITR) 483
Collins, Francis 494
coma, defined 537
combination medications, diabetes
treatment 261
combination oral medications,
defined 537
combination therapy, defined 537
"Complementary and Alternative
Medical Therapies for Diabetes"
(NDIC) 273n
complementary and alternative
medicine (CAM)
neuropathies 356
overview 273–82

comprehensive metabolic panel (CMP), described 196–97, 200
congestive heart failure, defined 537
Consolidated Omnibus Budget Reconciliation Act (COBRA) 589–90
continuous ambulatory peritoneal dialysis (CAPD), described 396, 403–5, 438
continuous cycler-assisted peritoneal dialysis (CCPD), described 396, 404–5, 437–38
conventional therapy, defined 537
Cooke, David A. 63n, 347n, 501n
corns, described 138
coronary artery disease (CAD), described 302
coronary heart disease, defined 537
corticosteroids, diabetes 63–65
counseling
   depression 383
   diabetes diagnosis 151
   monogenic diabetes 58–59
Cowie, Catherine 9
Coxsackie viruses, research 498–501
C-peptide, defined 537
creatinine
   defined 537
   kidney problems 86, 392
   test overview 199–203
"Creatinine: The Test Sample, The Test, Common Questions" (American Association for Clinical Chemistry) 199n
Cushing syndrome, described 64
Cygnus GlucoWatch Biographer 216
Cymbalta (duloxetine) 357

D

daclizumab 464–65, 480
DASP see Diabetes Autoantibody Standardization Program
Davis, Steve 571
dawn phenomenon, defined 538
DCCT see Diabetes Control and Complications Trial

DDAVP see desmopressin
decreased vaginal lubrication, nerve damage 339
dehydration, described 154
delayed gastric emptying see gastroparesis
dental disease, diabetes statistics 19–20
Department of Health and Human Services (DHHS; HHS) see US Department of Health and Human Services
Department of Veterans Affairs (VA) see US Department of Veterans Affairs
depression
   diabetes diagnosis 150
   overview 381–84
DERC see Diabetes Endocrinology Research Centers
desmopressin (DDAVP), diabetes insipidus 70
detemir insulin, described 218, *222*, 222–23
DGAP see Diabetes Genome Anatomy Project
DHHS see US Department of Health and Human Services
DiaBeta (glyburide) 259, 262
"Diabetes, Heart Disease, and Stroke" (NDIC) 297n
Diabetes Action Research and Education Foundation, contact information 560
"Diabetes and Alcohol: How to Stay Safe" (LifeMed Media, Inc.) 119n
"Diabetes and Depression" (LifeMed Media, Inc.) 381n
"Diabetes and High Blood Pressure: A Challenging Combination" (Michigan Diabetes Research and Training Center) 315n
"Diabetes and Incretin-Based Therapy" (Hormone Foundation) 264n
"Diabetes and Obesity" (International Diabetes Federation) 293n

Diabetes Autoantibody
Standardization Program
(DASP) 483
"Diabetes Clock Ticking for
Women" (Baker) 490n
Diabetes Control and Complications
Trial (DCCT) 369, 483, 538
Diabetes Dateline 479n
"Diabetes Dictionary" (NIDDK)
533n
diabetes educators
blood glucose meter 210–11
defined 538
described 190–91
see also certified diabetes educator
Diabetes Endocrinology Research
Centers (DERC) 573–75
Diabetes Exercise and
Sports Association,
contact information 561
Diabetes Food Pyramid 105–7
Diabetes Genome Anatomy
Project (DGAP) 484
Diabetes in America 484
diabetes insipidus
defined 538
overview 67–72
"Diabetes Insipidus" (NIH) 67n
diabetes mellitus
complications 18–21
cookbooks 555–58
costs 18
defined 335
everyday guidelines
overview 75–89
illnesses 145–48
monogenic forms 55–62
overview 3–6
research overview 469–87
see also gestational diabetes;
type 1 diabetes mellitus;
type 2 diabetes mellitus
Diabetes Prevention Program
(DPP) 484, 525–29
"Diabetes Prevention Program"
(NIDDK) 525n
Diabetes Prevention Program
Outcomes Study (DPPOS) 33,
484, 538

Diabetes Prevention Trial - Type 1
(DPT-1) 484
Diabetes Research and Education
Act 565
Diabetes Research and Training
Centers (DRTC) 565–73
Diabetes Research in Children
Network (DirecNet) 484–85
diabetes treatment plan,
hypoglycemia prevention 287
diabetic diarrhea, defined 538–39
diabetic eye disease, defined 335
diabetic ketoacidosis (DKA)
defined 539
type 1 diabetes mellitus 25
see also Kussmaul breathing
diabetic myelopathy, defined 539
diabetic nephropathy
described 390
nephrotic syndrome 327
"Diabetic Neuropathies: The Nerve
Damage of Diabetes" (NIDDK)
347n
diabetic neuropathy, described 136
see also nerve damage;
neuropathy
diabetic retinopathy
defined 539
overview 365–73
"Diabetic Retinopathy" (National
Eye Institute) 365n
Diabetic Retinopathy Clinical
Research Network (DRCR.net)
485
diabetogenic, defined 539
diabetologist, defined 539
Diabinese (chlorpropamide) 259
dialysis
defined 539
described 318
kidney failure 396–97
kidney problems 86
see also hemodialysis;
peritoneal dialysis
dialysis-related amyloidosis
(DRA) 325–26
dialyzer
depicted *401, 416*
described 400, 416–17

diet and nutrition
  buffet table tips 126
  creatinine 202
  fast food 124–25
  gastroparesis 362–63
  heart disease 299–300
  hemodialysis 429–33
  kidney disease 320, 395–96
  osteoporosis 379
  peritoneal dialysis 443
  sodium 122–23
  type 2 diabetes mellitus 44
dietary guidelines
  carbohydrate counting 109–19
  diabetics 91–101
dietary supplements
  hemodialysis 433
  type 2 diabetes 274–75
dietitians
  defined 539
  hemodialysis 430–31
  kidney disease 395
  meal plans 53, 76, 94–95
dilated eye exam, diabetic
  retinopathy 370
DirecNet *see* Diabetes Research
  in Children Network
distal symmetric neuropathy
  see peripheral neuropathy
diuretics
  diabetes insipidus 70
  kidney disease 324
DKA *see* diabetic ketoacidosis
docosahexaenoic acid 480
domperidone 362
Donahue, Richard 490
D-phenylalanine derivatives,
  defined 539, 549
DPP *see* Diabetes Prevention
  Program
DPP-IV inhibitors 266
DPPOS *see* Diabetes Prevention
  Program Outcomes Study
DPT-1 *see* Diabetes Prevention
  Trial - Type 1
DRA *see* dialysis-related
  amyloidosis
DRCR.net *see* Diabetic Retinopathy
  Clinical Research Network

driving
  diabetes 156–58
  hypoglycemia prevention 288
DRTC *see* Diabetes Research and
  Training Centers
dry skin, blood glucose levels 139
Duetact (glimepiride, pioglitazone)
  267
duloxetine 357
Dupuytren contracture defined 539
dwell time, described 436, 444

E

Easter Seals, contact information 591
Easter Seals Project ACTION,
  contact information 158
"Eat Right to Feel Right on
  Hemodialysis" (NDIC) 429n
edema
  defined 539
  described 330
EDIC *see* Epidemiology of Diabetes
  Interventions and Complications
EEOC *see* Equal Employment
  Opportunity Commission
Effexor (venlafaxine) 357
Albert Einstein College of
  Medicine DRTC 566–67, 572
elastic stockings, neuropathies
  356–57
ElderCare Locator,
  contact information 158
electromyography (EMG)
  defined 539
  neuropathies 354
EMG *see* electromyography
emotional concerns
  diabetes diagnosis 150–51
  stress 505–23
endocrine glands, defined 539
Endocrine Society, contact
  information 561
endocrinologists, incretin-based
  therapy 266
end-stage renal disease (ESRD)
  defined 540
  described 331–32, 396

entrapment syndromes,
  described 353
Entrez Gene, website address 60
The Environmental Determinant
  of Diabetes in the Young (TEDDY)
  485
Environmental Protection Agency
  (EPA) *see* US Environmental
  Protection Agency
EPA *see* US Environmental
  Protection Agency
Epidemiology of Diabetes
  Interventions and Complications
  (EDIC) 483, 485
Equal Employment Opportunity
  Commission (EEOC), workplace,
  diabetes publication 162n
erectile dysfunction,
  described 338
erythromycin 362
erythropoietin (EPO)
  anemia 334, 396
  defined 335
  described 388
  home hemodialysis 428
ESRD *see* end-stage renal disease
ethnic factors
  diabetes 16–17
  diabetes statistics 8–9,
    12–13
  insulin resistance 32
euglycemia, defined 540
euglycemic clamp, insulin
  resistance 32
exchange lists
  versus calorie counting 109–10
  carbohydrate counting 112
  defined 540
exenatide 223–24, 265–66
exercise
  foot care 313
  osteoporosis 379
  recommendations 179
  renal osteodystrophy 376–77
  summertime 155
  type 2 diabetes mellitus 44–45
  wintertime 153
  see also physical activity
eye, depicted 366

eye problems
  autonomic neuropathy 352
  daily guidelines 85–86
  focal neuropathy 353
  preventive care 21
  see also diabetic retinopathy

F

"Fact Sheet: Type 1 Diabetes"
  (NIH) 469n
"Fact Sheet: Type 2 Diabetes"
  (NIH) 469n
Family Investigation of
  Nephropathy of Diabetes
  (FIND) 485
fast foods, quick tips 124–25
fasting blood glucose test
  defined 540
  diabetes diagnosis 180
  gestational diabetes 49
  insulin resistance 32, 33
  results meanings *188*
fasting hypoglycemia,
  described 290–91
fats
  defined 540
  food pyramid 105, 106, *107*
  meal plans 98–99
FDA *see* US Food and Drug
  Administration
feeding tubes, gastroparesis 363
"Feelings about Diabetes"
  (Michigan Diabetes Research
  and Training Center) 150n
feet, nerve damage 87, 136, 138
  see also foot care
femoral neuropathy
  see proximal neuropathy
fertility issues
  polycystic ovary syndrome
    343–44
  retrograde ejaculation 338
fiber, blood glucose levels
  108–9
50/50 insulin, defined 540
fight-or-flight response,
  diabetes 63

financial considerations
  diabetes care assistance 587–93
  diabetes costs 18
  food and nutrition 592
  hemodialysis 418
  insulin 221
  kidney failure 411
  kidney failure assistance 593–97
  peritoneal dialysis 443
  prescription assistance 591–92, 596
  prosthetic care 591
  see also insurance coverage
"Financial Help for Diabetes Care"
  (NIDDK) 587n
"Financial Help for Treatment of
  Kidney Failure" (NIDDK) 587n
FIND *see* Family Investigation of
  Nephropathy of Diabetes
Fisher, Edwin B. 571
fludiazepam 517
flu shots
  overview 269–71
  recommendations 177, 179
focal neuropathy
  affected nerves 349
  described 349, 353
Food and Drug Administration
  (FDA) *see* US Food and Drug
  Administration
food pyramid
  depicted *94*
  described 93–95, 105
foot care
  daily guidelines 88
  neuropathies 355–56
  overview 135–40
  preventive care 21
  ulcers 309–14
  wintertime 153
"For Safety, NHLBI Changes
  Intensive Blood Sugar Treatment
  Strategy in Clinical Trial of
  Diabetes and Cardiovascular
  Disease" (NIH) 479n
Fortamet (metformin) 257–61
Fosrenol (lanthanum carbonate)
  377
"Frequently Asked Questions about
  Diabetes and Exercise" (CDC) 127n

"Frequently Asked Questions: Groups
  Especially Affected by Diabetes"
  (CDC) 15n
"Frequently Asked Questions:
  Staying Healthy with Diabetes"
  (CDC) 177n
Friedewald, William T. 482
fructosamine test, defined 540
fructose, defined 540
fruits
  food pyramid 105, 106, *107*
  meal plans 97

G

gabapentin 356
gangrene, defined 540
garlic 279
gastric manometry,
  gastroparesis 361
gastric neurostimulator,
  gastroparesis 363
gastrointestinal problems,
  neuropathies 356
gastroparesis
  defined 540
  described 352
  overview 359–64
"Gastroparesis and Diabetes"
  (NIDDK) 359n
GDM *see* gestational diabetes
  mellitus
genes
  diabetes 55–56
  diabetes research 494–96
  maturity-onset diabetes of the
    young *57*
  neonatal diabetes mellitus *57*
GeneTests, website address 60
Genetics Home Reference,
  website address 60
genetic testing, monogenic diabetes
  58–59
gestational diabetes mellitus (GDM)
  blood glucose test 185–86
  defined 540
  described 5, 15–16
  ethnic factors 16

gestational diabetes mellitus
(GDM), continued
insulin resistance 32
overview 47–53
"Getting Your Diabetes Ready
for Winter" (Michigan Diabetes
Research and Training Center)
152n
GFR *see* glomerular filtration rate
ginseng, blood pressure 274
glargine insulin
defined 540
described 218, *222*, 222–23
glaucoma, described 365
glimepiride 259, 261–64,
267, 541
glipizide 259, 261–64, 541
glomerular disease
described 390–91
overview 329–32
"Glomerular Diseases"
(NIDDK) 329n
glomerular filtration rate (GFR)
defined 541
kidney disease 392
overview 207–8
glomerulonephritis, described 329
glomerulosclerosis, described 329
glomerulus, defined 541
glucagon
defined 541
hypoglycemia 84–85
glucagon kits, hypoglycemia 83
glucocorticoids
diabetes 63–65
research 512
Glucophage (metformin) 258, 262,
525–28
glucose
defined 541
described 3, 23, 29, 39, 285
glucose challenge test, results
meanings *188*
glucose control
overview 172–77
statistics 20
"Glucose Meters and Diabetes
Management" (FDA) 209n
glucose tablets, defined 541

"Glucose: The Test Sample, Common
Questions" (American Association
for Clinical Chemistry) 184n
glucose tolerance test
insulin resistance 32, 33
overview 184–91
Glucotrol (glipizide) 259, 262
Glucovance (glyburide,
metformin) 261
glulisine insulin, described 217–18
glyburide 259, 261, 541
glycemic index
defined 541
overview 118–19
glycogen
defined 541
described 285
glycosuria, defined 541
glycosylated hemoglobin test,
defined 534
Glynase PresTab (glyburide) 259,
262
Glyset (miglitol) 257, 262
gums
daily guidelines 89
proper care 141–44

H

hair problems, dialysis 447–50
hammertoes, described 138
"Have Diabetes, Will Travel"
(NDEP) 159n
"Having Options: Home
Hemodialysis" (Blagg) 426n
"A Healthier You" (DHHS) 122n
health insurance
see insurance coverage
Health Insurance Portability Act
(1996) 589
heart attacks
diabetes 297–98
diabetes medications 267–68
heart disease
autonomic neuropathy 350
daily guidelines 84–85
diabetes 297–305
diabetes statistics 18

611

heart failure, described 303
heat exhaustion, described 154
hematocrit
  anemia 333
  blood glucose meter 213
  defined 335
hematuria, described 330
hemodialysis
  amyloidosis 325–26
  defined 539, 541
  depicted *401*
  dose, adequacy 422–26
  home administration 426–29
  overview 400–403, 414–18
  see also dialysis; peritoneal
    dialysis
"Hemodialysis Dose and
  Adequacy" (NIDDK) 422n
hemoglobin
  anemia 333
  defined 335
hemoglobin A1C test
  blood glucose levels *173*, 180
  defined 534
  described 80
  overview 191–94
  recommended frequency 80,
    176, 181
  wintertime 534
hepatitis C, diabetes research
  501–3
heredity
  diabetes 16
  insulin resistance 31
  maturity-onset diabetes of
    the young 57, *58*
  type 1 diabetes mellitus 24
HHNS *see* hyperosmolar
  hyperglycemic nonketotic
  syndrome
HHS *see* US Department of
  Health and Human Services
high blood pressure
  see hypertension
high blood sugar
  see hyperglycemia
Hill, Joan 581–82,
  584, 586
Hill, Lister 590

Hispanic Americans
  diabetes statistics 12–13
  foot ulcers 309
  gestational diabetes 48
  insulin resistance 32
  kidney disorders 318
  type 2 diabetes 41
HLA *see* human leukocyte antigens
home hemodialysis 426–29
honeymoon phase, defined 541–42
Hormone Foundation, incretins
  publication 264n
hormones
  defined 542
  gestational diabetes 47
Hospital Survey and Construction
  Act (1946) 590
Humalog (lispro insulin) 219
human leukocyte antigens (HLA),
  defined 542
Humulin (NPH insulin) 222–23
hyperglycemia
  blood glucose levels 184–85
  daily guidelines 82
  defined 542
hyperinsulinemia, defined 542
hyperlipidemia, defined 542
hyperosmolar coma, diabetes 20
hyperosmolar hyperglycemic
  nonketotic syndrome (HHNS),
  defined 542
hypertension (high blood pressure)
  defined 542
  diabetes 315–16
  diabetes statistics 18
  heart disease 299
  insulin resistance 32
  kidney damage 390
  kidney disease 319, 324
  research 504
hypertonic saline infusion test,
  diabetes insipidus 70
hypnosis, neuropathies 356
hypoglycemia
  autonomic neuropathy 350
  blood glucose levels 184–85,
    189–90
  daily guidelines 82–84
  defined 542–43

hypoglycemia, continued
  overview 285–92
  physical activity 130–31
  treatment 131
"Hypoglycemia" (NDIC) 285n
hypoglycemia unawareness,
  defined 543
hypoproteinemia, described 330
hypotension, hemodialysis 401

I

ibandronate 380
ICA *see* islet cell autoantibodies
ICR *see* Islet Cell Resource Centers
IDDM (insulin-dependent diabetes
  mellitus) *see* type 1 diabetes
  mellitus
IFG *see* impaired fasting glucose
IGT *see* impaired glucose tolerance
IHS *see* Indian Health Service
imipramine 356
impaired fasting glucose (IFG)
  defined 543, 550
  diabetes diagnosis 180
  statistics 8–10, 14, 30
impaired glucose tolerance (IGT)
  defined 543, 550
  diabetes diagnosis 180
  statistics 9–10, 14, 30
  see also pre-diabetes
implantable insulin pump,
  defined 543
incretin-based therapy,
  overview 264–66
incretin mimetics 265–66
Indian Health Service (IHS)
  contact information 561
  diabetes statistics 13
infants
  gestational diabetes 50
  hypoglycemia 291
ingrown toenails, described 138
inhaled insulin, defined 543
injection aids, overview 240–43
injection site rotation, defined 543
InnoLet 245–46
Innovo 246

insulin
  blood glucose levels 184
  defined 543
  described 3, 23, 29–30, 285, 461
  gestational diabetes 51
  overview 217–24
  see also aspart insulin; 50/50
    insulin; glargine insulin;
    glulisine insulin; implantable
    insulin pump; inhaled insulin;
    intermediate-acting insulin;
    lente insulin; lispro insulin;
    NPH insulin; premixed insulin;
    rapid-acting insulin; regular
    insulin; 70/30 insulin;
    short-acting insulin;
    ultralente insulin;
    very-long-acting insulin
insulin adjustment, defined 543
"Insulin Delivery" (American
  Diabetes Association) 226n
insulin delivery systems, visual
  impairments 246–49
insulin-dependent diabetes mellitus
  (IDDM) *see* type 1 diabetes mellitus
insulin pens
  defined 544
  described 219
  manufacturers 243–44
insulin pumps
  children 27
  defined 544
  manufacturers 233–38
  overview 232–40
  summertime 155
  supplies 238240
insulin reaction, defined 544
insulin receptors, defined 544
insulin resistance
  defined 544
  described 461
  overview 29–37
"Insulin Resistance and
  Pre-Diabetes" (NIDDK) 29n
insurance coverage
  diabetes care 587–93
  high quality care 577–78
  kidney failure 593–97
intensive therapy, defined 544

intermediate-acting insulin
 defined 544
 described 218, 222
intermittent claudication,
 defined 544
International Diabetes Federation
 contact information 561
 obesity, diabetes publication 293n
International Pemphigus and
 Pemphigoid Foundation,
 steroid-induced diabetes
 publication 63n
International Society for Pediatric
 and Adolescent Diabetes (ISPAD)
 website address 60
intramuscular injections,
 defined 544
islet cell autoantibodies (ICA),
 defined 544–45
Islet Cell Resource Centers (ICR)
 486
islets, defined 545
islet transplantation
 defined 545
 overview 461–65
Islet Transplantation Trials for
 Type 1 Diabetes 486
ISPAD *see* International Society for
 Pediatric and Adolescent Diabetes
Ivarsson, Sten 499

J

Jackson, Richard 580–82, 584
jejunostomy tube, described 363
jet injector, defined 545
Joslin, Elliott P. 579
Joslin Diabetes Center
 contact information 573
 publications
  carbohydrate counting 111n
  glycemic index 118n
  meal planning 109n
"Just the Facts: Skin and Hair
 Problems on Dialysis" (Life Options
 Rehabilitation Program) 447n
juvenile diabetes mellitus *see* type 1
 diabetes mellitus

Juvenile Diabetes Research
 Foundation International
 contact information 561

K

ketoacidosis
 described 79–80
 diabetes 20
ketones
 defined 545
 tests 194–95
 type 1 diabetes mellitus 25
ketonuria, defined 545
ketosis, defined 545
kidney disease
 anemia 333–34
 diabetes statistics 19
 overview 318–21
 preventive care 21
"Kidney Disease of Diabetes"
 (NIDDK) 318n
kidney disorders
 blood urea nitrogen 196–97
 creatinine 199
 glomerular filtration rate 207–8
kidney failure (renal failure)
 cookbooks 555–58
 defined 545
 described 318, 331
 treatment overview 399–411
 see also end-stage renal disease
"Kidney Failure: Choosing a
 Treatment That's Right for You"
 (NIDDK) 399n
kidney pancreas transplantation,
 overview 457–60
kidneys
 defined 545
 depicted *389*
 described 329–30
 overview 387–97
kidney transplantation
 depicted *409*
 kidney failure 397
 overview 407–10,
  451–56
Kordella, Terri 498n

Kt/V 423–26, 445
Kussmaul breathing, defined 545

L

LADA *see* latent autoimmune
diabetes in adults
lancets
blood glucose meter 211
defined 545
lanthanum carbonate 377
Lantus (glargine insulin) 218
laser surgery, diabetic
retinopathy 371–73
latent autoimmune diabetes in
adults (LADA), defined 545
latent diabetes *see* impaired
glucose tolerance
LEAP *see* Lower Extremity
Amputation Prevention Program
legislation
health insurance coverage 589
hospitalizations 590
lente insulin, defined 546
Lernmark, Åke 498–501
Levemir (detemir insulin) 218, 222
Levitra (vardenafil) 358
LifeMed Media, Inc.
contact information 561
publications
alcohol use 119n
depression 381n
peripheral vascular disease 307n
Life Options, contact information 561
Life Options Rehabilitation Program
contact information 597
dialysis side effects publication
447n
lifestyle changes
obesity 295
osteoporosis 379
physical activity 127–28
type 2 diabetes mellitus 40
L insulin, defined 546
lipid profile, defined 546
lipoatrophy, defined 546
lipodystrophy, defined 546
lipohypertrophy, defined 546

lipoic acid 277
lispro insulin
defined 546
described 217–19, *222*, 222–23
Lloyd, Cathy 505n
long-acting insulin
defined 546
described 218, 222
Look AHEAD *see* Action for
Health in Diabetes
losartan 320
low blood sugar *see* hypoglycemia
Lower Extremity Amputation
Prevention Program (LEAP),
contact information 591
lumbosacral plexus neuropathy
see proximal neuropathy
Lyrica (pregabalin) 357

M

macrosomia, defined 546
macular edema 370–72
magnesium 279–80
managed care, described 589
Massachusetts General Hospital
DERC, contact information 573–74
maturity-onset diabetes of the young
(MODY)
defined 546
described 55–57
genes *57*
McCarren, Marie 256n
meal plans
carbohydrate counting 109–19,
116
described 76, 94–95
diabetes control 175–76
gestational diabetes 51, 53
overview 104–26
meats, meal plans 98
Medicaid
described 588
kidney failure assistance 595
medical care, high quality 577–86
Medicare
described 587–88
kidney failure assistance 593–94

medications
  daily guidelines 78–79
  diabetes insipidus 70–71
  hypertension 320, 504
  hypoglycemia 286–87
  insulin resistance 36
  maturity-onset diabetes
    of the young 58
  osteoporosis 380
  overview 256–62
  peripheral vascular disease 308
  polycystic ovary syndrome 344
  stroke 305
  type 2 diabetes mellitus 45
meglitinides 36, 258, 546, 549
melphalan 325
membranous nephropathy,
  nephrotic syndrome 327
men
  androgen deprivation therapy
    492–93
  diabetes statistics 12
metabolic syndrome
  defined 546
  described 31, *300*
metabolism, defined 547
Metaglip (glipizide, metformin) 261
metformin 36–37, 258, 261–64, 267,
  525–28, 547
metoclopramide 362
Mexican Americans, diabetes
  statistics 9
mexiletine 356
mg/dL, defined 547
Michigan Diabetes Research
  and Training Center
  described 569
  publications
    emotional concerns 150n
    fast food 124n
    hypertension, diabetes 315n
    syringe reuse 250n
    winter preparations 152n
microalbumin, defined 547
"Microalbumin and
  Microalbumin/Creatinine Ratio"
  (American Association for Clinical
  Chemistry) 203n
microalbumin/creatinine ratio 203–6

microalbumin tests
  kidney problems 86, 391–92
  overview 203–6
microalbuminuria, described 319
Micronase (glyburide) 259, 262
miglitol 257, 262, 547
mild nonproliferative retinopathy,
  described 366
milk
  food pyramid 105, 106, *107*
  meal plans 97–98
minimally invasive glucose meters
  215–16
MiniMed Continuous Glucose
  Monitoring System 216
mixed dose, defined 547
mmol/L, defined 547
moderate nonproliferative
  retinopathy, described 366
MODY *see* maturity-onset diabetes
  of the young
"Mom's Antibodies: A Risk for
  Type 1?" (Kordella) 498n
monofilament
  defined 547
  neuropathy 309
"Monogenic Forms of Diabetes:
  Neonatal Diabetes Mellitus and
  Maturity-Onset Diabetes of the
  Young" (NIDDK) 55n
mononeuropathy, defined 547
mouth care, overview 141–44
mouth infections, diabetes 89
Muse (alprostadil) 358
mycophenolate mofetil 480

N

NAAC *see* National Anemia
  Action Council
Nabel, Elizabeth G. 481
nateglinide 258, 262, 547–48
National Anemia Action Council
  (NAAC), anemia publication 333n
National Center for Chronic Disease
  Prevention and Health Promotion,
  diabetes knowledge publication
  469n

National Center for Complementary and Alternative Medicine (NCCAM), diabetes CAM treatment publication 273n

National Certification Board for Diabetes Educators, contact information 561–62

National Committee for Quality Assurance (NCQA), contact information 589

National Diabetes Education Program (NDEP)
contact information 562
publications
meal planning guide 104n
travel information 159n

National Diabetes Information Clearinghouse (NDIC)
contact information 562
publications
CAM therapies 273n
diet and nutrition, hemodialysis 429n
heart disease, diabetes 297n
hypoglycemia 285n
stroke, diabetes 297n

"National Diabetes Statistics" (NIDDK) 11n, 18n

National Digestive Diseases Information Clearinghouse, contact information 562

National Eye Institute
contact information 562
diabetic retinopathy publication 365n

National Heart, Lung, and Blood Institute (NHLBI)
contact information 562
hypertension medications publication 504n

National Human Genome Research Institute, contact information 59–60

National Institute of Arthritis and Musculoskeletal and Skin Diseases (NIAMS), osteoporosis, diabetes publication 375n

National Institute of Child Health and Human Development (NICHD)
contact information 562
polycystic ovary syndrome publication 343n

National Institute of Diabetes and Digestive and Kidney Diseases (NIDDK)
contact information 562
publications
amyloidosis 324n
control measures 172n
costs, complications 18n
diabetes dictionary 533n
diabetes guidelines 75n
diabetes management 145n
diabetes overview 3n
diabetes prevention program 525n
diabetes research 479n
diabetes statistics 11n
diabetic neuropathies 347n
diet and nutrition, hemodialysis 429n
dietary guidelines 91n
financial assistance 587n
foot care 135n
gastroparesis 359n
gestational diabetes 47n
glomerular diseases 329n
hemodialysis 414n
hemodialysis dose, adequacy 422n
insulin resistance 29n
kidney damage 318n
kidney failure 399n
kidney transplantation 451n
monogenic forms 55n
nephrotic syndrome 327n
oral care 141n
pancreatic islet transplantation 461n
peritoneal dialysis 436n
peritoneal dialysis dose, adequacy 444n
pre-diabetes 29n
proteinuria 322n
renal osteodystrophy 375n

National Institute of Diabetes and
  Digestive and Kidney Diseases
  (NIDDK) publications, continued
    sexual problems 337n
    skin care 135n
    type 2 diabetes 39n
    urological problems 337n
    vascular access,
      hemodialysis 418n
National Institutes of Health
  (NIH), publications
  clinical trials 479n
  diabetes insipidus 67n
  diabetes knowledge 469n
National Kidney and Urologic
  Diseases Information
  Clearinghouse, contact
  information 563
National Kidney Disease
  Education Program
  contact information 563
  glomerular filtration rate
    publication 207n
National Kidney Foundation,
  contact information 563, 597
Native Americans
  foot ulcers 309
  kidney disorders 318
Native Hawaiians, diabetes
  statistics 13
NCQA *see* National Committee
  for Quality Assurance
NDEP *see* National Diabetes
  Education Program
NDIC *see* National Diabetes
  Information Clearinghouse
NDM *see* neonatal diabetes
  mellitus
necrobiosis lipoidica diabeticorum,
  defined 548
needle disposal 227, 232, 251–54
Nemours Foundation, type 1
  diabetes publication 23n
neonatal diabetes mellitus (NDM)
  described 55–56
  genes 57
nephrogenic diabetes insipidus,
  described 68–69
nephrologists, defined 548

nephrons
  depicted *389*
  described 387
  kidney failure 390
nephropathy
  defined 548
  described 318
nephrotic syndrome, overview
  327–28
"Nephrotic Syndrome in Adults"
  (NIDDK) 327n
nerve compressions, described 353
nerve conduction studies,
  defined 548
nerve damage
  decreased vaginal lubrication
    339
  feet 136, 138
  high blood glucose 87
  sweating 139, 352
nervous system disease, diabetes
  statistics 19
neurogenic bladder, described
  340–41
neurologists, defined 548
neuropathy
  alcohol use 314
  monofilament 309
  overview 347–49
  see also autonomic neuropathy;
    background neuropathy; focal
    neuropathy; mononeuropathy;
    peripheral neuropathy;
    proximal neuropathy
"News and Information: Diabetes
  Care Better Than 10 Years Ago,
  But More Improvement Needed"
  (National Center for Chronic
  Disease Prevention and Health
  Promotion) 469n
NHLBI *see* National Heart, Lung,
  and Blood Institute
"NHLBI Media Availability:
  Greater Diabetes Risk in Patients
  Taking High Blood Pressure
  Medications" (NHLBI) 504n
NHPCSG *see* Non-Human Primate
  Transplantation Tolerance
  Cooperative Study Group

NIAMS *see* National Institute of
Arthritis and Musculoskeletal
and Skin Diseases
NICHD *see* National Institute
of Child Health and Human
Development
NIDDK *see* National Institute
of Diabetes and Digestive and
Kidney Diseases
NIDDM (noninsulin-dependent
diabetes mellitus) *see* type 2
diabetes mellitus
NIH *see* National Institutes of Health
nitrogen production 196
Non-Human Primate
Transplantation Tolerance
Cooperative Study Group
(NHPCSG) 486
noninsulin-dependent diabetes
mellitus (NIDDM) *see* type 2
diabetes mellitus
noninvasive blood glucose
monitoring, defined 548
non-invasive glucose meters 215–16
nonsteroidal anti-inflammatory
drugs (NSAID), neuropathies 356
nortriptyline 356
NovoLog (aspart insulin) 219,
222–23
NPH insulin
defined 548
described 218–19, *222*, 222–23
NSAID *see* nonsteroidal anti-
inflammatory drugs
Nutritional Intervention to Prevent
Type 1 Diabetes (NIP) Trial 480
Nutrition Facts labels 122

O

obesity
defined 548
diabetes 293–95
insulin 29
Office of Minority Health Resource
Center, contact information 563
OGTT *see* oral glucose tolerance test
omega-3 fatty acids 280–81

"One-Third of Adults with Diabetes
Still Don't Know They Have It"
(DHHS) 8n
Online Mendelian Inheritance in
Man, website address 60
OPO *see* organ procurement
organizations
oral glucose tolerance test (OGTT)
defined 548–49
gestational diabetes 49
overview 184–91
results meanings *188*
oral hypoglycemic agents,
defined 549
oral insulin, research 479–80
"Ordering Fast-Food Wisely"
(Michigan Diabetes Research
and Training Center) 124n
organ donations, kidney
transplantation 455–56
organ procurement organizations
(OPO) 453
Orinase (tolbutamide) 552
osteoporosis, overview 377–80
overweight
defined 549
diabetes 293–95
diabetes control 178
foot ulcers 309
gestational diabetes 48
insulin 29
type 2 diabetes mellitus 41–42

P

Pacific Islanders
diabetes statistics 13
gestational diabetes 48
insulin resistance 32
type 2 diabetes 41
pain management,
neuropathies 356
pancreas
artificial 27
defined 549
depicted *462*
described 3, 285
insulin 29–30

619

pancreas, continued
  type 1 diabetes mellitus 24
  type 2 diabetes mellitus 39
pancreas kidney transplantation
  457–60
pancreatic islet transplantation
  defined 545
  overview 461–65
"Pancreatic Islet Transplantation"
  (NIDDK) 461n
parathyroid hormone (PTH) 376
parenteral nutrition,
  gastroparesis 363
PCOS *see* polycystic ovary
  syndrome
Pedorthic Footwear Association,
  contact information 563
pemphigus 64
pentoxifylline 308
periodontal disease, diabetes
  statistics 19–20
peripheral arterial disease (PAD),
  described 297, 303, 307
peripheral neuropathy
  affected nerves 349, *351*
  defined 549
  described 347, 349–50
peripheral vascular disease (PVD)
  defined 549
  described 136
  overview 307–8
"Peripheral Vascular Disease and
  Diabetes" (LifeMed Media, Inc.)
  307n
peritoneal dialysis
  defined 539, 549
  depicted *404*
  described 396–97
  dose, adequacy 444–46
  overview 403–6, 436–43
  see also dialysis; hemodialysis
"Peritoneal Dialysis Dose and
  Adequacy" (NIDDK) 444n
permanent neonatal diabetes
  mellitus (PNDM), genes *57*
perspiration
  autonomic neuropathy 352
  insulin pumps 155
  nerve damage 139

PhosLo (calcium acetate) 377
phosphorus
  hemodialysis 432
  renal osteodystrophy 376–77
physical activity
  daily guidelines 77, 92–93,
    127–34
  gestational diabetes 51
  insulin resistance 33–34
  summertime 154–55
  type 2 diabetes mellitus 44–45
  see also exercise
physicians, high quality care 578–81
Pichert, James 571
pioglitazone 260–64, 267, 549, 552
plantar warts, described 138
Pletal (cilostazol) 308
PNDM *see* permanent neonatal
  diabetes mellitus
pneumococcal vaccine,
  described 270
podiatrists
  defined 549
  described 138
  foot care 313–14
point system, defined 549
polycystic ovary syndrome (PCOS)
  overview 343–45
  type 2 diabetes mellitus 42
"Polycystic Ovary Syndrome
  (PCOS)" (NIDDK) 343n
polydipsia
  defined 549
  diabetes insipidus 68–69
polygenic forms of diabetes,
  described 55
polyphagia, defined 549
polyuria
  defined 550
  diabetes insipidus 68–69
postprandial blood glucose
  defined 550
  diabetes treatment 180
potassium
  hemodialysis 431
  kidney disease 395–96
pramlintide acetate 224
Prandin (repaglinide) 258, 262
Precose (acarbose) 257, 262

pre-diabetes
  defined 550
  described 3–4, 30
  gestational diabetes 48
  overview 29–37
  statistics 10
  type 2 diabetes mellitus 40
  see also impaired glucose
    tolerance
prednisone 325
pregabalin 357
pregnancy
  blood glucose meter 210
  blood glucose test 185–86
  diabetes care 148
  diabetes research 498–501
  gestational diabetes 5, 47–53
  ketone testing 195
pregnancy complications,
  diabetes statistics 20
premixed insulin, defined 550
preprandial blood glucose
  defined 550
  diabetes treatment 180
"Prevent Diabetes Problems: Keep
  You Feet and Skin Healthy"
  (NIDDK) 135n
"Prevent Diabetes Problems: Keep
  Your Diabetes Under Control"
  (NIDDK) 172n
"Prevent Diabetes Problems: Keep
  You Teeth and Gums Healthy"
  (NIDDK) 141n
primary amyloidosis 325
Prograf (tacrolimus) 464–65
proinsulin, defined 550
proliferative retinopathy
  defined 550
  described 367
prosthetics, financial
  considerations 591
"Protect Yourself, Protect Others:
  Safe Options for Home Needle
  Disposal" (EPA) 251n
protein
  defined 550
  hemodialysis 432
  kidney disease 391–92, 395
protein catabolism 197

proteinuria
  amyloidosis 325
  defined 550
  described 330, 391–92
  overview 322–24
"Proteinuria" (NIDDK) 322n
proximal neuropathy
  affected nerves 349
  described 349, 352
PTH *see* parathyroid hormone
PVD *see* peripheral vascular
  disease

Q

QST *see* quantitative sensory
  testing
quantitative sensory testing
  (QST), neuropathies 354
"Questions and Answers About
  Diabetes in the Workplace and the
  Americans with Disabilities Act
  (ADA)" (EEOC) 162n
Quickel, Kenneth E., Jr.
  579–81

R

racial factor
  diabetes 16–17
  diabetes statistics 8–9, 12–13
  insulin resistance 32
radioisotope gastric-emptying
  scan, gastroparesis 360–61
raloxifene 380
Rapamune (sirolimus) 464–65
rapid-acting insulin
  defined 550
  described 222
reactive hypoglycemia,
  described 289–90
reagents, test strips 213
reasonable accommodations,
  diabetes 164–65
rebound hyperglycemia,
  defined 550
  see also Somogyi effect

"Recipe and Meal Planner Guide" (NDEP) 104n
recipe planning guide 104–7
Recognized Diabetes Education Programs, defined 550
record keeping
  daily record page *81*
  diabetes control 175
reduced glomerular filtration rate, described 330
Reglan (metoclopramide) 362
regular insulin
  defined 550
  described 222
relaxation therapy
  neuropathies 356
  stress 515
Renagel (sevelamer hydrochloride) 377
renal, defined 551
renal failure *see* end-stage renal disease; kidney failure
renal function, described 389–90
"Renal Osteodystrophy" (NIDDK) 375n
renal osteodystrophy, described 375–77
renal rickets, described 375
renal threshold of glucose, defined 551
renin, described 388
repaglinide 258, 262, 551
research overview, diabetes mellitus 469–87
"Research Programs: Diabetes" (NIDDK) 479n
retina, defined 551
  see also diabetic retinopathy
retrograde ejaculation, described 338–39
R insulin, defined 550
Riomet (metformin) 258, 262
risedronate 380
rituximab 480
Rodgers, Griffin P. 496
rosiglitazone 260–64, 267, 551, 552
Royal Devon and Exeter Hospital, website address 60

S

SAD *see* seasonal affective disorder
safety considerations, needle disposal 251–54
St. John's wort 383
salt *see* sodium
Saudek, Christopher D. 63n
SCHIP *see* State Children's Health Insurance Program
Schlundt, David 571
screening glucose challenge test, gestational diabetes 49
SEARCH for Diabetes in Youth 486
seasonal affective disorder (SAD) 153
seasonal changes, diabetes 152–55
secondary diabetes, defined 551
selenium supplements, type 2 diabetes mellitus research 496–97
self-management
  defined 551
  diabetes care 15, 186
self-monitoring of blood glucose (SMBG)
  described 192–93
  overview 209–16
Sensipar (cinacalcet hydrochloride) 377
serving sizes, depicted *100*
sevelamer hydrochloride 377
70/30 insulin, defined 551
severe nonproliferative retinopathy, described 367
"Sexual and Urological Problems of Diabetes" (NIDDK) 337n
sexual problems
  autonomic neuropathy 352
  diabetes 337–39, 342
  neuropathies 357
sharps containers
  defined 551
  described 227, 232
  travel concerns 254
SHEP *see* Systolic Hypertension in the Elderly Program

shoes
  diabetics 137–38, *139*
  foot care 313–14
  neuropathies 356
short-acting insulin
  defined 551
  described 218
"Should I Count Calories or Use
  Exchanges for My Meal Planning
  Approach?" (Joslin Diabetes
  Center) 109n
sildenafil 358
sirolimus 464–65
sitagliptin 266
skin care
  dialysis 447–50
  overview 139–40
  wintertime 153
Skyler, Jay 480
sliding scale, defined 551
SMBG *see* self-monitoring of blood
  glucose
Smith, Julie 505n
smoking cessation
  diabetes control 174, 176
  foot care 313
  insulin resistance 36
Social Security Disability
  Insurance (SSDI), contact
  information 595
sodium (salt)
  hemodialysis 432
  kidney disease 395
  Nutrition Facts labels 122–23
Somogyi effect, defined 551
sorbitol, defined 552
split mixed dose, defined 552
SSDI *see* Social Security Disability
  Insurance
SSI *see* Supplemental Security
  Income
starches
  food pyramid 105, 106, *107*
  meal plans 95–96
Starlix (nateglinide) 258, 262,
  547–48
State Children's Health Insurance
  Program (SCHIP), contact
  information 588, 595

statistics
  anemia 333
  depression 381–82
  diabetes mellitus 8–21
  gestational diabetes 47
  kidney disorders 318
  neuropathies 347
  osteoporosis 377
Steiner, Donald 567
stents, peripheral vascular
  disease 308
"Steroid-Induced Diabetes"
  (Saudek) 63n
steroid-induced diabetes,
  overview 63–65
strength training, suggestions
  129–30
stress, diabetes research 505–23
"Stress and Diabetes: A Review
  of the Links" (Lloyd, et al.) 505n
stroke
  diabetes 297–305
  diabetes statistics 18
  see also transient ischemic attack
"Stronger Heart Warnings on
  Diabetes Drugs" (FDA) 267n
"Studies Test New Approaches to
  Islet Transplantation" (*Diabetes
  Dateline*) 479n
"Study Tests Oral Insulin to
  Prevent Type 1 Diabetes"
  (*Diabetes Dateline*) 479n
subclinical diabetes
  see impaired glucose tolerance
sucrose, defined 552
sugar diabetes *see* diabetes mellitus
sulfonylureas 36, 259–60, 549, 552
"Summaries for Patients:
  Long-Term Use of Selenium
  Supplements and Risk for Type 2
  Diabetes" (American College of
  Physicians) 496n
Supplemental Security Income
  (SSI), contact information 595
surgical procedures
  diabetic retinopathy 371–73
  erectile dysfunction 338
  foot ulcers 311
  peripheral vascular disease 308

sweets
  carbohydrate counting 118
  food pyramid 105, 106, *107*
  meal plans 98–99
Symlin (pramlintide acetate) 224
Syndrome X *see* metabolic syndrome
syringes
  defined 552
  manufacturers *228–31*
  overview 226–32
  reuse guidelines 250–51
  safe disposal 251–54
  U-500 insulin 220
Systolic Hypertension in the
  Elderly Program (SHEP) 504

T

T1DGC *see* Type 1 Diabetes
  Genetics Consortium
tacrolimus 464–65
tadalafil 358
"Take Charge of Your Diabetes"
  (CDC) 269n
Targeting Inflammation Using
  Salsalate for Type 2 Diabetes
  (TINSAL-T2D) 486–87
team management, defined 552
TEDDY *see* The Environmental
  Determinant of Diabetes
  in the Young
teeth
  daily guidelines 89
  proper care 141–44
TENS *see* transcutaneous
  electrical nerve stimulation
teriparatide 380
tests
  daily guidelines 79–80
  diabetes insipidus 69–70
  diabetic retinopathy 370–71
  gastroparesis 360–61
  gestational diabetes 49–50
  insulin resistance 32–33
  kidney disease 391–93
  kidney problems 86
  neuropathies 354
  peritoneal dialysis 445–46

tests, continued
  pre-diabetes 30
  questions and answers 177–79
  recommended frequency 176–77,
    181–82
  type 2 diabetes mellitus 41
  urinary tract infections
    341–42
  see also blood urea nitrogen;
    fasting blood glucose test;
    fructosamine test; glomerular
    filtration rate; glycosylated
    hemoglobin test; hemoglobin
    A1C test; impaired fasting
    glucose; lipid profile; nerve
    conduction studies;
    oral glucose tolerance test;
    urinalysis
test strips, blood glucose meter 211,
  213
tetanus/diphtheria (Td) toxoid
  270–71
thiazide 70
thiazolidinediones (TZD) 36, 260,
  549, 552
thioctic acid 277
thrifty gene, described 16
TINSAL-T2D *see* Targeting
  Inflammation Using Salsalate
  for Type 2 Diabetes
TNDM *see* transient neonatal
  diabetes mellitus
tobacco use
  diabetes control 174, 176
  heart disease 299
  kidney disease 395
TODAY (Treatment Options for
  type 2 Diabetes in Adolescents
  and Youth) Trial 487
tolazamide 260, 552
tolbutamide 260, 552
Tolinase (tolazamide) 552
tonometry, diabetic retinopathy
  371
Topamax (topiramate) 357
topiramate 357
transcutaneous electrical nerve
  stimulation (TENS)
  neuropathies 356

transient ischemic attack (TIA),
   described 301
   see also stroke
transient neonatal diabetes mellitus
   (TNDM), genes 57
Transportation Security
   Administration (TSA), website
   address 254
travel concerns
   automobile driving 156–58
   diabetes care 147–48
   needle disposal 254
   overview 159–61
"Treating Type 2 Diabetes
   with Dietary Supplements"
   (NCCAM) 273n
"Treatment Methods for
   Kidney Failure: Hemodialysis"
   (NIDDK) 414n
"Treatment Methods for Kidney
   Failure: Peritoneal Dialysis"
   (NIDDK) 436n
"Treatment Methods for Kidney
   Failure: Transplantation"
   (NIDDK) 451n
Trental (pentoxifylline) 308
TrialNet studies 479–80, 487
Trial to Reduce IDDM in the
   Genetically at Risk (TRIGR) 487
triglycerides, defined 552
TRIGR *see* Trial to Reduce
   IDDM in the Genetically at Risk
troglitazone 36
TSA *see* Transportation Security
   Administration
tubules, described 388
Tums (calcium carbonate) 377
Type 1 Diabetes Genetics
   Consortium (T1DGC) 487
type 1 diabetes mellitus
   children 17
   defined 553
   described 4
   heredity 16
   osteoporosis 378
   overview 23–27
   research 471–74
   see also latent autoimmune
      diabetes in adults
Type 1 Diabetes TrialNet 479–80,
   487
"Type 1 Diabetes: What Is It?"
   (Nemours Foundation) 23n
type 2 diabetes mellitus
   children 17
   defined 553
   described 4–5
   oral medications 257–61
   overview 39–45
   research 474–78
   selenium supplements 496–97
TZD *see* thiazolidinediones

U

UKPDS *see* United Kingdom
   Prospective Diabetes Study
ultralente insulin, defined 553
ultrasound
   gastroparesis 361
   neuropathies 354
"Understanding GFR: A Guide
   for Patients" (National Kidney
   Disease Education Program) 207n
United Kingdom Prospective
   Diabetes Study (UKPDS) 553
United Network for Organ Sharing
   (UNOS), contact information 596
unit of insulin, defined 553
University of Chicago DRTC 567–69,
   572
University of Colorado DERC,
   contact information 574
University of Iowa DERC, contact
   information 574
University of Massachusetts Medical
   School DERC, contact information
   574
University of Michigan DRTC 569,
   572
University of Pennsylvania DERC,
   contact information 574
University of Washington DERC,
   contact information 574
UNOS *see* United Network for
   Organ Sharing
upper endoscopy, gastroparesis 361

urea, defined 553
urea nitrogen 196
uremia, defined 553
urinalysis
  defined 553
  described 186, 190
urinary tract infections (UTI),
  described 341–42
urine osmolality test, diabetes
  insipidus 70
urine specific gravity test,
  diabetes insipidus 70
urine testing
  defined 553
  described 186, 190
  ketones 79
  kidney disease 393
  microalbumin 203–6
  retrograde ejaculation 339
urological problems, diabetes 340–42
URR (urea reduction result) 422–26
US Department of Health and
  Human Services (DHHS; HHS),
  publications
  physical activity guidelines 127n
  pre-diabetes 8n
  sodium intake 122n
US Department of Veterans
  Affairs (VA)
  A1C testing publication 191n
  contact information 560, 590
US Environmental Protection
  Agency (EPA), needle disposal
  safety publication 251n
US Food and Drug Administration
  (FDA), publications
  blood glucose self-monitoring 209n
  medication labels 267n
UTI *see* urinary tract infections

V

VA *see* US Department of
  Veterans Affairs
vaccinations, overview 269–71
vaginal yeast infections, type 1
  diabetes mellitus 25
vagus nerve, gastroparesis 359

vanadium, blood glucose 274
Vanderbilt University DRTC 569–71,
  572–73
vardenafil 358
vascular access
  hemodialysis 400–401, 415
  overview 418–22
"Vascular Access for Hemodialysis"
  (NIDDK) 418n
vasopressin, diabetes insipidus 67
vasopressin test, diabetes insipidus
  69–70
vegetables
  food pyramid 105, 106, *107*
  meal plans 96–97
venlafaxine 357
venous catheter
  depicted *420*
  described 420–21
very-long-acting insulin, defined 554
Viagra (sildenafil) 358
Vietnam veterans, diabetes
  mellitus 17
vildagliptin 266
visual acuity test, diabetic
  retinopathy 370
visual impairments, insulin
  delivery systems 246–49
vitrectomy, diabetic retinopathy
  371–73

W

waiting list
  kidney pancreas transplantation
    458
  kidney transplantation 452
Walker, Elizabeth A. 566
Washington University DRTC
  571–72, 573
water deprivation test, diabetes
  insipidus 69
water pills *see* diuretics
Weight-control Information Network
  (WIN), contact information 563
weight loss
  diabetes control 175–76
  foot care 313

weight loss, continued
   insulin resistance 33
   type 2 diabetes mellitus 39–40,
      44, 178
Weinger, Katie 505n
"What I Need to Know about Eating
   and Diabetes" (NIDDK) 91n
"What I Need to Know about
   Gestational Diabetes" (NIDDK) 47n
"What I Need to Know about
   Physical Activity and Diabetes"
   (NIDDK) 127n
"What Is a Kidney Pancreas
   Transplant?" (Cleveland Clinic)
   457n
"What Is the Glycemic Index and
   Is It a Helpful Tool?" (Joslin
   Diabetes Center) 118n
"What People with Diabetes Need
   to Know about Osteoporosis"
   (NIAMS) 375n
"While Most Diabetes Drugs
   Provide Similar Glucose Control,
   Some Offer Important Advantages,
   New Review Shows" (AHRQ) 262n
Whipple triad 186
WIC at FNS Headquarters, contact
   information 592

WIN *see* Weight-control Information
   Network
women
   diabetes, heart disease 297–98
   diabetes risk factors research
      490–91
   diabetes statistics 12, 15–16
workplace, diabetes 162–65
wound care
   defined 554
   foot ulcers 309–14

Y

Yale University School of Medicine
   DERC, contact information 575
"Your Guide to Diabetes: Type 1
   and Type 2" (NIDDK) 3n, 75n,
   145n
"Your Podiatric Physician Talks
   About Diabetic Wound Care"
   (APMA) 309n

Z

Zenapax (daclizumab) 464–65

Health Reference Series
COMPLETE CATALOG

List price $87 per volume. **School and library price $78 per volume.**

Adolescent Health Sourcebook, 2nd Edition

Basic Consumer Health Information about the Physical, Mental, and Emotional Growth and Development of Adolescents, Including Medical Care, Nutritional and Physical Activity Requirements, Puberty, Sexual Activity, Acne, Tanning, Body Piercing, Common Physical Illnesses and Disorders, Eating Disorders, Attention Deficit Hyperactivity Disorder, Depression, Bullying, Hazing, and Adolescent Injuries Related to Sports, Driving, and Work

Along with Substance Abuse Information about Nicotine, Alcohol, and Drug Use, a Glossary, and Directory of Additional Resources

Edited by Joyce Brennfleck Shannon. 683 pages. 2006. 978-0-7808-0943-7.

"It is written in clear, nontechnical language aimed at general readers. . . . Recommended for public libraries, community colleges, and other agencies serving health care consumers."
— *American Reference Books Annual, 2003*

"Recommended for school and public libraries. Parents and professionals dealing with teens will appreciate the easy-to-follow format and the clearly written text. This could become a 'must have' for every high school teacher." — *E-Streams, Jan '03*

"A good starting point for information related to common medical, mental, and emotional concerns of adolescents." — *School Library Journal, Nov '02*

"This book provides accurate information in an easy to access format. It addresses topics that parents and caregivers might not be aware of and provides practical, useable information."
— *Doody's Health Sciences Book Review Journal, Sep-Oct '02*

"Recommended reference source."
— *Booklist, American Library Association, Sep '02*

AIDS Sourcebook, 3rd Edition

Basic Consumer Health Information about Acquired Immune Deficiency Syndrome (AIDS) and Human Immunodeficiency Virus (HIV) Infection, Including Facts about Transmission, Prevention, Diagnosis, Treatment, Opportunistic Infections, and Other Complications, with a Section for Women and Children, Including Details about Associated Gynecological Concerns, Pregnancy, and Pediatric Care

Along with Updated Statistical Information, Reports on Current Research Initiatives, a Glossary, and Directories of Internet, Hotline, and Other Resources

Edited by Dawn D. Matthews. 664 pages. 2003. 978-0-7808-0631-3.

"The 3rd edition of the *AIDS Sourcebook*, part of Omnigraphics' *Health Reference Series*, is a welcome update. . . . This resource is highly recommended for academic and public libraries."
— *American Reference Books Annual, 2004*

"Excellent sourcebook. This continues to be a highly recommended book. There is no other book that provides as much information as this book provides."
— *AIDS Book Review Journal, Dec-Jan '00*

"Recommended reference source."
— *Booklist, American Library Association, Dec '99*

Alcoholism Sourcebook, 2nd Edition

Basic Consumer Health Information about Alcohol Use, Abuse, and Dependence, Featuring Facts about the Physical, Mental, and Social Health Effects of Alcohol Addiction, Including Alcoholic Liver Disease, Pancreatic Disease, Cardiovascular Disease, Neurological Disorders, and the Effects of Drinking during Pregnancy

Along with Information about Alcohol Treatment, Medications, and Recovery Programs, in Addition to Tips for Reducing the Prevalence of Underage Drinking, Statistics about Alcohol Use, a Glossary of Related Terms, and Directories of Resources for More Help and Information

Edited by Amy L. Sutton. 653 pages. 2006. 978-0-7808-0942-0.

"This title is one of the few reference works on alcoholism for general readers. For some readers this will be a welcome complement to the many self-help books on the market. Recommended for collections serving general readers and consumer health collections."
— *E-Streams, Mar '01*

"This book is an excellent choice for public and academic libraries."
— *American Reference Books Annual, 2001*

"Recommended reference source."
— *Booklist, American Library Association, Dec '00*

"Presents a wealth of information on alcohol use and abuse and its effects on the body and mind, treatment, and prevention." — *SciTech Book News, Dec '00*

"Important new health guide which packs in the latest consumer information about the problems of alcoholism." — *Reviewer's Bookwatch, Nov '00*

SEE ALSO Drug Abuse Sourcebook

Allergies Sourcebook, 3rd Edition

Basic Consumer Health Information about Allergic Disorders, Such as Anaphylaxis, Hives, Eczema, Rhinitis, Sinusitis, and Conjunctivitis, and Their Triggers, Including Pollen, Mold, Dust Mites, Animal Dander, Insects, Chemicals, Food, Food Additives, and Medications;

Along with Advice about the Diagnosis and Treatment of Allergy Symptoms, a Glossary of Related Terms, a Directory of Resources for Help and Information, and Suggestions for Additional Reading

Edited by Amy L. Sutton. 598 pages. 2007. 978-0-7808-0950-5.

"This book brings a great deal of useful material together. . . . This is an excellent addition to public and consumer health library collections."
— *American Reference Books Annual, 2003*

"This second edition would be useful to laypersons with little or advanced knowledge of the subject matter. This book would also serve as a resource for nursing and other health care professions students. It would be useful in public, academic, and hospital libraries with consumer health collections." — *E-Streams, Jul '02*

Alternative Medicine Sourcebook

SEE Complementary & Alternative Medicine Sourcebook

Alzheimer's Disease Sourcebook, 3rd Edition

Basic Consumer Health Information about Alzheimer's Disease, Other Dementias, and Related Disorders, Including Multi-Infarct Dementia, AIDS Dementia Complex, Dementia with Lewy Bodies, Huntington's Disease, Wernicke-Korsakoff Syndrome (Alcohol-Related Dementia), Delirium, and Confusional States

Along with Information for People Newly Diagnosed with Alzheimer's Disease and Caregivers, Reports Detailing Current Research Efforts in Prevention, Diagnosis, and Treatment, Facts about Long-Term Care Issues, and Listings of Sources for Additional Information

Edited by Karen Bellenir. 645 pages. 2003. 978-0-7808-0666-5.

"This very informative and valuable tool will be a great addition to any library serving consumers, students and health care workers."
— *American Reference Books Annual, 2004*

"This is a valuable resource for people affected by dementias such as Alzheimer's. It is easy to navigate and includes important information and resources."
— *Doody's Review Service, Feb '04*

"Recommended reference source."
— *Booklist, American Library Association, Oct '99*

***SEE ALSO** Brain Disorders Sourcebook*

Arthritis Sourcebook, 2nd Edition

Basic Consumer Health Information about Osteoarthritis, Rheumatoid Arthritis, Other Rheumatic Disorders, Infectious Forms of Arthritis, and Diseases with Symptoms Linked to Arthritis, Featuring Facts about Diagnosis, Pain Management, and Surgical Therapies

Along with Coping Strategies, Research Updates, a Glossary, and Resources for Additional Help and Information

Edited by Amy L. Sutton. 593 pages. 2004. 978-0-7808-0667-2.

"This easy-to-read volume is recommended for consumer health collections within public or academic libraries." — *E-Streams, May '05*

"As expected, this updated edition continues the excellent reputation of this series in providing sound, usable health information. . . . Highly recommended."
— *American Reference Books Annual, 2005*

"Excellent reference." — *The Bookwatch, Jan '05*

Asthma Sourcebook, 2nd Edition

Basic Consumer Health Information about the Causes, Symptoms, Diagnosis, and Treatment of Asthma in Infants, Children, Teenagers, and Adults, Including Facts about Different Types of Asthma, Common Co-Occurring Conditions, Asthma Management Plans, Triggers, Medications, and Medication Delivery Devices

Along with Asthma Statistics, Research Updates, a Glossary, a Directory of Asthma-Related Resources, and More

Edited by Karen Bellenir. 609 pages. 2006. 978-0-7808-0866-9.

"A worthwhile reference acquisition for public libraries and academic medical libraries whose readers desire a quick introduction to the wide range of asthma information." — *Choice, Association of College & Research Libraries, Jun '01*

"Recommended reference source."
— *Booklist, American Library Association, Feb '01*

"Highly recommended." — *The Bookwatch, Jan '01*

"There is much good information for patients and their families who deal with asthma daily."
— *American Medical Writers Association Journal, Winter '01*

"This informative text is recommended for consumer health collections in public, secondary school, and community college libraries and the libraries of universities with a large undergraduate population."
— *American Reference Books Annual, 2001*

Attention Deficit Disorder Sourcebook

Basic Consumer Health Information about Attention Deficit/Hyperactivity Disorder in Children and Adults,

Including Facts about Causes, Symptoms, Diagnostic Criteria, and Treatment Options Such as Medications, Behavior Therapy, Coaching, and Homeopathy

Along with Reports on Current Research Initiatives, Legal Issues, and Government Regulations, and Featuring a Glossary of Related Terms, Internet Resources, and a List of Additional Reading Material

Edited by Dawn D. Matthews. 470 pages. 2002. 978-0-7808-0624-5.

"Recommended reference source."
— Booklist, American Library Association, Jan '03

"This book is recommended for all school libraries and the reference or consumer health sections of public libraries." — American Reference Books Annual, 2003

Back & Neck Sourcebook, 2nd Edition

Basic Consumer Health Information about Spinal Pain, Spinal Cord Injuries, and Related Disorders, Such as Degenerative Disk Disease, Osteoarthritis, Scoliosis, Sciatica, Spina Bifida, and Spinal Stenosis, and Featuring Facts about Maintaining Spinal Health, Self-Care, Pain Management, Rehabilitative Care, Chiropractic Care, Spinal Surgeries, and Complementary Therapies

Along with Suggestions for Preventing Back and Neck Pain, a Glossary of Related Terms, and a Directory of Resources

Edited by Amy L. Sutton. 633 pages. 2004. 978-0-7808-0738-9.

"Recommended . . . an easy to use, comprehensive medical reference book." — E-Streams, Sep '05

"The strength of this work is its basic, easy-to-read format. Recommended." — Reference and User Services Quarterly, American Library Association, Winter '97

Blood & Circulatory Disorders Sourcebook, 2nd Edition

Basic Consumer Health Information about the Blood and Circulatory System and Related Disorders, Such as Anemia and Other Hemoglobin Diseases, Cancer of the Blood and Associated Bone Marrow Disorders, Clotting and Bleeding Problems, and Conditions That Affect the Veins, Blood Vessels, and Arteries, Including Facts about the Donation and Transplantation of Bone Marrow, Stem Cells, and Blood and Tips for Keeping the Blood and Circulatory System Healthy

Along with a Glossary of Related Terms and Resources for Additional Help and Information

Edited by Amy L. Sutton. 659 pages. 2005. 978-0-7808-0746-4.

"Highly recommended pick for basic consumer health reference holdings at all levels."
— The Bookwatch, Aug '05

"Recommended reference source."
— Booklist, American Library Association, Feb '99

"An important reference sourcebook written in simple language for everyday, non-technical users. "
— Reviewer's Bookwatch, Jan '99

Brain Disorders Sourcebook, 2nd Edition

Basic Consumer Health Information about Acquired and Traumatic Brain Injuries, Infections of the Brain, Epilepsy and Seizure Disorders, Cerebral Palsy, and Degenerative Neurological Disorders, Including Amyotrophic Lateral Sclerosis (ALS), Dementias, Multiple Sclerosis, and More

Along with Information on the Brain's Structure and Function, Treatment and Rehabilitation Options, Reports on Current Research Initiatives, a Glossary of Terms Related to Brain Disorders and Injuries, and a Directory of Sources for Further Help and Information

Edited by Sandra J. Judd. 625 pages. 2005. 978-0-7808-0744-0.

"Highly recommended pick for basic consumer health reference holdings at all levels."
— The Bookwatch, Aug '05

"Belongs on the shelves of any library with a consumer health collection." — E-Streams, Mar '00

"Recommended reference source."
— Booklist, American Library Association, Oct '99

SEE ALSO Alzheimer's Disease Sourcebook

Breast Cancer Sourcebook, 2nd Edition

Basic Consumer Health Information about Breast Cancer, Including Facts about Risk Factors, Prevention, Screening and Diagnostic Methods, Treatment Options, Complementary and Alternative Therapies, Post-Treatment Concerns, Clinical Trials, Special Risk Populations, and New Developments in Breast Cancer Research

Along with Breast Cancer Statistics, a Glossary of Related Terms, and a Directory of Resources for Additional Help and Information

Edited by Sandra J. Judd. 595 pages. 2004. 978-0-7808-0668-9.

"This book will be an excellent addition to public, community college, medical, and academic libraries."
— American Reference Books Annual, 2006

"It would be a useful reference book in a library or on loan to women in a support group."
— Cancer Forum, Mar '03

"Recommended reference source."
— Booklist, American Library Association, Jan '02

"This reference source is highly recommended. It is quite informative, comprehensive and detailed in nature, and yet it offers practical advice in easy-to-read language. It could be thought of as the 'bible' of breast cancer for the consumer." —*E-Streams, Jan '02*

"From the pros and cons of different screening methods and results to treatment options, *Breast Cancer Sourcebook* provides the latest information on the subject." —*Library Bookwatch, Dec '01*

"This thoroughgoing, very readable reference covers all aspects of breast health and cancer.... Readers will find much to consider here. Recommended for all public and patient health collections." —*Library Journal, Sep '01*

SEE ALSO Cancer Sourcebook for Women, Women's Health Concerns Sourcebook

---

Breastfeeding Sourcebook

Basic Consumer Health Information about the Benefits of Breastmilk, Preparing to Breastfeed, Breastfeeding as a Baby Grows, Nutrition, and More, Including Information on Special Situations and Concerns Such as Mastitis, Illness, Medications, Allergies, Multiple Births, Prematurity, Special Needs, and Adoption

Along with a Glossary and Resources for Additional Help and Information

Edited by Jenni Lynn Colson. 388 pages. 2002. 978-0-7808-0332-9.

"Particularly useful is the information about professional lactation services and chapters on breastfeeding when returning to work.... *Breastfeeding Sourcebook* will be useful for public libraries, consumer health libraries, and technical schools offering nurse assistant training, especially in areas where Internet access is problematic." —*American Reference Books Annual, 2003*

SEE ALSO Pregnancy & Birth Sourcebook

Burns Sourcebook

Basic Consumer Health Information about Various Types of Burns and Scalds, Including Flame, Heat, Cold, Electrical, Chemical, and Sun Burns

Along with Information on Short-Term and Long-Term Treatments, Tissue Reconstruction, Plastic Surgery, Prevention Suggestions, and First Aid

Edited by Allan R. Cook. 604 pages. 1999. 978-0-7808-0204-9.

"This is an exceptional addition to the series and is highly recommended for all consumer health collections, hospital libraries, and academic medical centers." —*E-Streams, Mar '00*

"This key reference guide is an invaluable addition to all health care and public libraries in confronting this ongoing health issue." —*American Reference Books Annual, 2000*

"Recommended reference source." —*Booklist, American Library Association, Dec '99*

SEE ALSO Dermatological Disorders Sourcebook

Cancer Sourcebook, 5th Edition

Basic Consumer Health Information about Major Forms and Stages of Cancer, Featuring Facts about Head and Neck Cancers, Lung Cancers, Gastrointestinal Cancers, Genitourinary Cancers, Lymphomas, Blood Cell Cancers, Endocrine Cancers, Skin Cancers, Bone Cancers, Metastatic Cancers, and More

Along with Facts about Cancer Treatments, Cancer Risks and Prevention, a Glossary of Related Terms, Statistical Data, and a Directory of Resources for Additional Information

Edited by Karen Bellenir. 1,133 pages. 2007. 978-0-7808-0947-5.

"With cancer being the second leading cause of death for Americans, a prodigious work such as this one, which locates centrally so much cancer-related information, is clearly an asset to this nation's citizens and others." —*Journal of the National Medical Association, 2004*

"This title is recommended for health sciences and public libraries with consumer health collections." —*E-Streams, Feb '01*

"... can be effectively used by cancer patients and their families who are looking for answers in a language they can understand. Public and hospital libraries should have it on their shelves." —*American Reference Books Annual, 2001*

"Recommended reference source." —*Booklist, American Library Association, Dec '00*

SEE ALSO Breast Cancer Sourcebook, Cancer Sourcebook for Women, Pediatric Cancer Sourcebook, Prostate Cancer Sourcebook

---

Cancer Sourcebook for Women, 3rd Edition

Basic Consumer Health Information about Leading Causes of Cancer in Women, Featuring Facts about Gynecologic Cancers and Related Concerns, Such as Breast Cancer, Cervical Cancer, Endometrial Cancer, Uterine Sarcoma, Vaginal Cancer, Vulvar Cancer, and Common Non-Cancerous Gynecologic Conditions, in Addition to Facts about Lung Cancer, Colorectal Cancer, and Thyroid Cancer in Women

Along with Information about Cancer Risk Factors, Screening and Prevention, Treatment Options, and Tips on Coping with Life after Cancer Treatment, a Glossary of Cancer Terms, and a Directory of Resources for Additional Help and Information

Edited by Amy L. Sutton. 715 pages. 2006. 978-0-7808-0867-6.

"An excellent addition to collections in public, consumer health, and women's health libraries." —*American Reference Books Annual, 2003*

"Overall, the information is excellent, and complex topics are clearly explained. As a reference book for the consumer it is a valuable resource to assist them to make informed decisions about cancer and its treatments." —*Cancer Forum, Nov '02*

Cancer Survivorship Sourcebook

Basic Consumer Health Information about the Physical, Educational, Emotional, Social, and Financial Needs of Cancer Patients from Diagnosis, through Cancer Treatment, and Beyond, Including Facts about Researching Specific Types of Cancer and Learning about Clinical Trials and Treatment Options, and Featuring Tips for Coping with the Side Effects of Cancer Treatments and Adjusting to Life after Cancer Treatment Concludes

Along with Suggestions for Caregivers, Friends, and Family Members of Cancer Patients, a Glossary of Cancer Care Terms, and Directories of Related Resources

Edited by Karen Bellenir. 6561 pages. 2007. 978-0-7808-0985-7.

Cardiovascular Diseases & Disorders Sourcebook, 3rd Edition

Basic Consumer Health Information about Heart and Vascular Diseases and Disorders, Such as Angina, Heart Attacks, Arrhythmias, Cardiomyopathy, Valve Disease, Atherosclerosis, and Aneurysms, with Information about Managing Cardiovascular Risk Factors and Maintaining Heart Health, Medications and Procedures Used to Treat Cardiovascular Disorders, and Concerns of Special Significance to Women

Along with Reports on Current Research Initiatives, a Glossary of Related Medical Terms, and a Directory of Sources for Further Help and Information

Edited by Sandra J. Judd. 713 pages. 2005. 978-0-7808-0739-6.

Caregiving Sourcebook

Basic Consumer Health Information for Caregivers, Including a Profile of Caregivers, Caregiving Responsibilities and Concerns, Tips for Specific Conditions, Care Environments, and the Effects of Caregiving

Along with Facts about Legal Issues, Financial Information, and Future Planning, a Glossary, and a Listing of Additional Resources

Edited by Joyce Brennfleck Shannon. 600 pages. 2001. 978-0-7808-0331-2.

Child Abuse Sourcebook

Basic Consumer Health Information about the Physical, Sexual, and Emotional Abuse of Children, with Additional Facts about Neglect, Munchausen Syndrome by Proxy (MSBP), Shaken Baby Syndrome, and Controversial Issues Related to Child Abuse, Such as Withholding Medical Care, Corporal Punishment, and Child Maltreatment in Youth Sports, and Featuring Facts about Child Protective Services, Foster Care, Adoption, Parenting Challenges, and Other Abuse Prevention Efforts

Along with a Glossary of Related Terms and Resources for Additional Help and Information

Edited by Dawn D. Matthews. 620 pages. 2004. 978-0-7808-0705-1.

Childhood Diseases & Disorders Sourcebook

Basic Consumer Health Information about Medical Problems Often Encountered in Pre-Adolescent Children, Including Respiratory Tract Ailments, Ear Infections, Sore Throats, Disorders of the Skin and Scalp, Digestive and Genitourinary Diseases, Infectious Diseases, Inflammatory Disorders, Chronic Physical and Developmental Disorders, Allergies, and More

Along with Information about Diagnostic Tests, Common Childhood Surgeries, and Frequently Used Medications, with a Glossary of Important Terms and Resource Directory

Edited by Chad T. Kimball. 662 pages. 2003. 978-0-7808-0458-6.

"This is an excellent book for new parents and should be included in all health care and public libraries."
—*American Reference Books Annual, 2004*

SEE ALSO: Healthy Children Sourcebook

■

Colds, Flu & Other Common Ailments Sourcebook

Basic Consumer Health Information about Common Ailments and Injuries, Including Colds, Coughs, the Flu, Sinus Problems, Headaches, Fever, Nausea and Vomiting, Menstrual Cramps, Diarrhea, Constipation, Hemorrhoids, Back Pain, Dandruff, Dry and Itchy Skin, Cuts, Scrapes, Sprains, Bruises, and More

Along with Information about Prevention, Self-Care, Choosing a Doctor, Over-the-Counter Medications, Folk Remedies, and Alternative Therapies, and Including a Glossary of Important Terms and a Directory of Resources for Further Help and Information

Edited by Chad T. Kimball. 638 pages. 2001. 978-0-7808-0435-7.

"A good starting point for research on common illnesses. It will be a useful addition to public and consumer health library collections."
—*American Reference Books Annual, 2002*

"Will prove valuable to any library seeking to maintain a current, comprehensive reference collection of health resources. . . . Excellent reference."
—*The Bookwatch, Aug '01*

"Recommended reference source."
—*Booklist, American Library Association, Jul '01*

■

Communication Disorders Sourcebook

Basic Information about Deafness and Hearing Loss, Speech and Language Disorders, Voice Disorders, Balance and Vestibular Disorders, and Disorders of Smell, Taste, and Touch

Edited by Linda M. Ross. 533 pages. 1996. 978-0-7808-0077-9.

"This is skillfully edited and is a welcome resource for the layperson. It should be found in every public and medical library." —*Booklist Health Sciences Supplement, American Library Association, Oct '97*

■

Complementary & Alternative Medicine Sourcebook, 3rd Edition

Basic Consumer Health Information about Complementary and Alternative Medical Therapies, Including Acupuncture, Ayurveda, Traditional Chinese Medicine, Herbal Medicine, Homeopathy, Naturopathy, Biofeedback, Hypnotherapy, Yoga, Art Therapy, Aromatherapy, Clinical Nutrition, Vitamin and Mineral Supplements, Chiropractic, Massage, Reflexology, Crystal Therapy, Therapeutic Touch, and More

Along with Facts about Alternative and Complementary Treatments for Specific Conditions Such as Cancer, Diabetes, Osteoarthritis, Chronic Pain, Menopause, Gastrointestinal Disorders, Headaches, and Mental Illness, a Glossary, and a Resource List for Additional Help and Information

Edited by Sandra J. Judd. 657 pages. 2006. 978-0-7808-0864-5.

"Recommended for public, high school, and academic libraries that have consumer health collections. Hospital libraries that also serve the public will find this to be a useful resource." —*E-Streams, Feb '03*

"Recommended reference source."
—*Booklist, American Library Association, Jan '03*

"An important alternate health reference."
—*MBR Bookwatch, Oct '02*

"A great addition to the reference collection of every type of library." —*American Reference Books Annual, 2000*

■

Congenital Disorders Sourcebook, 2nd Edition

Basic Consumer Health Information about Non-hereditary Birth Defects and Disorders Related to Prematurity, Gestational Injuries, Congenital Infections, and Birth Complications, Including Heart Defects, Hydrocephalus, Spina Bifida, Cleft Lip and Palate, Cerebral Palsy, and More

Along with Facts about the Prevention of Birth Defects, Fetal Surgery and Other Treatment Options, Research Initiatives, a Glossary of Related Terms, and Resources for Additional Information and Support

Edited by Sandra J. Judd. 647 pages. 2006. 978-0-7808-0945-1.

"Recommended reference source."
—*Booklist, American Library Association, Oct '97*

SEE ALSO Pregnancy & Birth Sourcebook

■

Contagious Diseases Sourcebook

Basic Consumer Health Information about Infectious Diseases Spread by Person-to-Person Contact through

Direct Touch, Airborne Transmission, Sexual Contact, or Contact with Blood or Other Body Fluids, Including Hepatitis, Herpes, Influenza, Lice, Measles, Mumps, Pinworm, Ringworm, Severe Acute Respiratory Syndrome (SARS), Streptococcal Infections, Tuberculosis, and Others

Along with Facts about Disease Transmission, Antimicrobial Resistance, and Vaccines, with a Glossary and Directories of Resources for More Information

Edited by Karen Bellenir. 643 pages. 2004. 978-0-7808-0736-5.

"This easy-to-read volume is recommended for consumer health collections within public or academic libraries." — E-Streams, May '05

"This informative book is highly recommended for public libraries, consumer health collections, and secondary schools and undergraduate libraries."
— American Reference Books Annual, 2005

"Excellent reference." — The Bookwatch, Jan '05

Death & Dying Sourcebook, 2nd Edition

Basic Consumer Health Information about End-of-Life Care and Related Perspectives and Ethical Issues, Including End-of-Life Symptoms and Treatments, Pain Management, Quality-of-Life Concerns, the Use of Life Support, Patients' Rights and Privacy Issues, Advance Directives, Physician-Assisted Suicide, Caregiving, Organ and Tissue Donation, Autopsies, Funeral Arrangements, and Grief

Along with Statistical Data, Information about the Leading Causes of Death, a Glossary, and Directories of Support Groups and Other Resources

Edited by Joyce Brennfleck Shannon. 653 pages. 2006. 978-0-7808-0871-3.

"Public libraries, medical libraries, and academic libraries will all find this sourcebook a useful addition to their collections."
— American Reference Books Annual, 2001

"An extremely useful resource for those concerned with death and dying in the United States."
— Respiratory Care, Nov '00

"Recommended reference source."
—Booklist, American Library Association, Aug '00

"This book is a definite must for all those involved in end-of-life care." — Doody's Review Service, 2000

Dental Care & Oral Health Sourcebook, 2nd Edition

Basic Consumer Health Information about Dental Care, Including Oral Hygiene, Dental Visits, Pain Management, Cavities, Crowns, Bridges, Dental Implants, and Fillings, and Other Oral Health Concerns, Such as Gum Disease, Bad Breath, Dry Mouth, Genetic and Developmental Abnormalities, Oral Cancers, Orthodontics, and Temporomandibular Disorders

Along with Updates on Current Research in Oral Health, a Glossary, a Directory of Dental and Oral Health Organizations, and Resources for People with Dental and Oral Health Disorders

Edited by Amy L. Sutton. 609 pages. 2003. 978-0-7808-0634-4.

"This book could serve as a turning point in the battle to educate consumers in issues concerning oral health."
— American Reference Books Annual, 2004

"Unique source which will fill a gap in dental sources for patients and the lay public. A valuable reference tool even in a library with thousands of books on dentistry. Comprehensive, clear, inexpensive, and easy to read and use. It fills an enormous gap in the health care literature." — Reference & User Services Quarterly, American Library Association, Summer '98

"Recommended reference source."
— Booklist, American Library Association, Dec '97

Depression Sourcebook

Basic Consumer Health Information about Unipolar Depression, Bipolar Disorder, Postpartum Depression, Seasonal Affective Disorder, and Other Types of Depression in Children, Adolescents, Women, Men, the Elderly, and Other Selected Populations

Along with Facts about Causes, Risk Factors, Diagnostic Criteria, Treatment Options, Coping Strategies, Suicide Prevention, a Glossary, and a Directory of Sources for Additional Help and Information

Edited by Karen Bellenir. 602 pages. 2002. 978-0-7808-0611-5.

"Depression Sourcebook is of a very high standard. Its purpose, which is to serve as a reference source to the lay reader, is very well served."
— Journal of the National Medical Association, 2004

"Invaluable reference for public and school library collections alike." — Library Bookwatch, Apr '03

"Recommended for purchase."
— American Reference Books Annual, 2003

Dermatological Disorders Sourcebook, 2nd Edition

Basic Consumer Health Information about Conditions and Disorders Affecting the Skin, Hair, and Nails, Such as Acne, Rosacea, Rashes, Dermatitis, Pigmentation Disorders, Birthmarks, Skin Cancer, Skin Injuries, Psoriasis, Scleroderma, and Hair Loss, Including Facts about Medications and Treatments for Dermatological Disorders and Tips for Maintaining Healthy Skin, Hair, and Nails

Along with Information about How Aging Affects the Skin, a Glossary of Related Terms, and a Directory of Resources for Additional Help and Information

Edited by Amy L. Sutton. 645 pages. 2005. 978-0-7808-0795-2.

"... comprehensive, easily read reference book."
    —Doody's Health Sciences Book Reviews, Oct '97

SEE ALSO Burns Sourcebook

■

Diabetes Sourcebook, 3rd Edition

Basic Consumer Health Information about Type 1 Diabetes (Insulin-Dependent or Juvenile-Onset Diabetes), Type 2 Diabetes (Noninsulin-Dependent or Adult-Onset Diabetes), Gestational Diabetes, Impaired Glucose Tolerance (IGT), and Related Complications, Such as Amputation, Eye Disease, Gum Disease, Nerve Damage, and End-Stage Renal Disease, Including Facts about Insulin, Oral Diabetes Medications, Blood Sugar Testing, and the Role of Exercise and Nutrition in the Control of Diabetes

Along with a Glossary and Resources for Further Help and Information

Edited by Dawn D. Matthews. 622 pages. 2003. 978-0-7808-0629-0.

"This edition is even more helpful than earlier versions. . . . It is a truly valuable tool for anyone seeking readable and authoritative information on diabetes."
    —American Reference Books Annual, 2004

"An invaluable reference." —Library Journal, May '00

Selected as one of the 250 "Best Health Sciences Books of 1999." —Doody's Rating Service, Mar-Apr '00

"Provides useful information for the general public."
    —Healthlines, University of Michigan Health Management Research Center, Sep/Oct '99

". . . provides reliable mainstream medical information . . . belongs on the shelves of any library with a consumer health collection." —E-Streams, Sep '99

"Recommended reference source."
    —Booklist, American Library Association, Feb '99

■

Diet & Nutrition Sourcebook, 3rd Edition

Basic Consumer Health Information about Dietary Guidelines and the Food Guidance System, Recommended Daily Nutrient Intakes, Serving Proportions, Weight Control, Vitamins and Supplements, Nutrition Issues for Different Life Stages and Lifestyles, and the Needs of People with Specific Medical Concerns, Including Cancer, Celiac Disease, Diabetes, Eating Disorders, Food Allergies, and Cardiovascular Disease

Along with Facts about Federal Nutrition Support Programs, a Glossary of Nutrition and Dietary Terms, and Directories of Additional Resources for More Information about Nutrition

Edited by Joyce Brennfleck Shannon. 633 pages. 2006. 978-0-7808-0800-3.

"This book is an excellent source of basic diet and nutrition information." —Booklist Health Sciences Supplement, American Library Association, Dec '00

"This reference document should be in any public library, but it would be a very good guide for beginning students in the health sciences. If the other books in this publisher's series are as good as this, they should all be in the health sciences collections."
    —American Reference Books Annual, 2000

"This book is an excellent general nutrition reference for consumers who desire to take an active role in their health care for prevention. Consumers of all ages who select this book can feel confident they are receiving current and accurate information." —Journal of Nutrition for the Elderly, Vol. 19, No. 4, 2000

SEE ALSO Digestive Diseases & Disorders Sourcebook, Eating Disorders Sourcebook, Gastrointestinal Diseases & Disorders Sourcebook, Vegetarian Sourcebook

■

Digestive Diseases & Disorders Sourcebook

Basic Consumer Health Information about Diseases and Disorders that Impact the Upper and Lower Digestive System, Including Celiac Disease, Constipation, Crohn's Disease, Cyclic Vomiting Syndrome, Diarrhea, Diverticulosis and Diverticulitis, Gallstones, Heartburn, Hemorrhoids, Hernias, Indigestion (Dyspepsia), Irritable Bowel Syndrome, Lactose Intolerance, Ulcers, and More

Along with Information about Medications and Other Treatments, Tips for Maintaining a Healthy Digestive Tract, a Glossary, and Directory of Digestive Diseases Organizations

Edited by Karen Bellenir. 335 pages. 2000. 978-0-7808-0327-5.

"This title would be an excellent addition to all public or patient-research libraries."
    —American Reference Books Annual, 2001

"This title is recommended for public, hospital, and health sciences libraries with consumer health collections." —E-Streams, Jul-Aug '00

"Recommended reference source."
    —Booklist, American Library Association, May '00

SEE ALSO Eating Disorders Sourcebook, Gastrointestinal Diseases & Disorders Sourcebook

■

Disabilities Sourcebook

Basic Consumer Health Information about Physical and Psychiatric Disabilities, Including Descriptions of Major Causes of Disability, Assistive and Adaptive Aids, Workplace Issues, and Accessibility Concerns

Along with Information about the Americans with Disabilities Act, a Glossary, and Resources for Additional Help and Information

Edited by Dawn D. Matthews. 616 pages. 2000. 978-0-7808-0389-3.

"It is a must for libraries with a consumer health section." —American Reference Books Annual, 2002

636

"A much needed addition to the Omnigraphics *Health Reference Series*. A current reference work to provide people with disabilities, their families, caregivers or those who work with them, a broad range of information in one volume, has not been available until now. . . . It is recommended for all public and academic library reference collections." — *E-Streams, May '01*

"An excellent source book in easy-to-read format covering many current topics; highly recommended for all libraries." — *Choice, Association of College & Research Libraries, Jan '01*

"Recommended reference source."
— *Booklist, American Library Association, Jul '00*

Domestic Violence Sourcebook, 2nd Edition

Basic Consumer Health Information about the Causes and Consequences of Abusive Relationships, Including Physical Violence, Sexual Assault, Battery, Stalking, and Emotional Abuse, and Facts about the Effects of Violence on Women, Men, Young Adults, and the Elderly, with Reports about Domestic Violence in Selected Populations, and Featuring Facts about Medical Care, Victim Assistance and Protection, Prevention Strategies, Mental Health Services, and Legal Issues

Along with a Glossary of Related Terms and Resources for Additional Help and Information

Edited by Dawn D. Matthews. 628 pages. 2004. 978-0-7808-0669-6.

"Educators, clergy, medical professionals, police, and victims and their families will benefit from this realistic and easy-to-understand resource."
— *American Reference Books Annual, 2005*

"Recommended for all collections supporting consumer health information. It should also be considered for any collection needing general, readable information on domestic violence." — *E-Streams, Jan '05*

"This sourcebook complements other books in its field, providing a one-stop resource . . . Recommended."
— *Choice, Association of College & Research Libraries, Jan '05*

"Interested lay persons should find the book extremely beneficial. . . . A copy of *Domestic Violence and Child Abuse Sourcebook* should be in every public library in the United States."
— *Social Science & Medicine, No. 56, 2003*

"This is important information. The Web has many resources but this sourcebook fills an important societal need. I am not aware of any other resources of this type." — *Doody's Review Service, Sep '01*

"Recommended reference source."
— *Booklist, American Library Association, Apr '01*

"Important pick for college-level health reference libraries." — *The Bookwatch, Mar '01*

"Because this problem is so widespread and because this book includes a lot of issues within one volume, this work is recommended for all public libraries."
— *American Reference Books Annual, 2001*

SEE ALSO *Child Abuse Sourcebook*

Drug Abuse Sourcebook, 2nd Edition

Basic Consumer Health Information about Illicit Substances of Abuse and the Misuse of Prescription and Over-the-Counter Medications, Including Depressants, Hallucinogens, Inhalants, Marijuana, Stimulants, and Anabolic Steroids

Along with Facts about Related Health Risks, Treatment Programs, Prevention Programs, a Glossary of Abuse and Addiction Terms, a Glossary of Drug-Related Street Terms, and a Directory of Resources for More Information

Edited by Catherine Ginther. 607 pages. 2004. 978-0-7808-0740-2.

"Commendable for organizing useful, normally scattered government and association-produced data into a logical sequence."
— *American Reference Books Annual, 2006*

"This easy-to-read volume is recommended for consumer health collections within public or academic libraries." — *E-Streams, Sep '05*

"An excellent library reference."
— *The Bookwatch, May '05*

"Containing a wealth of information, this book will be useful to the college student just beginning to explore the topic of substance abuse. This resource belongs in libraries that serve a lower-division undergraduate or community college clientele as well as the general public." — *Choice, Association of College & Research Libraries, Jun '01*

"Recommended reference source."
— *Booklist, American Library Association, Feb '01*

SEE ALSO *Alcoholism Sourcebook*

Ear, Nose & Throat Disorders Sourcebook, 2nd Edition

Basic Consumer Health Information about Disorders of the Ears, Hearing Loss, Vestibular Disorders, Nasal and Sinus Problems, Throat and Vocal Cord Disorders, and Otolaryngologic Cancers, Including Facts about Ear Infections and Injuries, Genetic and Congenital Deafness, Sensorineural Hearing Disorders, Tinnitus, Vertigo, Ménière Disease, Rhinitis, Sinusitis, Snoring, Sore Throats, Hoarseness, and More

Along with Reports on Current Research Initiatives, a Glossary of Related Medical Terms, and a Directory of Sources for Further Help and Information

Edited by Sandra J. Judd. 659 pages. 2006. 978-0-7808-0872-0.

"Overall, this sourcebook is helpful for the consumer seeking information on ENT issues. It is recommended for public libraries."
—*American Reference Books Annual, 1999*

"Recommended reference source."
—*Booklist, American Library Association, Dec '98*

◼

Eating Disorders Sourcebook, 2nd Edition

Basic Consumer Health Information about Anorexia Nervosa, Bulimia Nervosa, Binge Eating, Compulsive Exercise, Female Athlete Triad, and Other Eating Disorders, Including Facts about Body Image and Other Cultural and Age-Related Risk Factors, Prevention Efforts, Adverse Health Effects, Treatment Options, and the Recovery Process

Along with Guidelines for Healthy Weight Control, a Glossary, and Directories of Additional Resources

Edited by Joyce Brennfleck Shannon. 585 pages. 2007. 978-0-7808-0948-2.

"Recommended for health science libraries that are open to the public, as well as hospital libraries. This book is a good resource for the consumer who is concerned about eating disorders." —*E-Streams, Mar '02*

"This volume is another convenient collection of excerpted articles. Recommended for school and public library patrons; lower-division undergraduates; and two-year technical program students."
—*Choice, Association of College & Research Libraries, Jan '02*

"Recommended reference source."
—*Booklist, American Library Association, Oct '01*

SEE ALSO *Diet & Nutrition Sourcebook, Digestive Diseases & Disorders Sourcebook, Gastrointestinal Diseases & Disorders Sourcebook*

◼

Emergency Medical Services Sourcebook

Basic Consumer Health Information about Preventing, Preparing for, and Managing Emergency Situations, When and Who to Call for Help, What to Expect in the Emergency Room, the Emergency Medical Team, Patient Issues, and Current Topics in Emergency Medicine

Along with Statistical Data, a Glossary, and Sources of Additional Help and Information

Edited by Jenni Lynn Colson. 494 pages. 2002. 978-0-7808-0420-3.

"Handy and convenient for home, public, school, and college libraries. Recommended."
—*Choice, Association of College & Research Libraries, Apr '03*

"This reference can provide the consumer with answers to most questions about emergency care in the United States, or it will direct them to a resource where the answer can be found."
—*American Reference Books Annual, 2003*

"Recommended reference source."
—*Booklist, American Library Association, Feb '03*

◼

Endocrine & Metabolic Disorders Sourcebook

Basic Information for the Layperson about Pancreatic and Insulin-Related Disorders Such as Pancreatitis, Diabetes, and Hypoglycemia; Adrenal Gland Disorders Such as Cushing's Syndrome, Addison's Disease, and Congenital Adrenal Hyperplasia; Pituitary Gland Disorders Such as Growth Hormone Deficiency, Acromegaly, and Pituitary Tumors; Thyroid Disorders Such as Hypothyroidism, Graves' Disease, Hashimoto's Disease, and Goiter; Hyperparathyroidism; and Other Diseases and Syndromes of Hormone Imbalance or Metabolic Dysfunction

Along with Reports on Current Research Initiatives

Edited by Linda M. Shin. 574 pages. 1998. 978-0-7808-0207-0.

"Omnigraphics has produced another needed resource for health information consumers."
—*American Reference Books Annual, 2000*

"Recommended reference source."
—*Booklist, American Library Association, Dec '98*

◼

Environmental Health Sourcebook, 2nd Edition

Basic Consumer Health Information about the Environment and Its Effect on Human Health, Including the Effects of Air Pollution, Water Pollution, Hazardous Chemicals, Food Hazards, Radiation Hazards, Biological Agents, Household Hazards, Such as Radon, Asbestos, Carbon Monoxide, and Mold, and Information about Associated Diseases and Disorders, Including Cancer, Allergies, Respiratory Problems, and Skin Disorders

Along with Information about Environmental Concerns for Specific Populations, a Glossary of Related Terms, and Resources for Further Help and Information

Edited by Dawn D. Matthews. 673 pages. 2003. 978-0-7808-0632-0.

"This recently updated edition continues the level of quality and the reputation of the numerous other volumes in Omnigraphics' *Health Reference Series*."
—*American Reference Books Annual, 2004*

"An excellent updated edition."
—*The Bookwatch, Oct '03*

"Recommended reference source."
—*Booklist, American Library Association, Sep '98*

"This book will be a useful addition to anyone's library."
—*Choice Health Sciences Supplement, Association of College & Research Libraries, May '98*

". . . a good survey of numerous environmentally induced physical disorders . . . a useful addition to anyone's library."
—*Doody's Health Sciences Book Reviews, Jan '98*

Ethnic Diseases Sourcebook

Basic Consumer Health Information for Ethnic and Racial Minority Groups in the United States, Including General Health Indicators and Behaviors, Ethnic Diseases, Genetic Testing, the Impact of Chronic Diseases, Women's Health, Mental Health Issues, and Preventive Health Care Services

Along with a Glossary and a Listing of Additional Resources

Edited by Joyce Brennfleck Shannon. 664 pages. 2001. 978-0-7808-0336-7.

"Recommended for health sciences libraries where public health programs are a priority."
— *E-Streams, Jan '02*

"Not many books have been written on this topic to date, and the *Ethnic Diseases Sourcebook* is a strong addition to the list. It will be an important introductory resource for health consumers, students, health care personnel, and social scientists. It is recommended for public, academic, and large hospital libraries."
— *American Reference Books Annual, 2002*

"Recommended reference source."
— *Booklist, American Library Association, Oct '01*

"Will prove valuable to any library seeking to maintain a current, comprehensive reference collection of health resources.... An excellent source of health information about genetic disorders which affect particular ethnic and racial minorities in the U.S."
— *The Bookwatch, Aug '01*

Eye Care Sourcebook, 2nd Edition

Basic Consumer Health Information about Eye Care and Eye Disorders, Including Facts about the Diagnosis, Prevention, and Treatment of Common Refractive Problems Such as Myopia, Hyperopia, Astigmatism, and Presbyopia, and Eye Diseases, Including Glaucoma, Cataract, Age-Related Macular Degeneration, and Diabetic Retinopathy

Along with a Section on Vision Correction and Refractive Surgeries, Including LASIK and LASEK, a Glossary, and Directories of Resources for Additional Help and Information

Edited by Amy L. Sutton. 543 pages. 2003. 978-0-7808-0635-1.

". . . a solid reference tool for eye care and a valuable addition to a collection."
— *American Reference Books Annual, 2004*

Family Planning Sourcebook

Basic Consumer Health Information about Planning for Pregnancy and Contraception, Including Traditional Methods, Barrier Methods, Hormonal Methods, Permanent Methods, Future Methods, Emergency Contraception, and Birth Control Choices for Women at Each Stage of Life

Along with Statistics, a Glossary, and Sources of Additional Information

Edited by Amy Marcaccio Keyzer. 520 pages. 2001. 978-0-7808-0379-4.

"Recommended for public, health, and undergraduate libraries as part of the circulating collection."
— *E-Streams, Mar '02*

"Information is presented in an unbiased, readable manner, and the sourcebook will certainly be a necessary addition to those public and high school libraries where Internet access is restricted or otherwise problematic." — *American Reference Books Annual, 2002*

"Recommended reference source."
— *Booklist, American Library Association, Oct '01*

"Will prove valuable to any library seeking to maintain a current, comprehensive reference collection of health resources. . . . Excellent reference."
— *The Bookwatch, Aug '01*

SEE ALSO Pregnancy & Birth Sourcebook

Fitness & Exercise Sourcebook, 3rd Edition

Basic Consumer Health Information about the Physical and Mental Benefits of Fitness, Including Cardiorespiratory Endurance, Muscular Strength, Muscular Endurance, and Flexibility, with Facts about Sports Nutrition and Exercise-Related Injuries and Tips about Physical Activity and Exercises for People of All Ages and for People with Health Concerns

Along with Advice on Selecting and Using Exercise Equipment, Maintaining Exercise Motivation, a Glossary of Related Terms, and a Directory of Resources for More Help and Information

Edited by Amy L. Sutton. 663 pages. 2007. 978-0-7808-0946-8.

"This work is recommended for all general reference collections."
— *American Reference Books Annual, 2002*

"Highly recommended for public, consumer, and school grades fourth through college." — *E-Streams, Nov '01*

"Recommended reference source."
— *Booklist, American Library Association, Oct '01*

"The information appears quite comprehensive and is considered reliable. . . . This second edition is a welcomed addition to the series."
— *Doody's Review Service, Sep '01*

Food Safety Sourcebook

Basic Consumer Health Information about the Safe Handling of Meat, Poultry, Seafood, Eggs, Fruit Juices, and Other Food Items, and Facts about Pesticides, Drinking Water, Food Safety Overseas, and the Onset, Duration, and Symptoms of Foodborne Illnesses, Including Types of Pathogenic Bacteria, Parasitic Protozoa, Worms, Viruses, and Natural Toxins

Along with the Role of the Consumer, the Food Handler, and the Government in Food Safety; a Glossary, and Resources for Additional Help and Information

Edited by Dawn D. Matthews. 339 pages. 1999. 978-0-7808-0326-8.

"This book is recommended for public libraries and universities with home economic and food science programs." —*E-Streams, Nov '00*

"Recommended reference source."
—*Booklist, American Library Association, May '00*

"This book takes the complex issues of food safety and foodborne pathogens and presents them in an easily understood manner. [It does] an excellent job of covering a large and often confusing topic."
—*American Reference Books Annual, 2000*

Forensic Medicine Sourcebook

Basic Consumer Information for the Layperson about Forensic Medicine, Including Crime Scene Investigation, Evidence Collection and Analysis, Expert Testimony, Computer-Aided Criminal Identification, Digital Imaging in the Courtroom, DNA Profiling, Accident Reconstruction, Autopsies, Ballistics, Drugs and Explosives Detection, Latent Fingerprints, Product Tampering, and Questioned Document Examination

Along with Statistical Data, a Glossary of Forensics Terminology, and Listings of Sources for Further Help and Information

Edited by Annemarie S. Muth. 574 pages. 1999. 978-0-7808-0232-2.

"Given the expected widespread interest in its content and its easy to read style, this book is recommended for most public and all college and university libraries."
—*E-Streams, Feb '01*

"Recommended for public libraries."
—*Reference & User Services Quarterly, American Library Association, Spring 2000*

"Recommended reference source."
—*Booklist, American Library Association, Feb '00*

"A wealth of information, useful statistics, references are up-to-date and extremely complete. This wonderful collection of data will help students who are interested in a career in any type of forensic field. It is a great resource for attorneys who need information about types of expert witnesses needed in a particular case. It also offers useful information for fiction and nonfiction writers whose work involves a crime. A fascinating compilation. All levels."
—*Choice, Association of College & Research Libraries, Jan '00*

"There are several items that make this book attractive to consumers who are seeking certain forensic data. . . . This is a useful current source for those seeking general forensic medical answers."
—*American Reference Books Annual, 2000*

Gastrointestinal Diseases & Disorders Sourcebook, 2nd Edition

Basic Consumer Health Information about the Upper and Lower Gastrointestinal (GI) Tract, Including the Esophagus, Stomach, Intestines, Rectum, Liver, and Pancreas, with Facts about Gastroesophageal Reflux Disease, Gastritis, Hernias, Ulcers, Celiac Disease, Diverticulitis, Irritable Bowel Syndrome, Hemorrhoids, Gastrointestinal Cancers, and Other Diseases and Disorders Related to the Digestive Process

Along with Information about Commonly Used Diagnostic and Surgical Procedures, Statistics, Reports on Current Research Initiatives and Clinical Trials, a Glossary, and Resources for Additional Help and Information

Edited by Sandra J. Judd. 681 pages. 2006. 978-0-7808-0798-3.

". . . very readable form. The successful editorial work that brought this material together into a useful and understandable reference makes accessible to all readers information that can help them more effectively understand and obtain help for digestive tract problems."
—*Choice, Association of College & Research Libraries, Feb '97*

SEE ALSO *Diet & Nutrition Sourcebook, Digestive Diseases & Disorders Sourcebook, Eating Disorders Sourcebook*

Genetic Disorders Sourcebook, 3rd Edition

Basic Consumer Health Information about Hereditary Diseases and Disorders, Including Facts about the Human Genome, Genetic Inheritance Patterns, Disorders Associated with Specific Genes, Such as Sickle Cell Disease, Hemophilia, and Cystic Fibrosis, Chromosome Disorders, Such as Down Syndrome, Fragile X Syndrome, and Turner Syndrome, and Complex Diseases and Disorders Resulting from the Interaction of Environmental and Genetic Factors, Such as Allergies, Cancer, and Obesity

Along with Facts about Genetic Testing, Suggestions for Parents of Children with Special Needs, Reports on Current Research Initiatives, a Glossary of Genetic Terminology, and Resources for Additional Help and Information

Edited by Karen Bellenir. 777 pages. 2004. 978-0-7808-0742-6.

"This text is recommended for any library with an interest in providing consumer health resources."
—*E-Streams, Aug '05*

"This is a valuable resource for anyone wishing to have an understandable description of any of the topics or disorders included. The editor succeeds in making complex genetic issues understandable."
—*Doody's Book Review Service, May '05*

"A good acquisition for public libraries."
—*American Reference Books Annual, 2005*

Head Trauma Sourcebook

Basic Information for the Layperson about Open-Head and Closed-Head Injuries, Treatment Advances, Recovery, and Rehabilitation

Along with Reports on Current Research Initiatives

Edited by Karen Bellenir. 414 pages. 1997. 978-0-7808-0208-7.

Headache Sourcebook

Basic Consumer Health Information about Migraine, Tension, Cluster, Rebound and Other Types of Headaches, with Facts about the Cause and Prevention of Headaches, the Effects of Stress and the Environment, Headaches during Pregnancy and Menopause, and Childhood Headaches

Along with a Glossary and Other Resources for Additional Help and Information

Edited by Dawn D. Matthews. 362 pages. 2002. 978-0-7808-0337-4.

Healthy Aging Sourcebook

Basic Consumer Health Information about Maintaining Health through the Aging Process, Including Advice on Nutrition, Exercise, and Sleep, Help in Making Decisions about Midlife Issues and Retirement, and Guidance Concerning Practical and Informed Choices in Health Consumerism

Along with Data Concerning the Theories of Aging, Different Experiences in Aging by Minority Groups, and Facts about Aging Now and Aging in the Future; and Featuring a Glossary, a Guide to Consumer Help, Additional Suggested Reading, and Practical Resource Directory

Edited by Jenifer Swanson. 536 pages. 1999. 978-0-7808-0390-9.

SEE ALSO *Physical & Mental Issues in Aging Sourcebook*

Healthy Children Sourcebook

Basic Consumer Health Information about the Physical and Mental Development of Children between the Ages of 3 and 12, Including Routine Health Care, Preventative Health Services, Safety and First Aid,

Healthy Sleep, Dental Care, Nutrition, and Fitness, and Featuring Parenting Tips on Such Topics as Bedwetting, Choosing Day Care, Monitoring TV and Other Media, and Establishing a Foundation for Substance Abuse Prevention

Along with a Glossary of Commonly Used Pediatric Terms and Resources for Additional Help and Information.

Edited by Chad T. Kimball. 647 pages. 2003. 978-0-7808-0247-6.

SEE ALSO *Childhood Diseases & Disorders Sourcebook*

Healthy Heart Sourcebook for Women

Basic Consumer Health Information about Cardiac Issues Specific to Women, Including Facts about Major Risk Factors and Prevention, Treatment and Control Strategies, and Important Dietary Issues

Along with a Special Section Regarding the Pros and Cons of Hormone Replacement Therapy and Its Impact on Heart Health, and Additional Help, Including Recipes, a Glossary, and a Directory of Resources

Edited by Dawn D. Matthews. 336 pages. 2000. 978-0-7808-0329-9.

SEE ALSO *Cardiovascular Diseases & Disorders Sourcebook, Women's Health Concerns Sourcebook*

Hepatitis Sourcebook

Basic Consumer Health Information about Hepatitis A, Hepatitis B, Hepatitis C, and Other Forms of Hepatitis, Including Autoimmune Hepatitis, Alcoholic Hepatitis, Nonalcoholic Steatohepatitis, and Toxic Hepatitis, with

Facts about Risk Factors, Screening Methods, Diagnostic Tests, and Treatment Options

Along with Information on Liver Health, Tips for People Living with Chronic Hepatitis, Reports on Current Research Initiatives, a Glossary of Terms Related to Hepatitis, and a Directory of Sources for Further Help and Information

Edited by Sandra J. Judd. 597 pages. 2005. 978-0-7808-0749-5.

"Highly recommended."
— *American Reference Books Annual, 2006*

■

Household Safety Sourcebook

Basic Consumer Health Information about Household Safety, Including Information about Poisons, Chemicals, Fire, and Water Hazards in the Home

Along with Advice about the Safe Use of Home Maintenance Equipment, Choosing Toys and Nursery Furniture, Holiday and Recreation Safety, a Glossary, and Resources for Further Help and Information

Edited by Dawn D. Matthews. 606 pages. 2002. 978-0-7808-0338-1.

"This work will be useful in public libraries with large consumer health and wellness departments."
— *American Reference Books Annual, 2003*

"As a sourcebook on household safety this book meets its mark. It is encyclopedic in scope and covers a wide range of safety issues that are commonly seen in the home." — *E-Streams, Jul '02*

■

Hypertension Sourcebook

Basic Consumer Health Information about the Causes, Diagnosis, and Treatment of High Blood Pressure, with Facts about Consequences, Complications, and Co-Occurring Disorders, Such as Coronary Heart Disease, Diabetes, Stroke, Kidney Disease, and Hypertensive Retinopathy, and Issues in Blood Pressure Control, Including Dietary Choices, Stress Management, and Medications

Along with Reports on Current Research Initiatives and Clinical Trials, a Glossary, and Resources for Additional Help and Information

Edited by Dawn D. Matthews and Karen Bellenir. 613 pages. 2004. 978-0-7808-0674-0.

"Academic, public, and medical libraries will want to add the *Hypertension Sourcebook* to their collections."
— *E-Streams, Aug '05*

"The strength of this source is the wide range of information given about hypertension."
— *American Reference Books Annual, 2005*

■

Immune System Disorders Sourcebook, 2nd Edition

Basic Consumer Health Information about Disorders of the Immune System, Including Immune System Function and Response, Diagnosis of Immune Disorders, Information about Inherited Immune Disease, Acquired Immune Disease, and Autoimmune Diseases, Including Primary Immune Deficiency, Acquired Immunodeficiency Syndrome (AIDS), Lupus, Multiple Sclerosis, Type 1 Diabetes, Rheumatoid Arthritis, and Graves' Disease

Along with Treatments, Tips for Coping with Immune Disorders, a Glossary, and a Directory of Additional Resources.

Edited by Joyce Brennfleck Shannon. 671 pages. 2005. 978-0-7808-0748-8.

"Highly recommended for academic and public libraries." — *American Reference Books Annual, 2006*

"The updated second edition is a 'must' for any consumer health library seeking a solid resource covering the treatments, symptoms, and options for immune disorder sufferers. . . . An excellent guide."
— *MBR Bookwatch, Jan '06*

■

Infant & Toddler Health Sourcebook

Basic Consumer Health Information about the Physical and Mental Development of Newborns, Infants, and Toddlers, Including Neonatal Concerns, Nutrition Recommendations, Immunization Schedules, Common Pediatric Disorders, Assessments and Milestones, Safety Tips, and Advice for Parents and Other Caregivers

Along with a Glossary of Terms and Resource Listings for Additional Help

Edited by Jenifer Swanson. 585 pages. 2000. 978-0-7808-0246-9.

"As a reference for the general public, this would be useful in any library." — *E-Streams, May '01*

"Recommended reference source."
— *Booklist, American Library Association, Feb '01*

"This is a good source for general use."
— *American Reference Books Annual, 2001*

■

Infectious Diseases Sourcebook

Basic Consumer Health Information about Non-Contagious Bacterial, Viral, Prion, Fungal, and Parasitic Diseases Spread by Food and Water, Insects and Animals, or Environmental Contact, Including Botulism, E. Coli, Encephalitis, Legionnaires' Disease, Lyme Disease, Malaria, Plague, Rabies, Salmonella, Tetanus, and Others, and Facts about Newly Emerging Diseases, Such as Hantavirus, Mad Cow Disease, Monkeypox, and West Nile Virus

Along with Information about Preventing Disease Transmission, the Threat of Bioterrorism, and Current Research Initiatives, with a Glossary and Directory of Resources for More Information

Edited by Karen Bellenir. 634 pages. 2004. 978-0-7808-0675-7.

"This reference continues the excellent tradition of the *Health Reference Series* in consolidating a wealth of information on a selected topic into a format that is easy to use and accessible to the general public."
— *American Reference Books Annual, 2005*

"Recommended for public and academic libraries."
— *E-Streams, Jan '05*

■

Injury & Trauma Sourcebook

Basic Consumer Health Information about the Impact of Injury, the Diagnosis and Treatment of Common and Traumatic Injuries, Emergency Care, and Specific Injuries Related to Home, Community, Workplace, Transportation, and Recreation

Along with Guidelines for Injury Prevention, a Glossary, and a Directory of Additional Resources

Edited by Joyce Brennfleck Shannon. 696 pages. 2002. 978-0-7808-0421-0.

"This publication is the most comprehensive work of its kind about injury and trauma."
— *American Reference Books Annual, 2003*

"This sourcebook provides concise, easily readable, basic health information about injuries. . . . This book is well organized and an easy to use reference resource suitable for hospital, health sciences and public libraries with consumer health collections."
— *E-Streams, Nov '02*

"Practitioners should be aware of guides such as this in order to facilitate their use by patients and their families." — *Doody's Health Sciences Book Review Journal, Sep-Oct '02*

"Recommended reference source."
— *Booklist, American Library Association, Sep '02*

"Highly recommended for academic and medical reference collections." — *Library Bookwatch, Sep '02*

■

Kidney & Urinary Tract Diseases & Disorders Sourcebook

SEE Urinary Tract & Kidney Diseases & Disorders Sourcebook

■

Learning Disabilities Sourcebook, 2nd Edition

Basic Consumer Health Information about Learning Disabilities, Including Dyslexia, Developmental Speech and Language Disabilities, Non-Verbal Learning Disorders, Developmental Arithmetic Disorder, Developmental Writing Disorder, and Other Conditions That Impede Learning Such as Attention Deficit/Hyperactivity Disorder, Brain Injury, Hearing Impairment, Klinefelter Syndrome, Dyspraxia, and Tourette's Syndrome

Along with Facts about Educational Issues and Assistive Technology, Coping Strategies, a Glossary of Related Terms, and Resources for Further Help and Information

Edited by Dawn D. Matthews. 621 pages. 2003. 978-0-7808-0626-9.

"The second edition of Learning Disabilities Sourcebook far surpasses the earlier edition in that it is more focused on information that will be useful as a consumer health resource."
— *American Reference Books Annual, 2004*

"Teachers as well as consumers will find this an essential guide to understanding various syndromes and their latest treatments. [An] invaluable reference for public and school library collections alike."
— *Library Bookwatch, Apr '03*

Named "Outstanding Reference Book of 1999."
— *New York Public Library, Feb '00*

"An excellent candidate for inclusion in a public library reference section. It's a great source of information. Teachers will also find the book useful. Definitely worth reading."
— *Journal of Adolescent & Adult Literacy, Feb 2000*

"Readable . . . provides a solid base of information regarding successful techniques used with individuals who have learning disabilities, as well as practical suggestions for educators and family members. Clear language, concise descriptions, and pertinent information for contacting multiple resources add to the strength of this book as a useful tool." — *Choice, Association of College & Research Libraries, Feb '99*

"Recommended reference source."
— *Booklist, American Library Association, Sep '98*

"A useful resource for libraries and for those who don't have the time to identify and locate the individual publications." — *Disability Resources Monthly, Sep '98*

■

Leukemia Sourcebook

Basic Consumer Health Information about Adult and Childhood Leukemias, Including Acute Lymphocytic Leukemia (ALL), Chronic Lymphocytic Leukemia (CLL), Acute Myelogenous Leukemia (AML), Chronic Myelogenous Leukemia (CML), and Hairy Cell Leukemia, and Treatments Such as Chemotherapy, Radiation Therapy, Peripheral Blood Stem Cell and Marrow Transplantation, and Immunotherapy

Along with Tips for Life During and After Treatment, a Glossary, and Directories of Additional Resources

Edited by Joyce Brennfleck Shannon. 587 pages. 2003. 978-0-7808-0627-6.

"Unlike other medical books for the layperson, . . . the language does not talk down to the reader. . . . This volume is highly recommended for all libraries."
— *American Reference Books Annual, 2004*

". . . a fine title which ranges from diagnosis to alternative treatments, staging, and tips for life during and after diagnosis." — *The Bookwatch, Dec '03*

Liver Disorders Sourcebook

Basic Consumer Health Information about the Liver and How It Works, Liver Diseases, Including Cancer, Cirrhosis, Hepatitis, and Toxic and Drug Related Diseases; Tips for Maintaining a Healthy Liver; Laboratory Tests, Radiology Tests, and Facts about Liver Transplantation

Along with a Section on Support Groups, a Glossary, and Resource Listings

Edited by Joyce Brennfleck Shannon. 591 pages. 2000. 978-0-7808-0383-1.

"A valuable resource."
—American Reference Books Annual, 2001

"This title is recommended for health sciences and public libraries with consumer health collections."
—E-Streams, Oct '00

"Recommended reference source."
—Booklist, American Library Association, Jun '00

Lung Disorders Sourcebook

Basic Consumer Health Information about Emphysema, Pneumonia, Tuberculosis, Asthma, Cystic Fibrosis, and Other Lung Disorders, Including Facts about Diagnostic Procedures, Treatment Strategies, Disease Prevention Efforts, and Such Risk Factors as Smoking, Air Pollution, and Exposure to Asbestos, Radon, and Other Agents

Along with a Glossary and Resources for Additional Help and Information

Edited by Dawn D. Matthews. 678 pages. 2002. 978-0-7808-0339-8.

"This title is a great addition for public and school libraries because it provides concise health information on the lungs."
—American Reference Books Annual, 2003

"Highly recommended for academic and medical reference collections." *—Library Bookwatch, Sep '02*

SEE ALSO *Respiratory Diseases & Disorders Sourcebook*

Medical Tests Sourcebook, 2nd Edition

Basic Consumer Health Information about Medical Tests, Including Age-Specific Health Tests, Important Health Screenings and Exams, Home-Use Tests, Blood and Specimen Tests, Electrical Tests, Scope Tests, Genetic Testing, and Imaging Tests, Such as X-Rays, Ultrasound, Computed Tomography, Magnetic Resonance Imaging, Angiography, and Nuclear Medicine

Along with a Glossary and Directory of Additional Resources

Edited by Joyce Brennfleck Shannon. 654 pages. 2004. 978-0-7808-0670-2.

"Recommended for hospital and health sciences

libraries with consumer health collections."
—E-Streams, Mar '00

"This is an overall excellent reference with a wealth of general knowledge that may aid those who are reluctant to get vital tests performed."
—Today's Librarian, Jan '00

"A valuable reference guide."
—American Reference Books Annual, 2000

Men's Health Concerns Sourcebook, 2nd Edition

Basic Consumer Health Information about the Medical and Mental Concerns of Men, Including Theories about the Shorter Male Lifespan, the Leading Causes of Death and Disability, Physical Concerns of Special Significance to Men, Reproductive and Sexual Concerns, Sexually Transmitted Diseases, Men's Mental and Emotional Health, and Lifestyle Choices That Affect Wellness, Such as Nutrition, Fitness, and Substance Use

Along with a Glossary of Related Terms and a Directory of Organizational Resources in Men's Health

Edited by Robert Aquinas McNally. 644 pages. 2004. 978-0-7808-0671-9.

"A very accessible reference for non-specialist general readers and consumers." *— The Bookwatch, Jun '04*

"This comprehensive resource and the series are highly recommended."
—American Reference Books Annual, 2000

"Recommended reference source."
—Booklist, American Library Association, Dec '98

Mental Health Disorders Sourcebook, 3rd Edition

Basic Consumer Health Information about Mental and Emotional Health and Mental Illness, Including Facts about Depression, Bipolar Disorder, and Other Mood Disorders, Phobias, Post-Traumatic Stress Disorder (PTSD), Obsessive-Compulsive Disorder, and Other Anxiety Disorders, Impulse Control Disorders, Eating Disorders, Personality Disorders, and Psychotic Disorders, Including Schizophrenia and Dissociative Disorders

Along with Statistical Information, a Special Section Concerning Mental Health Issues in Children and Adolescents, a Glossary, and Directories of Resources for Additional Help and Information

Edited by Karen Bellenir. 661 pages. 2005. 978-0-7808-0747-1.

"Recommended for public libraries and academic libraries with an undergraduate program in psychology."
—American Reference Books Annual, 2006

"Recommended reference source."
—Booklist, American Library Association, Jun '00

Mental Retardation Sourcebook

Basic Consumer Health Information about Mental Retardation and Its Causes, Including Down Syndrome, Fetal Alcohol Syndrome, Fragile X Syndrome, Genetic Conditions, Injury, and Environmental Sources

Along with Preventive Strategies, Parenting Issues, Educational Implications, Health Care Needs, Employment and Economic Matters, Legal Issues, a Glossary, and a Resource Listing for Additional Help and Information

Edited by Joyce Brennfleck Shannon. 642 pages. 2000. 978-0-7808-0377-0.

"Public libraries will find the book useful for reference and as a beginning research point for students, parents, and caregivers."
— American Reference Books Annual, 2001

"The strength of this work is that it compiles many basic fact sheets and addresses for further information in one volume. It is intended and suitable for the general public. This sourcebook is relevant to any collection providing health information to the general public."
— E-Streams, Nov '00

"From preventing retardation to parenting and family challenges, this covers health, social and legal issues and will prove an invaluable overview."
— Reviewer's Bookwatch, Jul '00

■

Movement Disorders Sourcebook

Basic Consumer Health Information about Neurological Movement Disorders, Including Essential Tremor, Parkinson's Disease, Dystonia, Cerebral Palsy, Huntington's Disease, Myasthenia Gravis, Multiple Sclerosis, and Other Early-Onset and Adult-Onset Movement Disorders, Their Symptoms and Causes, Diagnostic Tests, and Treatments

Along with Mobility and Assistive Technology Information, a Glossary, and a Directory of Additional Resources

Edited by Joyce Brennfleck Shannon. 655 pages. 2003. 978-0-7808-0628-3.

". . . a good resource for consumers and recommended for public, community college and undergraduate libraries." *— American Reference Books Annual, 2004*

■

Muscular Dystrophy Sourcebook

Basic Consumer Health Information about Congenital, Childhood-Onset, and Adult-Onset Forms of Muscular Dystrophy, Such as Duchenne, Becker, Emery-Dreifuss, Distal, Limb-Girdle, Facioscapulohumeral (FSHD), Myotonic, and Ophthalmoplegic Muscular Dystrophies, Including Facts about Diagnostic Tests, Medical and Physical Therapies, Management of Co-Occurring Conditions, and Parenting Guidelines

Along with Practical Tips for Home Care, a Glossary, and Directories of Additional Resources

Edited by Joyce Brennfleck Shannon. 577 pages. 2004. 978-0-7808-0676-4.

"This book is highly recommended for public and academic libraries as well as health care offices that support the information needs of patients and their families."
— E-Streams, Apr '05

"Excellent reference."   *— The Bookwatch, Jan '05*

■

Obesity Sourcebook

Basic Consumer Health Information about Diseases and Other Problems Associated with Obesity, and Including Facts about Risk Factors, Prevention Issues, and Management Approaches

Along with Statistical and Demographic Data, Information about Special Populations, Research Updates, a Glossary, and Source Listings for Further Help and Information

Edited by Wilma Caldwell and Chad T. Kimball. 376 pages. 2001. 978-0-7808-0333-6.

"The book synthesizes the reliable medical literature on obesity into one easy-to-read and useful resource for the general public."
— American Reference Books Annual, 2002

"This is a very useful resource book for the lay public."
— Doody's Review Service, Nov '01

"Well suited for the health reference collection of a public library or an academic health science library that serves the general population."   *— E-Streams, Sep '01*

"Recommended reference source."
– Booklist, American Library Association, Apr '01

"Recommended pick both for specialty health library collections and any general consumer health reference collection."   *— The Bookwatch, Apr '01*

■

Oral Health Sourcebook

SEE Dental Care & Oral Health Sourcebook

■

Osteoporosis Sourcebook

Basic Consumer Health Information about Primary and Secondary Osteoporosis and Juvenile Osteoporosis and Related Conditions, Including Fibrous Dysplasia, Gaucher Disease, Hyperthyroidism, Hypophosphatasia, Myeloma, Osteopetrosis, Osteogenesis Imperfecta, and Paget's Disease

Along with Information about Risk Factors, Treatments, Traditional and Non-Traditional Pain Management, a Glossary of Related Terms, and a Directory of Resources

Edited by Allan R. Cook. 584 pages. 2001. 978-0-7808-0239-1.

"This would be a book to be kept in a staff or patient library. The targeted audience is the layperson, but the therapist who needs a quick bit of information on a particular topic will also find the book useful."
— Physical Therapy, Jan '02

"This resource is recommended as a great reference source for public, health, and academic libraries, and is another triumph for the editors of Omnigraphics."
— *American Reference Books Annual, 2002*

"Recommended for all public libraries and general health collections, especially those supporting patient education or consumer health programs."
— *E-Streams, Nov '01*

"Will prove valuable to any library seeking to maintain a current, comprehensive reference collection of health resources. . . . From prevention to treatment and associated conditions, this provides an excellent survey."
— *The Bookwatch, Aug '01*

"Recommended reference source."
— *Booklist, American Library Association, Jul '01*

SEE ALSO *Healthy Aging Sourcebook, Physical & Mental Issues in Aging Sourcebook, Women's Health Concerns Sourcebook*

Pain Sourcebook, 2nd Edition

Basic Consumer Health Information about Specific Forms of Acute and Chronic Pain, Including Muscle and Skeletal Pain, Nerve Pain, Cancer Pain, and Disorders Characterized by Pain, Such as Fibromyalgia, Shingles, Angina, Arthritis, and Headaches

Along with Information about Pain Medications and Management Techniques, Complementary and Alternative Pain Relief Options, Tips for People Living with Chronic Pain, a Glossary, and a Directory of Sources for Further Information

Edited by Karen Bellenir. 670 pages. 2002. 978-0-7808-0612-2.

"A source of valuable information. . . . This book offers help to nonmedical people who need information about pain and pain management. It is also an excellent reference for those who participate in patient education."
— *Doody's Review Service, Sep '02*

"Highly recommended for academic and medical reference collections." — *Library Bookwatch, Sep '02*

"The text is readable, easily understood, and well indexed. This excellent volume belongs in all patient education libraries, consumer health sections of public libraries, and many personal collections."
— *American Reference Books Annual, 1999*

"The information is basic in terms of scholarship and is appropriate for general readers. Written in journalistic style . . . intended for non-professionals. Quite thorough in its coverage of different pain conditions and summarizes the latest clinical information regarding pain treatment." — *Choice, Association of College and Research Libraries, Jun '98*

"Recommended reference source."
— *Booklist, American Library Association, Mar '98*

Pediatric Cancer Sourcebook

Basic Consumer Health Information about Leukemias, Brain Tumors, Sarcomas, Lymphomas, and Other Cancers in Infants, Children, and Adolescents, Including Descriptions of Cancers, Treatments, and Coping Strategies

Along with Suggestions for Parents, Caregivers, and Concerned Relatives, a Glossary of Cancer Terms, and Resource Listings

Edited by Edward J. Prucha. 587 pages. 1999. 978-0-7808-0245-2.

"An excellent source of information. Recommended for public, hospital, and health science libraries with consumer health collections." — *E-Streams, Jun '00*

"Recommended reference source."
— *Booklist, American Library Association, Feb '00*

"A valuable addition to all libraries specializing in health services and many public libraries."
— *American Reference Books Annual, 2000*

SEE ALSO *Childhood Diseases & Disorders Sourcebook, Healthy Children Sourcebook*

Physical & Mental Issues in Aging Sourcebook

Basic Consumer Health Information on Physical and Mental Disorders Associated with the Aging Process, Including Concerns about Cardiovascular Disease, Pulmonary Disease, Oral Health, Digestive Disorders, Musculoskeletal and Skin Disorders, Metabolic Changes, Sexual and Reproductive Issues, and Changes in Vision, Hearing, and Other Senses

Along with Data about Longevity and Causes of Death, Information on Acute and Chronic Pain, Descriptions of Mental Concerns, a Glossary of Terms, and Resource Listings for Additional Help

Edited by Jenifer Swanson. 660 pages. 1999. 978-0-7808-0233-9.

"This is a treasure of health information for the layperson." — *Choice Health Sciences Supplement, Association of College & Research Libraries, May '00*

"Recommended for public libraries."
— *American Reference Books Annual, 2000*

"Recommended reference source."
— *Booklist, American Library Association, Oct '99*

SEE ALSO *Healthy Aging Sourcebook*

Podiatry Sourcebook, 2nd Edition

Basic Consumer Health Information about Disorders, Diseases, Deformities, and Injuries that Affect the Foot and Ankle, Including Sprains, Corns, Calluses, Bunions, Plantar Warts, Plantar Fasciitis, Neuromas, Clubfoot, Flat Feet, Achilles Tendonitis, and Much More

Along with Information about Selecting a Foot Care Specialist, Foot Fitness, Shoes and Socks, Diagnostic Tests and Corrective Procedures, Financial Assistance for Corrective Devices, a Glossary of Related Terms, and a *Directory of Resources for Additional Help and Information*

Edited by Ivy L. Alexander. 543 pages. 2007. 978-0-7808-0944-4.

"**Recommended reference source.**"
— *Booklist, American Library Association, Feb '02*

"**There is a lot of information presented here on a topic that is usually only covered sparingly in most larger comprehensive medical encyclopedias.**"
— *American Reference Books Annual, 2002*

■

Pregnancy & Birth Sourcebook, 2nd Edition

Basic Consumer Health Information about Conception and Pregnancy, Including Facts about Fertility, Infertility, Pregnancy Symptoms and Complications, Fetal Growth and Development, Labor, Delivery, and the Postpartum Period, as Well as Information about Maintaining Health and Wellness during Pregnancy and Caring for a Newborn

Along with Information about Public Health Assistance for Low-Income Pregnant Women, a Glossary, and Directories of Agencies and Organizations Providing Help and Support

Edited by Amy L. Sutton. 626 pages. 2004. 978-0-7808-0672-6.

"**Will appeal to public and school reference collections strong in medicine and women's health. . . . Deserves a spot on any medical reference shelf.**"
— *The Bookwatch, Jul '04*

"**A well-organized handbook. Recommended.**"
— *Choice, Association of College & Research Libraries, Apr '98*

"**Recommended reference source.**"
— *Booklist, American Library Association, Mar '98*

"**Recommended for public libraries.**"
— *American Reference Books Annual, 1998*

SEE ALSO *Breastfeeding Sourcebook, Congenital Disorders Sourcebook, Family Planning Sourcebook*

■

Prostate & Urological Disorders Sourcebook

Basic Consumer Health Information about Urogenital and Sexual Disorders in Men, Including Prostate and Other Andrological Cancers, Prostatitis, Benign Prostatic Hyperplasia, Testicular and Penile Trauma, Cryptorchidism, Peyronie Disease, Erectile Dysfunction, and Male Factor Infertility, and Facts about Commonly Used Tests and Procedures, Such as Prostatectomy, Vasectomy, Vasectomy Reversal, Penile Implants, and Semen Analysis

Along with a Glossary of Andrological Terms and a Directory of Resources for Additional Information

Edited by Karen Bellenir. 631 pages. 2005. 978-0-7808-0797-6.

Prostate Cancer Sourcebook

Basic Consumer Health Information about Prostate Cancer, Including Information about the Associated Risk Factors, Detection, Diagnosis, and Treatment of Prostate Cancer

Along with Information on Non-Malignant Prostate Conditions, and Featuring a Section Listing Support and Treatment Centers and a Glossary of Related Terms

Edited by Dawn D. Matthews. 358 pages. 2001. 978-0-7808-0324-4.

"**Recommended reference source.**"
— *Booklist, American Library Association, Jan '02*

"**A valuable resource for health care consumers seeking information on the subject. . . . All text is written in a clear, easy-to-understand language that avoids technical jargon. Any library that collects consumer health resources would strengthen their collection with the addition of the *Prostate Cancer Sourcebook*.**"
— *American Reference Books Annual, 2002*

SEE ALSO *Men's Health Concerns Sourcebook*

■

Reconstructive & Cosmetic Surgery Sourcebook

Basic Consumer Health Information on Cosmetic and Reconstructive Plastic Surgery, Including Statistical Information about Different Surgical Procedures, Things to Consider Prior to Surgery, Plastic Surgery Techniques and Tools, Emotional and Psychological Considerations, and Procedure-Specific Information

Along with a Glossary of Terms and a Listing of Resources for Additional Help and Information

Edited by M. Lisa Weatherford. 374 pages. 2001. 978-0-7808-0214-8.

"**An excellent reference that addresses cosmetic and medically necessary reconstructive surgeries. . . . The style of the prose is calm and reassuring, discussing the many positive outcomes now available due to advances in surgical techniques.**"
— *American Reference Books Annual, 2002*

"**Recommended for health science libraries that are open to the public, as well as hospital libraries that are open to the patients. This book is a good resource for the consumer interested in plastic surgery.**"
— *E-Streams, Dec '01*

"**Recommended reference source.**"
— *Booklist, American Library Association, Jul '01*

■

Rehabilitation Sourcebook

Basic Consumer Health Information about Rehabilitation for People Recovering from Heart Surgery, Spinal Cord Injury, Stroke, Orthopedic Impairments, Amputation, Pulmonary Impairments, Traumatic Injury, and More, Including Physical Therapy, Occupational Therapy, Speech/Language Therapy, Massage Therapy, Dance Therapy, Art Therapy, and Recreational Therapy

Along with Information on Assistive and Adaptive Devices, a Glossary, and Resources for Additional Help and Information

Edited by Dawn D. Matthews. 531 pages. 1999. 978-0-7808-0236-0.

"This is an excellent resource for public library reference and health collections."
— *American Reference Books Annual, 2001*

"Recommended reference source."
— *Booklist, American Library Association, May '00*

■

Respiratory Diseases & Disorders Sourcebook

Basic Information about Respiratory Diseases and Disorders, Including Asthma, Cystic Fibrosis, Pneumonia, the Common Cold, Influenza, and Others, Featuring Facts about the Respiratory System, Statistical and Demographic Data, Treatments, Self-Help Management Suggestions, and Current Research Initiatives

Edited by Allan R. Cook and Peter D. Dresser. 771 pages. 1995. 978-0-7808-0037-3.

"Designed for the layperson and for patients and their families coping with respiratory illness. . . . an extensive array of information on diagnosis, treatment, management, and prevention of respiratory illnesses for the general reader." — *Choice, Association of College & Research Libraries, Jun '96*

"A highly recommended text for all collections. It is a comforting reminder of the power of knowledge that good books carry between their covers."
— *Academic Library Book Review, Spring '96*

"A comprehensive collection of authoritative information presented in a nontechnical, humanitarian style for patients, families, and caregivers."
— *Association of Operating Room Nurses, Sep/Oct '95*

SEE ALSO *Lung Disorders Sourcebook*

■

Sexually Transmitted Diseases Sourcebook, 3rd Edition

Basic Consumer Health Information about Chlamydial Infections, Gonorrhea, Hepatitis, Herpes, HIV/AIDS, Human Papillomavirus, Pubic Lice, Scabies, Syphilis, Trichomoniasis, Vaginal Infections, and Other Sexually Transmitted Diseases, Including Facts about Risk Factors, Symptoms, Diagnosis, Treatment, and the Prevention of Sexually Transmitted Infections

Along with Updates on Current Research Initiatives, a Glossary of Related Terms, and Resources for Additional Help and Information

Edited by Amy L. Sutton. 629 pages. 2006. 978-0-7808-0824-9.

"Recommended for consumer health collections in public libraries, and secondary school and community college libraries."
— *American Reference Books Annual, 2002*

"Every school and public library should have a copy of this comprehensive and user-friendly reference book."
— *Choice, Association of College & Research Libraries, Sep '01*

"This is a highly recommended book. This is an especially important book for all school and public libraries."
— *AIDS Book Review Journal, Jul-Aug '01*

"Recommended reference source."
— *Booklist, American Library Association, Apr '01*

■

Sleep Disorders Sourcebook, 2nd Edition

Basic Consumer Health Information about Sleep and Sleep Disorders, Including Insomnia, Sleep Apnea, Restless Legs Syndrome, Narcolepsy, Parasomnias, and Other Health Problems That Affect Sleep, Plus Facts about Diagnostic Procedures, Treatment Strategies, Sleep Medications, and Tips for Improving Sleep Quality

Along with a Glossary of Related Terms and Resources for Additional Help and Information

Edited by Amy L. Sutton. 567 pages. 2005. 978-0-7808-0743-3.

"This book will be useful for just about everybody, especially the 40 million Americans with sleep disorders."
— *American Reference Books Annual, 2006*

"Recommended for public libraries and libraries supporting health care professionals." — *E-Streams, Sep '05*

". . . key medical library acquisition."
— *The Bookwatch, Jun '05*

■

Smoking Concerns Sourcebook

Basic Consumer Health Information about Nicotine Addiction and Smoking Cessation, Featuring Facts about the Health Effects of Tobacco Use, Including Lung and Other Cancers, Heart Disease, Stroke, and Respiratory Disorders, Such as Emphysema and Chronic Bronchitis

Along with Information about Smoking Prevention Programs, Suggestions for Achieving and Maintaining a Smoke-Free Lifestyle, Statistics about Tobacco Use, Reports on Current Research Initiatives, a Glossary of Related Terms, and Directories of Resources for Additional Help and Information

Edited by Karen Bellenir. 621 pages. 2004. 978-0-7808-0323-7.

"Provides everything needed for the student or general reader seeking practical details on the effects of tobacco use." — *The Bookwatch, Mar '05*

"Public libraries and consumer health care libraries will find this work useful."
— *American Reference Books Annual, 2005*

Sports Injuries Sourcebook, 3rd Edition

Basic Consumer Health Information about Sprains and Strains, Fractures, Growth Plate Injuries, Overtraining Injuries, and Injuries to the Head, Face, Shoulders, Elbows, Hands, Spinal Column, Knees, Ankles, and Feet, and with Facts about Heat-Related Illness, Steroids and Sport Supplements, Protective Equipment, Diagnostic Procedures, Treatment Options, and Rehabilitation

Along with a Glossary of Related Terms and a Directory of Resources for Additional Help and Information

Edited by Sandra J. Judd. 651 pages. 2007. 978-0-7808-0949-9.

"This is an excellent reference for consumers and it is recommended for public, community college, and undergraduate libraries."
— *American Reference Books Annual, 2003*

"Recommended reference source."
— *Booklist, American Library Association, Feb '03*

Stress-Related Disorders Sourcebook

Basic Consumer Health Information about Stress and Stress-Related Disorders, Including Stress Origins and Signals, Environmental Stress at Work and Home, Mental and Emotional Stress Associated with Depression, Post-Traumatic Stress Disorder, Panic Disorder, Suicide, and the Physical Effects of Stress on the Cardiovascular, Immune, and Nervous Systems

Along with Stress Management Techniques, a Glossary, and a Listing of Additional Resources

Edited by Joyce Brennfleck Shannon. 610 pages. 2002. 978-0-7808-0560-6.

"Well written for a general readership, the *Stress-Related Disorders Sourcebook* is a useful addition to the health reference literature."
— *American Reference Books Annual, 2003*

"I am impressed by the amount of information. It offers a thorough overview of the causes and consequences of stress for the layperson. . . . A well-done and thorough reference guide for professionals and nonprofessionals alike." — *Doody's Review Service, Dec '02*

Stroke Sourcebook

Basic Consumer Health Information about Stroke, Including Ischemic, Hemorrhagic, Transient Ischemic Attack (TIA), and Pediatric Stroke, Stroke Triggers and Risks, Diagnostic Tests, Treatments, and Rehabilitation Information

Along with Stroke Prevention Guidelines, Legal and Financial Information, a Glossary, and a Directory of Additional Resources

Edited by Joyce Brennfleck Shannon. 606 pages. 2003. 978-0-7808-0630-6.

"This volume is highly recommended and should be in every medical, hospital, and public library."
— *American Reference Books Annual, 2004*

"Highly recommended for the amount and variety of topics and information covered." — *Choice, Nov '03*

Surgery Sourcebook

Basic Consumer Health Information about Inpatient and Outpatient Surgeries, Including Cardiac, Vascular, Orthopedic, Ocular, Reconstructive, Cosmetic, Gynecologic, and Ear, Nose, and Throat Procedures and More

Along with Information about Operating Room Policies and Instruments, Laser Surgery Techniques, Hospital Errors, Statistical Data, a Glossary, and Listings of Sources for Further Help and Information

Edited by Annemarie S. Muth and Karen Bellenir. 596 pages. 2002. 978-0-7808-0380-0.

"Large public libraries and medical libraries would benefit from this material in their reference collections."
— *American Reference Books Annual, 2004*

"Invaluable reference for public and school library collections alike." — *Library Bookwatch, Apr '03*

Thyroid Disorders Sourcebook

Basic Consumer Health Information about Disorders of the Thyroid and Parathyroid Glands, Including Hypothyroidism, Hyperthyroidism, Graves Disease, Hashimoto Thyroiditis, Thyroid Cancer, and Parathyroid Disorders, Featuring Facts about Symptoms, Risk Factors, Tests, and Treatments

Along with Information about the Effects of Thyroid Imbalance on Other Body Systems, Environmental Factors That Affect the Thyroid Gland, a Glossary, and a Directory of Additional Resources

Edited by Joyce Brennfleck Shannon. 599 pages. 2005. 978-0-7808-0745-7.

"Recommended for consumer health collections."
— *American Reference Books Annual, 2006*

"Highly recommended pick for basic consumer health reference holdings at all levels."
— *The Bookwatch, Aug '05*

Transplantation Sourcebook

Basic Consumer Health Information about Organ and Tissue Transplantation, Including Physical and Financial Preparations, Procedures and Issues Relating to Specific Solid Organ and Tissue Transplants, Rehabilitation, Pediatric Transplant Information, the Future of Transplantation, and Organ and Tissue Donation

Along with a Glossary and Listings of Additional Resources

Edited by Joyce Brennfleck Shannon. 628 pages. 2002. 978-0-7808-0322-0.

"Along with these advances [in transplantation technology] have come a number of daunting questions for potential transplant patients, their families, and their health care providers. This reference text is the best single tool to address many of these questions. . . . It will be a much-needed addition to the reference collections in health care, academic, and large public libraries."
— *American Reference Books Annual*, 2003

"Recommended for libraries with an interest in offering consumer health information." — *E-Streams, Jul '02*

"This is a unique and valuable resource for patients facing transplantation and their families."
— *Doody's Review Service, Jun '02*

Traveler's Health Sourcebook

Basic Consumer Health Information for Travelers, Including Physical and Medical Preparations, Transportation Health and Safety, Essential Information about Food and Water, Sun Exposure, Insect and Snake Bites, Camping and Wilderness Medicine, and Travel with Physical or Medical Disabilities

Along with International Travel Tips, Vaccination Recommendations, Geographical Health Issues, Disease Risks, a Glossary, and a Listing of Additional Resources

Edited by Joyce Brennfleck Shannon. 613 pages. 2000. 978-0-7808-0384-8.

"Recommended reference source."
— *Booklist, American Library Association, Feb '01*

"This book is recommended for any public library, any travel collection, and especially any collection for the physically disabled."
— *American Reference Books Annual, 2001*

SEE ALSO *Worldwide Health Sourcebook*

Urinary Tract & Kidney Diseases & Disorders Sourcebook, 2nd Edition

Basic Consumer Health Information about the Urinary System, Including the Bladder, Urethra, Ureters, and Kidneys, with Facts about Urinary Tract Infections, Incontinence, Congenital Disorders, Kidney Stones, Cancers of the Urinary Tract and Kidneys, Kidney Failure, Dialysis, and Kidney Transplantation

Along with Statistical and Demographic Information, Reports on Current Research in Kidney and Urologic Health, a Summary of Commonly Used Diagnostic Tests, a Glossary of Related Terms, and a Directory of Resources for Additional Help and Information

Edited by Ivy L. Alexander. 649 pages. 2005. 978-0-7808-0750-1.

"A good choice for a consumer health information library or for a medical library needing information to refer to their patients."
— *American Reference Books Annual, 2006*

Vegetarian Sourcebook

Basic Consumer Health Information about Vegetarian Diets, Lifestyle, and Philosophy, Including Definitions of Vegetarianism and Veganism, Tips about Adopting Vegetarianism, Creating a Vegetarian Pantry, and Meeting Nutritional Needs of Vegetarians, with Facts Regarding Vegetarianism's Effect on Pregnant and Lactating Women, Children, Athletes, and Senior Citizens

Along with a Glossary of Commonly Used Vegetarian Terms and Resources for Additional Help and Information

Edited by Chad T. Kimball. 360 pages. 2002. 978-0-7808-0439-5.

"Organizes into one concise volume the answers to the most common questions concerning vegetarian diets and lifestyles. This title is recommended for public and secondary school libraries." — *E-Streams, Apr '03*

"Invaluable reference for public and school library collections alike." — *Library Bookwatch, Apr '03*

"The articles in this volume are easy to read and come from authoritative sources. The book does not necessarily support the vegetarian diet but instead provides the pros and cons of this important decision. The Vegetarian Sourcebook is recommended for public libraries and consumer health libraries."
— *American Reference Books Annual, 2003*

SEE ALSO *Diet & Nutrition Sourcebook*

Women's Health Concerns Sourcebook, 2nd Edition

Basic Consumer Health Information about the Medical and Mental Concerns of Women, Including Maintaining Health and Wellness, Gynecological Concerns, Breast Health, Sexuality and Reproductive Issues, Menopause, Cancer in Women, Leading Causes of Death and Disability among Women, Physical Concerns of Special Significance to Women, and Women's Mental and Emotional Health

Along with a Glossary of Related Terms and Directories of Resources for Additional Help and Information

Edited by Amy L. Sutton. 746 pages. 2004. 978-0-7808-0673-3.

"This is a useful reference book, which makes the reader knowledgeable about several issues that concern women's health. It is recommended for public libraries and home library collections." — *E-Streams, May '05*

"A useful addition to public and consumer health library collections."
— *American Reference Books Annual, 2005*

"A highly recommended title."
— *The Bookwatch, May '04*

"Handy compilation. There is an impressive range of diseases, devices, disorders, procedures, and other physical and emotional issues covered . . . well organized, illustrated, and indexed." — *Choice, Association of College & Research Libraries, Jan '98*

SEE ALSO Breast Cancer Sourcebook, Cancer Sourcebook for Women, Healthy Heart Sourcebook for Women, Osteoporosis Sourcebook

Workplace Health & Safety Sourcebook

Basic Consumer Health Information about Workplace Health and Safety, Including the Effect of Workplace Hazards on the Lungs, Skin, Heart, Ears, Eyes, Brain, Reproductive Organs, Musculoskeletal System, and Other Organs and Body Parts

Along with Information about Occupational Cancer, Personal Protective Equipment, Toxic and Hazardous Chemicals, Child Labor, Stress, and Workplace Violence

Edited by Chad T. Kimball. 626 pages. 2000. 978-0-7808-0231-5

"As a reference for the general public, this would be useful in any library." *— E-Streams, Jun '01*

"Provides helpful information for primary care physicians and other caregivers interested in occupational medicine. . . . General readers; professionals."
— Choice, Association of College & Research Libraries, May '01

"Recommended reference source."
— Booklist, American Library Association, Feb '01

"Highly recommended." *— The Bookwatch, Jan '01*

Worldwide Health Sourcebook

Basic Information about Global Health Issues, Including Malnutrition, Reproductive Health, Disease Dispersion and Prevention, Emerging Diseases, Risky Health Behaviors, and the Leading Causes of Death

Along with Global Health Concerns for Children, Women, and the Elderly, Mental Health Issues, Research and Technology Advancements, and Economic, Environmental, and Political Health Implications, a Glossary, and a Resource Listing for Additional Help and Information

Edited by Joyce Brennfleck Shannon. 614 pages. 2001. 978-0-7808-0330-5.

"Named an Outstanding Academic Title."
— Choice, Association of College & Research Libraries, Jan '02

"Yet another handy but also unique compilation in the extensive *Health Reference Series*, this is a useful work because many of the international publications reprinted or excerpted are not readily available. Highly recommended." *— Choice, Association of College & Research Libraries, Nov '01*

"Recommended reference source."
— Booklist, American Library Association, Oct '01

SEE ALSO Traveler's Health Sourcebook

Teen Health Series

Helping Young Adults Understand, Manage, and Avoid Serious Illness

List price $65 per volume. **School and library price $58 per volume.**

Alcohol Information for Teens
Health Tips about Alcohol and Alcoholism

Including Facts about Underage Drinking, Preventing Teen Alcohol Use, Alcohol's Effects on the Brain and the Body, Alcohol Abuse Treatment, Help for Children of Alcoholics, and More

Edited by Joyce Brennfleck Shannon. 370 pages. 2005. 978-0-7808-0741-9.

"Boxed facts and tips add visual interest to the well-researched and clearly written text."
— *Curriculum Connection, Apr '06*

Allergy Information for Teens
Health Tips about Allergic Reactions Such as Anaphylaxis, Respiratory Problems, and Rashes

Including Facts about Identifying and Managing Allergies to Food, Pollen, Mold, Animals, Chemicals, Drugs, and Other Substances

Edited by Karen Bellenir. 410 pages. 2006. 978-0-7808-0799-0.

Asthma Information for Teens
Health Tips about Managing Asthma and Related Concerns

Including Facts about Asthma Causes, Triggers, Symptoms, Diagnosis, and Treatment

Edited by Karen Bellenir. 386 pages. 2005. 978-0-7808-0770-9.

"Highly recommended for medical libraries, public school libraries, and public libraries."
— *American Reference Books Annual, 2006*

"It is so clearly written and well organized that even hesitant readers will be able to find the facts they need, whether for reports or personal information. . . . A succinct but complete resource."
— *School Library Journal, Sep '05*

Body Information for Teens
Health Tips about Maintaining Well-Being for a Lifetime

Including Facts about the Development and Functioning of the Body's Systems, Organs, and Structures and the Health Impact of Lifestyle Choices

Edited by Sandra Augustyn Lawton. 458 pages. 2007. 978-0-7808-0443-2.

Cancer Information for Teens
Health Tips about Cancer Awareness, Prevention, Diagnosis, and Treatment

Including Facts about Frequently Occurring Cancers, Cancer Risk Factors, and Coping Strategies for Teens Fighting Cancer or Dealing with Cancer in Friends or Family Members

Edited by Wilma R. Caldwell. 428 pages. 2004. 978-0-7808-0678-8.

"Recommended for school libraries, or consumer libraries that see a lot of use by teens."
— *E-Streams, May '05*

"A valuable educational tool."
— *American Reference Books Annual, 2005*

"Young adults and their parents alike will find this new addition to the *Teen Health Series* an important reference to cancer in teens."
— *Children's Bookwatch, Feb '05*

Complementary and Alternative Medicine Information for Teens
Health Tips about Non-Traditional and Non-Western Medical Practices

Including Information about Acupuncture, Chiropractic Medicine, Dietary and Herbal Supplements, Hypnosis, Massage Therapy, Prayer and Spirituality, Reflexology, Yoga, and More

Edited by Sandra Augustyn Lawton. 405 pages. 2006. 978-0-7808-0966-6.

Diabetes Information for Teens
Health Tips about Managing Diabetes and Preventing Related Complications

Including Information about Insulin, Glucose Control, Healthy Eating, Physical Activity, and Learning to Live with Diabetes

Edited by Sandra Augustyn Lawton. 410 pages. 2006. 978-0-7808-0811-9.

Diet Information for Teens, 2nd Edition

Health Tips about Diet and Nutrition

Including Facts about Dietary Guidelines, Food Groups, Nutrients, Healthy Meals, Snacks, Weight Control, Medical Concerns Related to Diet, and More

Edited by Karen Bellenir. 432 pages. 2006. 978-0-7808-0820-1.

"Full of helpful insights and facts throughout the book. ... An excellent resource to be placed in public libraries or even in personal collections."
— *American Reference Books Annual, 2002*

"Recommended for middle and high school libraries and media centers as well as academic libraries that educate future teachers of teenagers. It is also a suitable addition to health science libraries that serve patrons who are interested in teen health promotion and education." — *E-Streams, Oct '01*

"This comprehensive book would be beneficial to collections that need information about nutrition, dietary guidelines, meal planning, and weight control. ... This reference is so easy to use that its purchase is recommended." — *The Book Report, Sep-Oct '01*

"This book is written in an easy to understand format describing issues that many teens face every day, and then provides thoughtful explanations so that teens can make informed decisions. This is an interesting book that provides important facts and information for today's teens." — *Doody's Health Sciences Book Review Journal, Jul-Aug '01*

"A comprehensive compendium of diet and nutrition. The information is presented in a straightforward, plain-spoken manner. This title will be useful to those working on reports on a variety of topics, as well as to general readers concerned about their dietary health."
— *School Library Journal, Jun '01*

Drug Information for Teens, 2nd Edition

Health Tips about the Physical and Mental Effects of Substance Abuse

Including Information about Marijuana, Inhalants, Club Drugs, Stimulants, Hallucinogens, Opiates, Prescription and Over-the-Counter Drugs, Herbal Products, Tobacco, Alcohol, and More

Edited by Sandra Augustyn Lawton. 468 pages. 2006. 978-0-7808-0862-1.

"A clearly written resource for general readers and researchers alike." — *School Library Journal*

"This book is well-balanced. ... a must for public and school libraries."
— *VOYA: Voice of Youth Advocates, Dec '03*

"The chapters are quick to make a connection to their teenage reading audience. The prose is straightforward and the book lends itself to spot reading. It should be useful both for practical information and for research, and it is suitable for public and school libraries."
— *American Reference Books Annual, 2003*

"Recommended reference source."
— *Booklist, American Library Association, Feb '03*

"This is an excellent resource for teens and their parents. Education about drugs and substances is key to discouraging teen drug abuse and this book provides this much needed information in a way that is interesting and factual." — *Doody's Review Service, Dec '02*

Eating Disorders Information for Teens

Health Tips about Anorexia, Bulimia, Binge Eating, and Other Eating Disorders

Including Information on the Causes, Prevention, and Treatment of Eating Disorders, and Such Other Issues as Maintaining Healthy Eating and Exercise Habits

Edited by Sandra Augustyn Lawton. 337 pages. 2005. 978-0-7808-0783-9.

"An excellent resource for teens and those who work with them."
— *VOYA: Voice of Youth Advocates, Apr '06*

"A welcome addition to high school and undergraduate libraries." — *American Reference Books Annual, 2006*

"This book covers the topic in a lucid manner but delves deeper into every aspect of an eating disorder. A solid addition for any nonfiction or reference collection." — *School Library Journal, Dec '05*

Fitness Information for Teens

Health Tips about Exercise, Physical Well-Being, and Health Maintenance

Including Facts about Aerobic and Anaerobic Conditioning, Stretching, Body Shape and Body Image, Sports Training, Nutrition, and Activities for Non-Athletes

Edited by Karen Bellenir. 425 pages. 2004. 978-0-7808-0679-5.

"Another excellent offering from Omnigraphics in their *Teen Health Series*. ... This book will be a great addition to any public, junior high, senior high, or secondary school library."
— *American Reference Books Annual, 2005*

Learning Disabilities Information for Teens

Health Tips about Academic Skills Disorders and Other Disabilities That Affect Learning

Including Information about Common Signs of Learning Disabilities, School Issues, Learning to Live with a Learning Disability, and Other Related Issues

Edited by Sandra Augustyn Lawton. 337 pages. 2005. 978-0-7808-0796-9.

"This book provides a wealth of information for any reader interested in the signs, causes, and consequences of learning disabilities, as well as related legal rights and educational interventions.... Public and academic libraries should want this title for both students and general readers."

—American Reference Books Annual, 2006

■

Mental Health Information for Teens, 2nd Edition

Health Tips about Mental Wellness and Mental Illness

Including Facts about Mental and Emotional Health, Depression and Other Mood Disorders, Anxiety Disorders, Behavior Disorders, Self-Injury, Psychosis, Schizophrenia, and More

Edited by Karen Bellenir. 400 pages. 2006. 978-0-7808-0863-8.

"In both language and approach, this user-friendly entry in the *Teen Health Series* is on target for teens needing information on mental health concerns."

—Booklist, American Library Association, Jan '02

"Readers will find the material accessible and informative, with the shaded notes, facts, and embedded glossary insets adding appropriately to the already interesting and succinct presentation."

—School Library Journal, Jan '02

"This title is highly recommended for any library that serves adolescents and parents/caregivers of adolescents."

—E-Streams, Jan '02

"Recommended for high school libraries and young adult collections in public libraries. Both health professionals and teenagers will find this book useful."

—American Reference Books Annual, 2002

"This is a nice book written to enlighten the society, primarily teenagers, about common teen mental health issues. It is highly recommended to teachers and parents as well as adolescents."

—Doody's Review Service, Dec '01

■

Sexual Health Information for Teens

Health Tips about Sexual Development, Human Reproduction, and Sexually Transmitted Diseases

Including Facts about Puberty, Reproductive Health, Chlamydia, Human Papillomavirus, Pelvic Inflammatory Disease, Herpes, AIDS, Contraception, Pregnancy, and More

Edited by Deborah A. Stanley. 391 pages. 2003. 978-0-7808-0445-6.

"This work should be included in all high school libraries and many larger public libraries.... highly recommended."

—American Reference Books Annual, 2004

"*Sexual Health* approaches its subject with appropriate seriousness and offers easily accessible advice and information."

—School Library Journal, Feb '04

Skin Health Information for Teens

Health Tips about Dermatological Concerns and Skin Cancer Risks

Including Facts about Acne, Warts, Hives, and Other Conditions and Lifestyle Choices, Such as Tanning, Tattooing, and Piercing, That Affect the Skin, Nails, Scalp, and Hair

Edited by Robert Aquinas McNally. 429 pages. 2003. 978-0-7808-0446-3.

"This volume, as with others in the series, will be a useful addition to school and public library collections."

—American Reference Books Annual, 2004

"There is no doubt that this reference tool is valuable."

—VOYA: Voice of Youth Advocates, Feb '04

"This volume serves as a one-stop source and should be a necessity for any health collection."

—Library Media Connection

■

Sports Injuries Information for Teens

Health Tips about Sports Injuries and Injury Protection

Including Facts about Specific Injuries, Emergency Treatment, Rehabilitation, Sports Safety, Competition Stress, Fitness, Sports Nutrition, Steroid Risks, and More

Edited by Joyce Brennfleck Shannon. 405 pages. 2003. 978-0-7808-0447-0.

"This work will be useful in the young adult collections of public libraries as well as high school libraries."

—American Reference Books Annual, 2004

■

Suicide Information for Teens

Health Tips about Suicide Causes and Prevention

Including Facts about Depression, Risk Factors, Getting Help, Survivor Support, and More

Edited by Joyce Brennfleck Shannon. 368 pages. 2005. 978-0-7808-0737-2.

■

Tobacco Information for Teens

Health Tips about the Hazards of Using Cigarettes, Smokeless Tobacco, and Other Nicotine Products

Including Facts about Nicotine Addiction, Immediate and Long-Term Health Effects of Tobacco Use, Related Cancers, Smoking Cessation, Tobacco Use Prevention, and Tobacco Use Statistics

Edited by Karen Bellenir. 440 pages. 2007. 978-0-7808-0976-5.

655

Health Reference Series

Adolescent Health Sourcebook, 2nd Edition

Adult Health Concerns Sourcebook

AIDS Sourcebook, 4th Edition

Alcoholism Sourcebook, 2nd Edition

Allergies Sourcebook, 3rd Edition

Alzheimer Disease Sourcebook, 4th Edition

Arthritis Sourcebook, 2nd Edition

Asthma Sourcebook, 2nd Edition

Attention Deficit Disorder Sourcebook

Autism & Pervasive Developmental Disorders
  Sourcebook

Back & Neck Sourcebook, 2nd Edition

Blood & Circulatory Disorders Sourcebook,
  2nd Edition

Brain Disorders Sourcebook, 2nd Edition

Breast Cancer Sourcebook, 2nd Edition

Breastfeeding Sourcebook

Burns Sourcebook

Cancer Sourcebook, 5th Edition

Cancer Sourcebook for Women, 3rd Edition

Cancer Survivorship Sourcebook

Cardiovascular Diseases & Disorders
  Sourcebook, 3rd Edition

Caregiving Sourcebook

Child Abuse Sourcebook

Childhood Diseases & Disorders Sourcebook

Colds, Flu & Other Common Ailments
  Sourcebook

Communication Disorders Sourcebook

Complementary & Alternative Medicine
  Sourcebook, 3rd Edition

Congenital Disorders Sourcebook, 2nd
  Edition

Contagious Diseases Sourcebook

Cosmetic & Reconstructive Surgery
  Sourcebook, 2nd Edition

Death & Dying Sourcebook, 2nd Edition

Dental Care and Oral Health Sourcebook,
  3rd Edition

Depression Sourcebook, 2nd Edition

Dermatological Disorders Sourcebook, 2nd
  Edition

Diabetes Sourcebook, 4th Edition

Diet & Nutrition Sourcebook, 3rd Edition

Digestive Diseases & Disorder Sourcebook

Disabilities Sourcebook

Disease Management Sourcebook

Domestic Violence Sourcebook, 2nd Edition

Drug Abuse Sourcebook, 2nd Edition

Ear, Nose & Throat Disorders Sourcebook,
  2nd Edition

Eating Disorders Sourcebook, 2nd Edition

Emergency Medical Services Sourcebook

Endocrine & Metabolic Disorders
  Sourcebook, 2nd Edition

EnvironmentalHealth Sourcebook, 2nd Edition

Ethnic Diseases Sourcebook

Eye Care Sourcebook, 3rd Edition

Family Planning Sourcebook

Fitness & Exercise Sourcebook, 3rd Edition

Food Safety Sourcebook

Forensic Medicine Sourcebook

Gastrointestinal Diseases & Disorders
  Sourcebook, 2nd Edition

Genetic Disorders Sourcebook, 3rd Edition

Head Trauma Sourcebook

Headache Sourcebook

Health Insurance Sourcebook

Healthy Aging Sourcebook

Healthy Children Sourcebook

Healthy Heart Sourcebook for Women

Hepatitis Sourcebook

Household Safety Sourcebook

Hypertension Sourcebook

Immune System Disorders Sourcebook, 2nd
  Edition

Infant & Toddler Health Sourcebook

Infectious Diseases Sourcebook